When *Roe* Fell

Critical Issues in Health and Medicine

Edited by
Rima D. Apple, University of Wisconsin–Madison;
Janet Golden, Rutgers University–Camden; and
Rana A. Hogarth, University of Illinois at Urbana–Champaign

Growing criticism of the U.S. healthcare system is coming from consumers, politicians, the media, activists, and healthcare professionals. Critical Issues in Health and Medicine is a collection of books that explores these contemporary dilemmas from a variety of perspectives, among them political, legal, historical, sociological, and comparative, and with attention to crucial dimensions such as race, gender, ethnicity, sexuality, and culture.

For a complete list of titles in the series, please see the last page of the book.

When *Roe* Fell

How Barriers, Inequities, and Systemic Failures of Justice in Abortion Became Visible

EDITED BY KATRINA KIMPORT

RUTGERS UNIVERSITY PRESS

NEW BRUNSWICK, CAMDEN, AND NEWARK, NEW JERSEY

LONDON AND OXFORD

Rutgers University Press is a department of Rutgers, The State University of New Jersey, one of the leading public research universities in the nation. By publishing worldwide, it furthers the University's mission of dedication to excellence in teaching, scholarship, research, and clinical care.

Library of Congress Cataloging-in-Publication Data

Names: Kimport, Katrina, 1978– editor
Title: When Roe fell: how barriers, inequities, and systemic failures
   of justice in abortion became visible / edited by Katrina Kimport.
Description: New Brunswick: Rutgers University Press, 2025. |
   Includes bibliographical references and index.
Identifiers: LCCN 2025004731 (print) | LCCN 2025004732 (ebook) |
   ISBN 9781978841925 paperback | ISBN 9781978841932 hardcover |
   ISBN 9781978841949 epub | ISBN 9781978841956 pdf
Subjects: LCSH: Abortion—Law and legislation—United States | Roe, Jane,
   1947–2017—Trials, litigation, etc. | Wade, Henry—Trials, litigation, etc.
Classification: LCC KF3771 .W44 2025 (print) | LCC KF3771 (ebook) |
   DDC 342.7308/78—dc23/eng/20250211
LC record available at https://lccn.loc.gov/2025004731
LC ebook record available at https://lccn.loc.gov/2025004732

A British Cataloging-in-Publication record for this book is available from the British Library.

References to internet websites (URLs) were accurate at the time of writing. Neither the author nor Rutgers University Press is responsible for URLs that may have expired or changed since the manuscript was prepared.

♾ The paper used in this publication meets the requirements of the American National Standard for Information Sciences—Permanence of Paper for Printed Library Materials, ANSI Z39.48-1992.

rutgersuniversitypress.org

Contents

PART II

What the Fall of Roe *Revealed About Abortion Provision*

PART III

What the Fall of Roe *Revealed About Advocacy
For and Against Abortion*

When *Roe* Fell

Introduction

WHAT LOSING CONSTITUTIONAL PROTECTION DID AND DIDN'T CHANGE ABOUT ABORTION IN THE UNITED STATES

Katrina Kimport

Major moments in history do not always appear as such to the people living them. Others are obvious. The June 2022 majority decision of the U.S. Supreme Court in *Dobbs v. Jackson Women's Health Organization* was not a sleeper moment in history.[1] The majority ruled that there is no constitutional right to abortion, overturning a federal protection the same court had established in its 1973 *Roe v. Wade* decision and subsequently upheld in its 1992 *Planned Parenthood v. Casey* decision.[2] Ostensibly, *Dobbs* returned jurisdiction over abortion to the states with no federal check. State governments were free to create their own laws around abortion, however they wanted. In practice, the *Dobbs* decision paved the way for U.S. state governments to ban or severely restrict abortion.

The effects were immediate, visible, and consequential. Within hours of the decision, facilities that provided abortions suspended their services, and people seeking abortions were turned away. Within weeks, some facilities closed, unable to sustain operations when they were legally prohibited from conducting business, or they substantially reduced their services, offering general family planning care but not abortion. More significant changes followed, many of which came as a surprise and shock to the general public.

From a legal perspective, *Dobbs* was a bombshell, dramatically altering the geographical landscape of abortion legality and availability. But it did not occur in a vacuum. It is worth pointing out an obvious but regularly overlooked fact: *Dobbs* would have little to no impact if it did not leverage existing social and political contention over (the meaning of) abortion. If state governments, for example, did not take up the mantle of abortion opponents to impose bans and severe restrictions on abortion, no clinics would have stopped providing care, no abortion seekers would have been turned away. *Dobbs* occurred in a context: specifically, in a history of abortion care that had (already) failed to ensure reproductive autonomy in pregnancy for all.

In this volume, the chapter authors start from the premise that to understand the implications of a decision like *Dobbs*, we must first understand what abortion looked like historically, politically, and practically leading up to the Supreme Court's ruling. To do so requires a subtle shift: instead of focusing on the impacts of *Dobbs*—that is, what happened and continues to happen afterward—this volume places *Dobbs* in a longer history of abortion in the United States.

Such a framework positions *Dobbs* not just as a decision that did things but also as a decision centrally about *undoing*. Specifically, *Dobbs* overturned *Roe* and the cases since *Roe* that had upheld constitutional protection for abortion. It was the absence of a federal right to abortion—established in *Roe* in 1973 and overturned by *Dobbs* in 2022—that enabled state governments to implement severely restrictive laws and ban abortion. *Roe*, however, was far from an uncritical success. As reproductive justice advocates pointed out decades ago,[3] countless people faced significant and often insurmountable barriers to accessing abortion care under *Roe*.

Among the ways *Dobbs* is historically noteworthy is for what it did not change—and, perhaps, for what it made more visible about who the *Roe* legal regime served and who it failed. Indeed, understanding how abortion care was organized and the lived experiences of abortion seekers and providers as well as abortion technologies, advocacy, and the intersections of race, class, gender, and nation under *Roe* is integral to understanding the impact of overturning *Roe*. In this volume, the chapter authors interrogate whether and how *Dobbs* failed to impact the practical experience of seeking and providing abortion. It may have been a legal bombshell, but *Dobbs* might also be of only marginal consequence to the people who had been already left out under *Roe*.

Moreover, positioning *Dobbs* as an undoing enables scholars to think beyond the logic of *Roe* and explore what the elimination of its precedent can afford. As readers will discover, the fall of *Roe* revealed long-standing—yet untested—assumptions about abortion and opened new opportunities to think about abortion, abortion seekers, abortion provision, and abortion advocacy. Recognizing this and its consequences at this historical moment is essential for anticipating what might happen next in the ongoing social and political contention over reproductive autonomy and freedom.

I hope readers will find another opportunity in this volume: the opportunity to think about abortion *as a case*—and perhaps even as a case to examine in their future scholarship. Just as *Dobbs* did not occur in a vacuum, neither is the scholarly topic of abortion isolated from the interests, concepts, and challenges of academic fields and disciplines. As Tracy Weitz and I (2024) have argued, abortion is a rich and underutilized case for the exploration of a range of questions of theoretical and methodological interest to scholars from many disciplines. It is both exceptionalized and an exemplar, it is at the nexus of myriad social forces, and it is dually intimate and quite public. Although this volume is organized as an examination of abortion in a specific historical moment, each of the chapters can also be read for how the case of abortion can advance theory and method. I encourage readers to attend not only to the nuances of abortion but also to how the case of abortion connects to other aspects of the social world, including meaning-making, work, advocacy, and more.

In this introduction, I will expound on the premise of this volume, providing an overview of state restrictions and service reductions in the immediate aftermath of *Dobbs*, an accounting of the failures of *Roe* to ensure reproductive autonomy, and a description of some of the political and individual efforts to contest abortion bans. Readers well-versed in these topics may prefer to skim or skip those sections. I then briefly summarize the chapters in this volume. I encourage readers to read from cover to cover, but each chapter can stand alone.

RESTRICTIONS ON ABORTION AFTER *DOBBS*

The *Dobbs* decision had an immediate effect because several states already had laws dramatically restricting and even banning abortion on the books. Known as "trigger laws," these gestation-based bans were unenforceable under *Roe* but would go into effect should *Roe* be overturned. Other state governments soon leveraged the opportunity *Dobbs* offered to pass new legislation constraining abortion rights. Within three months, fourteen states had banned abortion and an additional four restricted abortion after a gestation earlier than *Roe* allowed (KFF 2023).[4] Millions of women and other people who could become pregnant now lived in states where legal abortion was unavailable or severely restricted (Shepherd, Roubein, and Kitchener 2022). Some state laws were contested in state courts, with varying results. Other states introduced new legislation aimed at restricting the movement of abortion seekers across state lines. Assessments of the state-level political climate anticipated that, when the dust finally settled, twenty-four states would ban or severely restrict the provision of abortion within their borders (Jones and Chiu 2023). Abortion was illegal and unavailable in the formal healthcare system in large swaths of the country. And chaos ensued as state laws were implemented, then sometimes enjoined, and again enforced within short time periods.

The effects of *Dobbs*, in other words, were neither invisible to nor unnoticed by those living through the moment. *Dobbs* immediately established itself as momentous and consequential. It demanded its place in history, quickly ushering in language that oriented time, society, and lives around it: there was "pre-*Dobbs*" and there was "post-*Dobbs*." Broadly, the public narrative of *Dobbs* was characterized by the injustice it wrought: the state-level bans, the clinic closures, the people who would be denied abortions, and the loss of a constitutional right that had been protected for almost fifty years. Extrapolating from demographic data collected before *Dobbs* and anticipating abortion bans in states with a pre-*Dobbs* track record of hostility to abortion rights, scholars found that the populations most likely to be subject to abortion bans—to have their access to abortion eliminated—were disproportionately women of color and low income (Jones and Chiu 2023), suggesting an extension of the injustices and inequalities that already characterized their lives. The story of *Dobbs* was a continued story of reproductive injustice.

ABORTION UNDER *ROE*

This story is factually true, but it is only partial. For many pregnant people, abortion was already unavailable under *Roe* (Kimport 2022a). Although *Roe* and subsequent Supreme Court decisions on abortion asserted a right to abortion, they also allowed for limits on that right (Hull and Hoffer 2010). *Roe* itself permitted states to severely restrict access to abortion after assumed fetal "viability," when the fetus is believed to have the potential to survive outside the pregnant person's body (Kimport and Weitz 2025). In 1976, Congress first enacted the Hyde Amendment, which prevented federal tax dollars from being spent on abortion care.

Many states mirrored this language to apply to their state tax dollars, with the upshot being that people with public insurance (aka Medicaid) must pay for their abortions out of pocket. The Supreme Court judged these prohibitions constitutional in their 1980 decision in *Harris v. McRae*.[5] Later, in 1992, the Supreme Court in *Planned Parenthood of Southeastern Pennsylvania v. Casey* allowed states to pass laws requiring specific actions of abortion seekers and providers so long as those actions were not judged to be an "undue burden" on patients' ability to access abortion care, as evaluated by the courts and never fully resolved.

The subsequent Supreme Court decision in *Gonzales v. Carhart* (2007) allowed a federal prohibition on a kind of abortion technique (although the legal language did not precisely match any clinical procedures, making the overall ban ambiguous).[6] When the 2010 midterm elections swept Republicans—the party with an antiabortion platform (Schlozman 2015)—into legislative majorities in twenty-five states, state laws restricting abortion began a dramatic rise. Even as the Supreme Court's 2016 decision in *Whole Woman's Health v. Hellerstedt* and 2020 decision in *June Medical Services v. Russo* found some restrictions unconstitutional, the litany of regulation continued.[7] By 2022, there were hundreds of state-level restrictions on the books throughout the United States.

Specifically, at the time of the *Dobbs* decision, among other limits, states already severely restricted access to abortion at gestations before the generally accepted point of fetal "viability." By 2021, sixteen states had laws banning abortion after twenty weeks' gestation (aka twenty-week bans; Guttmacher Institute 2021). Texas's Senate Bill 8 banned abortion after fetal heart tones were detectable, typically around six weeks' gestation, starting in September 2021. Numerous states required abortion seekers under age eighteen to involve their parents or guardians in their abortion decision, and thirty-four states, mimicking the federally approved language, prohibited the use of state public monies to pay for abortion care thereby forcing abortion seekers who rely on public insurance (i.e., Medicaid) to pay out of pocket for care.

These restrictions had consequences for abortions seekers' ability to enact their reproductive desires. In a 2014 study—that is, pre-*Dobbs*—researchers estimated that at least 4,000 abortion seekers a year were unable to obtain a wanted abortion because of gestational limits (Upadhyay et al. 2014). Minors who could not involve their parents in their abortion decision were regularly denied abortions (Stevenson and Coleman-Minahan 2023). And abortion seekers who were financially struggling had to forego basic necessities in order to afford abortion care (Roberts et al. 2014) or resign themselves to continuing their pregnancy despite not wanting a baby (Cook et al. 1999; Roberts et al. 2019).

Under *Roe*, states could also legally require abortion-providing facilities and health professionals to meet arbitrary standards, even when they did not require such standards for similar or higher risk medical procedures. The upshot of these laws—commonly called TRAP laws, for "targeted regulation of abortion providers"—was to complicate abortion facilities' ability to remain in business, leading to clinic closures and, in turn, large geographical areas that lacked an abortion clinic (Cartwright et al. 2018). All this occurred in the absence of robust evidence of any benefit to these requirements (Roberts et al. 2018). Yet even with these numerous obstacles to abortion, there were over 930,000 abortions in 2020, representing an increase from 2017 and suggesting a reversal of a decades-long trend of decreases in annual abortions in the United States (Jones, Kirstein, and Philbin 2022).

Although not all states enacted all possible restrictions on abortion, nearly every state restricted abortion in at least one way. In parallel to restriction by state governments, social stigmatization and medical institutions and organizations limited healthcare providers' ability to provide abortion care, thereby reducing the number of willing and able abortion providers (Freedman 2010). As a result, many abortion seekers experienced no real right to abortion under *Roe*.

The impediments to abortion were more acute in some states than others. Republican-led states were generally more hostile to abortion and established more barriers to care than Democrat-led and split-leadership states. It also bears noting that the effects of these obstacles to abortion were more significant for some populations than others. People without the financial resources, mobility, and time to work around these barriers—including people who were financially struggling, adolescents, incarcerated people, undocumented people, refugees and asylum seekers, and military personnel—were particularly vulnerable and thus were more likely to continue an unwanted pregnancy (Kimport 2022a; Sufrin et al. 2023; Stevenson and Coleman-Minahan 2023; Seymour et al. 2020). For these people, abortion pre-*Dobbs* was essentially a right in name only. Pregnant people continued their pregnancies not necessarily because they wanted to have a baby but because they could not get an abortion.

Recognizing how abortion was unchooseable or unobtainable for people before *Dobbs* suggests *Dobbs* may not have had a meaningful effect on people's ability to choose or obtain abortion—and that *Roe* had not meaningfully protected all people's right to abortion. Such a recognition is hardly novel. For decades before *Roe* fell, reproductive justice advocates identified and critiqued the limits of *Roe*, documenting who it failed and how it failed (see Nelson 2003; Ross et al. 2017; Ross and Solinger 2017; Silliman et al. 2004). For large portions of the country and for several specific populations, *Dobbs* did not change their material experiences. *Dobbs* entered into an already grossly unequal abortion landscape wherein abortion was formally legal but often unavailable or difficult to access—at least for some. This landscape was the result of a social history littered with missed opportunities, concessions to opponents of abortion, and willful ignorance of the needs of socially marginalized groups by mainstream abortion rights organizations, advocates, and politicians.

ABORTION ADVOCACY AFTER *DOBBS*

In addition to state bans and closed abortion services, part of the legacy of *Dobbs* is how it shined a light on the failure to ensure reproductive justice under *Roe*— and, at last, compelled large-scale responses. Even as *Dobbs* enabled state legislatures to curtail abortion rights, advocates for abortion rights mounted their own political campaigns. Just weeks after the *Dobbs* decision eliminated federal protection for abortion, voters in Kansas rejected a proposed state constitutional amendment that would deny a state-level right to abortion. Other states, including California, Vermont, and Ohio, codified protections for abortion rights in their state constitutions in the wake of *Dobbs*. Legislatures in New York and Massachusetts passed "shield laws" that protected licensed physicians in their state who provided care to out-of-state residents from prosecution efforts originating in other states. Money poured into advocacy organizations that support abortion rights, including ones that target politics and ones that provide direct service and support for abortion seekers.

The insights and critiques of reproductive justice advocates gained greater recognition on ever bigger stages. Loretta Ross, one of the founders of the reproductive justice movement, was awarded a MacArthur fellowship, often referred to as a "genius award," in the fall 2022. Healthcare workers, particularly physicians, publicly expressed their frustration with the constraints the law enacted on their ability to practice medicine. Professional associations of healthcare workers, such as the American College of Obstetricians and Gynecologists, publicly decried *Dobbs* as "a direct blow to bodily autonomy, reproductive health, patient safety, and health equity in the United States" (ACOG 2022). Obstetric patients denied timely abortion care after pregnancy complications sued their states. Democrats made abortion a central part of their campaigning, discovering that abortion rights could be a winning issue.

As this political wrangling occurred, abortion seekers traveled from states where abortion was banned to states where it remained legal. Initially, this meant long waits for an appointment and overwhelmed staff at the abortion-providing facilities that remained open. Eventually, facilities were largely able to adjust their operations to support this increase in patients and shift in their patient population to more out-of-state clients. New abortion providers, including telehealth medication abortion-only providers, entered the market, serving patients without requiring them to travel. Some abortion seekers turned to mutual aid and direct orders from international pharmacies to obtain and use medication abortion pills in their home state even as abortion provision there was criminalized. After an initial post-*Dobbs* drop, the number of abortions provided through the formal healthcare system (including telehealth) increased compared with before *Dobbs* (Society of Family Planning 2023). This number did not even include abortions completed outside the healthcare system (known as "self-managed abortions"). Perhaps this increase reflected that innovations in abortion service delivery following the *Dobbs* decision meant that (at least some) people who previously would not have been able to implement an abortion decision (because of cost, difficulty traveling, or any number of reasons) were now able to determine whether and when they continued a pregnancy.

This possibility underscores the shortcomings of thinking only about pre-*Dobbs* and post-*Dobbs*. *Dobbs* was not a singular event, bringing into effect abortion bans and abortion advocacy. It was also the removal—some might say loss—of the constraints of the *Roe* framework. By only focusing on *Dobbs* and its impact, scholars miss the opportunity to examine what the fall of *Roe* means—or could mean. Moreover, only focusing on *Dobbs* renders invisible the experiences of populations who were already excluded from abortion care under *Roe*. In the absence of federal protection for abortion in the United States, scholars can and must ask, What was foreclosed and who was underserved when *Roe* was the precedent?

Chapters in This Volume

This volume is a collective, multi- and interdisciplinary effort to examine *Dobbs* in its social, political, and historical context. Chapter authors hail from many disciplines, with some chapters even boasting multidisciplinary author teams. They come from and study different geographies and are at different stages of their careers. For some, studying abortion is a primary focus of their research; for others, it is less so. They share in common an interest in making sense of this key moment in history and insisting on a deep understanding of abortion seekers, providers, advocates, and opponents.

But they do not do so using the same presentation voices, formats, and styles. Some chapters draw on years of empirical research and experience, providing a big picture perspective. Some chapters follow the format of an empirical research article, with a specific research question and method. Others do a bit of both. Some provide case studies of specific geographies; others have a national lens. Collectively, these chapters demystify abortion and abortion research, laying bare common misunderstandings and misinformation about the topic and belying claims that *Dobbs* "changed everything." The social world is rarely so simple.

Following this introductory chapter, the volume is divided into three sections. In the first, the chapters focus on what the fall of *Roe* revealed about people who have abortions. Diana Greene Foster's chapter opens the section with a response to the oft-made assertion that the abortion rate could be reduced or even eliminated if only people were better at using contraception. Noting the underlying premise of this assertion, that abortion is generally bad and should be avoided, Foster breaks down this claim and shows the flaws in its assumptions. From inevitable contraceptive failures to the reasonableness of not contracepting to the fallacy that only unintended pregnancies end in abortion, Foster weaves together data from multiple disciplines and studies to puncture claims that (better use of) contraception could allay the negative effects of abortion bans. In so doing, her chapter contests the perennial talking point that abortion is never necessary, a talking point whose salience is more acute in the absence of a nationwide legal right to abortion.

In the next chapter, Whitney Arey and Klaira Lerma draw on the experiences of people who had abortions pre-*Dobbs* in North Carolina and Texas to explore how the narrative of legitimacy and "exceptional" abortions matters in how people make sense of their abortions. Specifically, they show how the idea that some abortions are more acceptable—the exceptions to general social disapproval of abortion—permeates abortion patients' own accounts of their abortions in these two states. Since *Dobbs*, Texas has banned abortion and North Carolina, after some contentious politicking, banned abortions after twelve weeks' gestation. These states, in other words, fall into the category of restrictive states. Understanding the pre-*Dobbs* presence of the abortion legitimacy framing for abortion seekers in these (and perhaps other) states is integral to understanding who seeks abortion and how they make sense of their experiences after *Dobbs*.

The volume's third chapter, by Lindsay Ruhr, employs in-depth methods to empirically examine the effects of one abortion restriction in one state—an extension of the mandatory waiting period in Missouri from twenty-four to seventy-two hours in 2015—to illustrate the presence of constraints on abortion availability long before *Dobbs*. Using surveys, medical record analysis, and elicitation interviews, Ruhr shows how this waiting period extension, though consequential from a legal perspective, had little material impact on patients' experience of care. Because Missouri already lacked abortion availability, even under the shorter waiting period the patients typically waited more than twenty-four hours for their second appointment. The extension did not meaningfully change that delay. Ruhr's case shows the resilience of abortion seekers in navigating barriers to abortion and, moreover, how poor abortion access had been under *Roe*. *Dobbs* thus did not render a remade abortion landscape. Abortion seekers had long successfully navigated barrier after barrier, making the question of how, whether, and whom current *Dobbs*-related bans will affect an open one.

Next, Jenny O'Donnell tackles the question of measurement and of measuring change in depth. Detailing the history behind the #WeCount effort by the Society of Family Planning to capture and share nearly real-time abortion census data in the United States, O'Donnell walks through the "how" of designing and implementing this ambitious, time-sensitive, nationwide project and bringing accurate scientific evidence to the public conversation. Along the way, her chapter probes some of the challenges of abortion research, including gatekeeping and lack of resources, as well as how the #WeCount project overcame them. In addition, this chapter documents why such projects are necessary—noting that real post-*Dobbs* data diverged in significant ways from pre-*Dobbs* predictions—and why they are not enough to tell us all of consequence in this post-*Dobbs* landscape. Readers interested in abortion research methods will find this examination of particular interest.

In the last chapter of this section, Jane Seymour and Jenny Higgins offer an immensely practical conceptual contribution to thinking about the abortion seeker experience while also introducing precision to a concept used in the research literature to mean broad and sometimes incompatible things: abortion access. With a focus on advocacy and clinical attention, "abortion access" often operates as a catchall in discussions of abortion. Seymour and Higgins present a six-domain framing of the concept that uses Wisconsin as an exemplar state for how these domains are consequential and how research could measure them. In so doing, they offer researchers tools to compare evaluations of "access" across studies as well as a framework for measuring consequential change—for better or for worse—to whether an individual pregnant person can get a desired abortion.

In the volume's second section, the chapters explore what the fall of *Roe* revealed about abortion provision. The section begins with a chapter by Kelly Ward and Barbara Alvarez that reviews the history of abortion workers, charting the push and pull of professionalization and deprofessionalization in the abortion care workforce. They usefully summarize the literature on the topic as well as analyze their own empirical qualitative data from an ethnography of a clinic in California, then and now a state considered abortion supportive. From midwives to homeopaths to physicians to, most recently, greater use of less skilled professions like medical assistants, abortion provision both has a dynamic, unique history and is reflective of broader shifts in healthcare provision. Ward and Alvarez point to how *Dobbs* and the ensuing state bans on abortion will likely shepherd in new types of abortion workers and challenge existing ideas about who is and can be an abortion provider, the latest in a longer history of shifts in work.

Lori Freedman's chapter examines Catholic hospitals, a workplace that, even before the *Dobbs* decision, ostensibly was abortion-free. Based on their official prohibition on abortion stemming from Catholic precepts, these religiously affiliated hospitals have been cited as examples of successful health care without abortion, suggesting that abortion bans are medically safe. Freedman synthesizes more than a decade of her research on Catholic health care to expose the fallacy of these claims, showing how abortion provision has always been part of Catholic hospital practice and troubling the assertion that the absence of abortion without significant health compromises is possible. The pushback from doctors in states that have banned abortion and lawsuits by patients who challenge abortion bans as compromising their obstetric care suggest that *Dobbs* indeed is revealing the claims of care without abortion as false.

Next, Tracy Weitz traces the history of regulation and practice of medication abortion in the United States, arguing that the actions of not only antiabortion activists but also abortion rights supporters—specifically through their lack of imagination for the possibilities of medication abortion—collectively limited the promise of medication abortion to fundamentally change abortion access and provision for decades. Weitz shows how this promise, a potential boon to people who do not want to be pregnant, was interpreted as a risk to broader pro-choice goals and institutional structure. It took the dual shocks of the COVID-19 pandemic and *Dobbs* to dislodge a business-as-usual approach to medication abortion and afford the opportunity to think beyond the status quo toward the liberatory possibilities of this technology. With the hindsight afforded by innovations to medication abortion provision that have scaled following *Dobbs* and the state bans on abortion, the institutional neglect of and opposition to the possibilities of medication abortion have become clear.

Danielle Bessett, Jessie Hill, Meredith Pensak, and Michelle McGowan investigate the efforts by abortion-trained physicians to navigate the shifts—and decreases—in their professional authority, a process occurring across health care. Using the case of Ohio, Bessett and colleagues offer an empirical study that focuses on how legislation restricting abortion in specific has tread on obstetrician-gynecologists' cultural authority and how they have responded. Invoking claims to their authority because of their training and medical expertise, physicians in the state contest abortion restrictions through recourse to claims that center their authority and power, with unexamined consequences for efforts to center pregnant people in their reproductive decision-making. Bessett and colleagues show how the case of abortion is an example of professional authority negotiation, with effects that reverberate beyond the medical profession.

Finally in this section, Alexandra Woodcock and Jessica Sanders's empirical chapter zeroes in on the decision-making of physicians on their preferred geographical practice location—and how the (il)legality of abortion in those settings plays into their preferences. Using a national survey, they find that state bans on abortion were salient to many obstetrician-gynecologists' future practice location preferences, but, drawing on a survey of all graduating medical residents at the University of Utah, they also find that this relationship did not hold for physicians in other specialties. Likely an effect of greater awareness and sensitivity to how abortion bans constrain obstetrician-gynecologists' medical practice—that is, their ability to do their job—these results also highlight the historical disconnect between abortion care and mainstream medicine. Abortion care has been siloed in more ways than one, enabling physicians outside the obstetrics-gynecology specialty to remain largely ignorant of the potential consequences of abortion bans for their patients and, indeed, themselves and their loved ones.

Finally, in the book's third section, the chapters examine what the fall of *Roe* revealed about advocacy for and against abortion. Sara Matthiesen provides a history of advocacy related to crisis pregnancy centers and, more pointedly, how abortion rights advocates have characterized them over the years. Noting the singularity of the critiques levied against these centers over decades, Matthiesen shows how the centers themselves have pivoted to deflect these critiques and ultimately have benefited from the abortion rights gaze. She asks abortion rights supporters what it means to rehash a critique that has only marginal evidence to support it and, perhaps more importantly, has failed to meaningfully affect pregnant people's lives. Coming into a world without *Roe*, Matthiesen challenges advocates—and researchers—to think critically about their assumptions and the long histories some carry.

Next, Micki Burdick offers an ethnographic account of an overlooked wing of the anti-abortion movement: evangelical white women. With archival, historical, and observational data, Burdick weaves the raced and gendered expectations that characterize evangelical white women, highlighting the association of this population with emotionality. This emotionality, Burdick writes, is leveraged in anti-abortion pregnancy resource centers (also known as crisis pregnancy centers) to launder pro-life frames through medical technologies and to construct them as science and truth, obscuring their ideological origins and underpinnings. Their chapter points to the deep history outside of politics that characterizes how advocates have and will continue to make sense of abortion in the United States.

In the volume's last chapter, Ophra Leyser-Whalen and Erin Johnson examine abortion funds, nonprofit advocacy organizations that work to eliminate barriers to accessing abortion. Always a part of abortion service delivery, especially for abortion seekers who were financially struggling, abortion funds took on an increased role after the fall of *Roe*. Leyser-Whalen and Johnson draw on interviews with abortion fund workers from local, regional, and national funds to gain insight into how the funds have navigated these changes. They document how new public attention, an influx of donations and offers to volunteer, and dramatically larger client bases requiring more complex support have pushed the funds to innovate and collaborate. In the process, they find, these changes and the funds' responses reveal the substantial obstacles to direct-action efforts to enable abortion seekers to get care that they faced before *Dobbs* and the ongoing consequences of—and opportunities to innovate from—that structure.

The chapters in this volume situate the post-*Dobbs* moment in a history that began well before, offering context for what *Dobbs* leveraged and how the fall of *Roe* matters. The volume does not do it all. No volume can, of course, but I think it is useful to highlight some of the gaps that remain. This volume does not explore the implications of U.S. abortion policy globally (see, for example, Suh 2021). It does not examine public opinion, including whether *Dobbs* has shifted public support for abortion. Emerging evidence suggests that *Dobbs* did not change people's attitudes toward abortion but may have shifted their willingness to be vocal about their attitudes and act politically on them (Jozkowski et al. 2023). It does not draw connections between pre-*Dobbs* experiences of abortion travel (e.g., Kimport 2022b; Kimport and Rasidjan 2023) and post-*Dobbs* travel, which may be different largely in number of people affected and scale. While this volume includes chapters with both national and state- or region-specific lenses, not all geographical communities are represented, nor are the throughlines from abortion under *Roe* to the present for communities defined not (only) by geography (e.g., adolescents, undocumented people, indigenous people) explored. I hope readers will consider this volume a beginning, not the decisive conclusion of understanding what the fall of *Roe* means.

In this way, this volume represents an opportunity. To the extent that political and cultural imaginations about abortion have failed to reflect the lived experience of abortion (Bruce, Hutchens, and Cowan 2024; Kimport and McLemore 2022), scholars have a chance in the aftermath of *Dobbs* to reorient our scholarship and understanding to center lived experience. These chapters describe what was already true before *Dobbs* and how losing the protections of *Roe* forced, enabled, and perhaps even facilitated a new era of abortion. Indeed, the fact that *Dobbs* already has had an impact on politics, medicine, and family formation is evidence of the importance of understanding the political, social, and cultural landscape into which the decision was released. Ultimately, this edited volume offers crucial historical, organizational, and social context for understanding the public moment when *Roe* was overturned and the implications of the fall of *Roe* on abortion care, abortion seekers, abortion providers, and abortion advocates in the United States.

ACKNOWLEDGMENTS

I am deeply indebted to Tracy Weitz for being a thought partner in conceptualizing this volume and for her excellent feedback on earlier versions of this chapter.

NOTES

1. Dobbs v. Jackson Women's Health Organization, 597 U.S. 215 (2022).

2. Roe v. Wade, 410 U.S. 113 (1973); Planned Parenthood of Southeastern Pennsylvania v. Casey, 505 U.S. 833 (1992).

3. The reproductive justice movement was founded a group of Black women in 1994 after years of their concerns being overlooked and ignored by the mainstream reproductive rights movement in the United States (see Luna 2020 for a comprehensive history). Intentionally centering the lives of Black people, reproductive justice insists on every person's right to have children, to not have children, and to raise the children they have in safe and sustainable communities (Ross and Solinger 2017). In contrast to the mainstream reproductive rights movement, reproductive justice recognizes that abortion rights alone are insufficient to ensure reproductive autonomy. It starts from the acknowledgment that some populations face more significant barriers—including social, financial, and political barriers—to achieving their reproductive desires.

4. Informed readers will note that even before *Dobbs* many states had laws that were unconstitutional under *Roe*. As discussed later in this chapter, as of 2021, sixteen states had laws banning abortion after twenty weeks' gestation (aka twenty-week bans; Guttmacher Institute 2021). This point in pregnancy is before the *Roe* threshold of viability, rendering these bans likely unconstitutional (Calhoun 2012). However, these laws were never litigated, so the Supreme Court never weighed in on their constitutionality. The post-*Dobbs* laws referenced here were at six (n = 2), fifteen, and eighteen weeks' gestation.

5. Harris v. McRae, 448 U. S. 297 (1980).

6. Gonzales v. Carhart, 550 U.S. 124 (2007).

7. Whole Woman's Health v. Hellerstedt, 579 U.S. 582 (2016); June Medical Services L.L.C. v. Russo, 591 U. S. 299 (2020).

REFERENCES

American College of Obstetricians and Gynecologists (ACOG). 2022. "ACOG Statement on the Decision in *Dobbs v. Jackson*." Accessed April 24, 2024. https://www.acog.org/news/news-releases/2022/06/acog-statement-on-the-decision-in-dobbs-v-jackson.

Bruce, Tricia C., Kendra Hutchens, and Sarah K. Cowan. 2024. "The 'Abortion Imaginary': Shared Perceptions and Personal Representations among Everyday Americans." *Science Advances* 10 (9): eadj3135.

Calhoun, Lindsay J. 2012. "The Painless Truth: Challenging Fetal Pain-based Abortion Bans." *Tulane Law Review* 87 (1): 141–167.

Cartwright, Alice F., Mihiri Karunaratne, Jill Barr-Walker, Nicole E. Johns, and Ushma D. Upadhyay. 2018. "Identifying National Availability of Abortion Care and Distance from Major US Cities: Systematic Online Search." *Journal of Medical Internet Research* 20 (5): e186.

Cook, Philip J., Allan M. Parnell, Michael J. Moore, and Deanna Pagnini. 1999. "The Effects of Short-Term Variation in Abortion Funding on Pregnancy Outcomes." *Journal of Health Economics* 18 (2): 241–257.

Freedman, Lori. 2010. *Willing and Unable: Doctors' Constraints in Abortion Care.* Vanderbilt University Press.

Guttmacher Institute. 2021. "State Bans on Abortion throughout Pregnancy." Last modified October 1, 2021. https://www.guttmacher.org/state-policy/explore/state-policies-later -abortions#.

Hull, N.E.H., and Peter Charles Hoffer. 2010. *Roe v. Wade: The Abortion Rights Controversy in American History.* 2nd ed. University of Kansas.

Jones, Rachel K., and Doris W. Chiu. 2023. "Characteristics of Abortion Patients in Protected and Restricted States Accessing Clinic-based Care 12 Months prior to the Elimination of the Federal Constitutional Right to Abortion in the United States." *Perspectives on Sexual and Reproductive Health* 55 (2): 80–85.

Jones, Rachel K., Marielle Kirstein, and Jesse Philbin. 2022. "Abortion Incidence and Service Availability in the United States, 2020." *Perspectives on Sexual and Reproductive Health* 54 (4): 128–141.

Jozkowski, Kristen N., Xiana Bueno, Ronna C. Turner, Brandon L. Crawford, and Wen-Juo Lo. 2023. "People's Knowledge of and Attitudes toward Abortion Laws before and after the Dobbs v. Jackson decision." *Sexual and Reproductive Health Matters* 31 (1): 2233794.

KFF. 2023. "Abortion Policy Tracker." Accessed April 23, 2024. https://www.kff.org/other /state-indicator/abortion-policy-tracker/?currentTimeframe=0&sortModel=%7B.

Kimport, Katrina. 2022a. *No Real Choice: How Culture and Politics Matter for Reproductive Autonomy.* Rutgers University Press.

———. 2022b. "Reducing the Burdens of Forced Abortion Travel: Referrals, Financial and Emotional Support, and Opportunities for Positive Experiences in Traveling for Third-Trimester Abortion Care." *Social Science & Medicine* 293: 114667.

Kimport, Katrina, and Monica R. McLemore. 2022. "The Problem with 'Justifying' Abortion: Why Real Reproductive Justice Cannot Be Achieved by Theorizing the Legitimacy of Abortion." *Women's Reproductive Health* 9 (1): 27–31.

Kimport, Katrina, and Maryani Palupy Rasidjan. 2023. "Exploring the Emotional Costs of Abortion Travel in the United States due to Legal Restriction." *Contraception* 120: 109956.

Kimport, Katrina, and Tracy A. Weitz. 2024. "Abortion as a Sociological Case." *Sociological Forum* 39 (1): 7–21.

———. 2025. "Regulating Abortion Later in Pregnancy: Fetal-centric Laws and the Erasure of Women's Subjectivity." *Journal of Health Politics, Policy and Law* 50 (1): 47–68.

Luna, Zakiya. 2020. *Reproductive Rights as Human Rights: Women of Color and the Fight for Reproductive Justice.* NYU Press.

Nelson, Jennifer. 2003. *Women of Color and the Reproductive Rights Movement.* NYU Press.

Roberts, Sarah C. M., Heather Gould, Katrina Kimport, Tracy A. Weitz, and Diana Greene Foster. 2014. "Out-of-Pocket Costs and Insurance Coverage for Abortion in the United States." *Women's Health Issues* 24 (2): e211–e218.

Roberts, Sarah C. M., Nicole E. Johns, Valerie Williams, Erin Wingo, and Ushma D. Upadhyay. 2019. "Estimating the Proportion of Medicaid-eligible Pregnant Women in Louisiana Who Do Not Get Abortions When Medicaid Does Not Cover Abortion." *BMC Women's Health* 19 (1): 78.

Roberts, Sarah C. M., Ushma D. Upadhyay, Guodong Liu, Jennifer L. Kerns, Djibril Ba, Nancy Beam, and Douglas L. Leslie. 2018. "Association of Facility Type with Procedural-related Morbidities and Adverse Events among Patients Undergoing Induced Abortions." *JAMA* 319 (24): 2497–2506.

Ross, Loretta, Erika Derkas, Whitney Peoples, Lynn Roberts, and Pamela Bridgewater. 2017. *Radical Reproductive Justice: Foundation, Theory, Practice, Critique.* Feminist Press at CUNY.

Ross, Loretta, and Rickie Solinger. 2017. *Reproductive Justice: An Introduction.* University of California Press.

Schlozman, Daniel. 2015. *When Movements Anchor Parties: Electoral Alignments in American History.* Princeton University Press.

Seymour, Jane W, Laura Fix, Daniel Grossman, and Kate Grindlay. 2020. "Pregnancy and Abortion: Experiences and Attitudes of Deployed US Servicewomen." *Military Medicine* 185 (9–10): e1390–e1390.

Shepherd, Katie, Rachel Roubein, and Carolyn Kitchener. 2022. "1 in 3 American Women Have Already Lost Abortion Access. More Restrictive Laws Are Coming." *Washington Post,* August 22, 2022. https://www.washingtonpost.com/nation/2022/08/22/more-trigger-bans-loom-1-3-women-lose-most-abortion-access-post-roe/.

Silliman, Jael, Marlene Gerber Fried, Loretta Ross, and Elena R. Gutierrez. 2004. *Undivided Rights: Women of Color Organize for Reproductive Justice.* South End Press.

Society of Family Planning. 2023. "April 2022 to September 2023." *#WeCount Public Report,* February 28, 2024. https://doi.org/10.46621/675707thmfmv.

Stevenson, Amanda Jean, and Kate Coleman-Minahan. 2023. "Use of Judicial Bypass of Mandatory Parental Consent to Access Abortion and Judicial Bypass Denials, Florida and Texas, 2018–2021." *American Journal of Public Health* 113 (3): 316–319.

Sufrin, Carolyn B, Ashley Devon-Williamston, Lauren Beal, Crystal M. Hayes, and Camille Kramer. 2023. "'I Mean, I Didn't Really Have a Choice of Anything': How Incarceration Influences Abortion Decision-Making and Precludes Access in the United States." *Perspectives on Sexual and Reproductive Health* 55 (3): 165–177.

Suh, Siri. 2021. *Dying to Count: Post-abortion Care and Global Reproductive Health Politics in Senegal.* Rutgers University Press.

Upadhyay, Ushma D., Tracy A. Weitz, Rachel K. Jones, Rana E. Barar, and Diana Greene Foster. 2014. "Denial of Abortion because of Provider Gestational Age Limits in the United States." *American Journal of Public Health* 104 (9): 1687–1694.

PART I

What the Fall of *Roe* Revealed About People Who Have Abortions

CHAPTER 1

Contraception Is Not Enough

Diana Greene Foster

I did my first ever TED talk in the fall of 2023. It was about the consequences of receiving versus being denied an abortion, based on a study I led at the University of California, San Francisco called the Turnaway Study. When the talk was posted online in January 2024, the counter on the video registered hundreds of thousands of views. It's hard to imagine reaching such a large number of people. And really, my only way to know if I have reached bots versus a new audience is to scan my email inbox for the people who were moved to look me up after watching to offer their kudos or critiques. If I have really reached people who haven't previously read our scientific papers or the Turnaway Study book, I expect some critiques. Based on emails, I did reach new people, and here's proof:

> I listened to your Ted Talk with interest. You brought up some very valuable points, some of which most people have never heard. However, you left off one important part, in my opinion. . . . I did not hear anything about the responsibility of the woman and man to take the necessary steps to not get pregnant. I understand there are circumstances where women get raped and, therefore, own no responsibility of the pregnancy. I am sure there are other circumstances as well. Your talk included what seemed to me to be excuses for not taking the personal responsibility for becoming pregnant.

The correspondent is correct: I did not talk about all the reasons why people become pregnant when they don't intend to. For a fifteen-minute talk on a national stage, it seemed to me to be enough to start with the fact that they do and consider what should happen next. Should they be able to decide about whether to have a child, or should they carry a pregnancy to term against their will?

However, it is clearly important to some people, in deciding whether they personally support abortion rights, to understand the context. If someone doesn't want to have a baby and there are multiple, very effective ways to prevent pregnancy, why not contracept instead of becoming pregnant and having an abortion? Before we talk about access to abortion (let alone abortion rights), the question is whether the couple was "responsible" when they ended up in that situation—why couldn't they simply prevent pregnancy?[1]

This chapter addresses the question of whether or how often abortions could be prevented by contraception. That is, how often could contraception prevent a pregnancy that would end in abortion? Before I begin, I have to note that the data I draw on here about causes of unwanted pregnancy and reasons for abortion are far from complete. There is no national dataset on why people have abortions or whether they were trying to prevent conception, or even if they willingly had sex at the time they became pregnant. But in examining the data we do have, perhaps we can understand how it happens that nearly a million people seek abortions each year in the United States.

PREVENTED PREGNANCIES

First of all, from a demographic perspective, there's no doubt about it: the vast majority of unwanted pregnancies are prevented through contraception rather than ended through abortion. Based on historical data, we estimate that people at risk of pregnancy might have about eleven children each over a lifetime. The highest observed fertility was among the Hutterites, a Protestant group in the midwestern United States, who were observed in the 1920s to have an average of 10.9 children per woman (Coale 1965, 1971). Further examination showed that even the Hutterites were doing some things that reduced their maximum possible childbearing, such as delaying marriage to their early twenties, breastfeeding children (Chao 1987), and reducing the frequency of coitus toward the end of childbearing ages (Robinson 1986). If we all began having heterosexual sex as teenagers, did not nurse our children, and kept up the pace of date nights, we might achieve about fifteen children on average. Abortion, contraception, and not universal or constant heterosexual intercourse all help explain why we have fewer children than that: an average of 1.66 children per woman in the United States in 2021 (Hamilton, Martin, and Osterman 2021).

It's worth underscoring that abortion is only one contributor to that number. We don't have an average of over thirteen abortions, which is what we would need to yield just 1.6 children per woman if abortion was the only method used for preventing births. In fact, the average number of lifetime abortions in the United States is significantly less than one per woman (Hamilton, Martin, and Osterman 2024).[2] It's not easy to determine how much of the reduction from fifteen children to our current average is due to contraception versus abstinence, but it is likely that contraception explains the vast majority of pregnancy prevention among heterosexual women. And it is clear is that abortion accounts for only a tiny fraction. However, the observation that most unwanted pregnancies are averted rather than aborted doesn't answer the question about how many more could have been prevented.

Unpreventable Pregnancies

My email correspondent asserts that there are some people who bear no responsibility for becoming pregnant. He gives people who have been raped as the example. A rough estimate, based on surveys of people seeking abortion in clinics, is that the pregnancy was a result of rape for 1 in 100 patients (Finer et al. 2005). In addition to self-reported victims of rape, other patients may not have chosen to have sex. One in twenty-five abortions are to women under age eighteen (Jerman, Jones, and Onda 2016). Some who are very young and whose partners were older are victims of statutory rape. There is clearly a level of development below which someone cannot truly consent to intercourse, though the line is not likely marked by a specific age. Even the estimate of one in twenty-five abortions being to minors based on surveys of abortion patients undercounts the number of young women who become pregnant against their will. Young women have greater barriers to accessing abortion care and are less likely to be able to get a wanted abortion (Upadhyay et al. 2014). We don't know the true magnitude of unwanted pregnancy among very young people if they don't show up at an abortion clinic to be counted in abortion surveys.

There's a whole other set of pregnancies ending in abortion that could not have been prevented—those that are wanted. Some fraction of abortions are to women whose intended pregnancies went wrong—either due to a developing health problem in the pregnancy or a concern about the health of the fetus. From the national data of abortion patients, approximately one in eight say they are seeking abortions because of a concern about fetal health and an equal fraction because of a concern for the pregnant person's health (Finer et al. 2005).

We don't know how many of these were intended pregnancies terminated for maternal or fetal health reasons alone or unintended pregnancies for which health was just one of the deciding factors. I do know that these estimates don't count all *intended* pregnancies that end in abortion. These data are partial. They come from high volume, primarily outpatient providers. So they don't count those who get care for an emergency—such as ruptured membranes, eclampsia, or cardiovascular emergency—who are more likely to get abortions in hospitals. They also may undercount those who receive a diagnosis of a fetal anomaly. Such diagnoses occur later in pregnancy, and therefore are more likely to be treated in smaller abortion practices that specialize in people later in pregnancy. These estimates of the fetal and maternal health indications for abortion also don't count selective reduction abortions for multiple gestation pregnancies, where some fetuses are removed from the uterus to give the others and the pregnant person a greater chance of health and survival (Sam et al. 2022).

For many reasons—maternal and fetal—not all wanted pregnancies are carried to term, and sometimes an abortion enables people to regain their health and deliver children who have the greatest chance at survival.

SEX

This brings us to people who knowingly, willingly had the kind of sex that can lead to conception despite not actively seeking pregnancy. I hope it is not news to readers that this is not a rare occurrence. We've all heard the joke about the young child first learning about sexual intercourse from their older sibling who says to their parents, "You've done this TWICE?" Most people do not have sex for the chance at conception but for many other reasons including pleasure, emotional bonding, and joy.

It is not just children and a few religious groups who might envision a world where people have sex only for reproduction. I have a story about this. My sister, Lesley Greene, wrote a funny and smart play about the Turnaway Study. It tells the story of the science and also shares the words of women who participated in the study, telling their own experiences. One step in developing a play is to host readings of the play with actors reading from scripts and afterward provide a chance for the audience to give feedback. Lesley hosted a reading at the end of 2022 in a very small theater in Hartford, Connecticut. After the reading, the actors, my sister, and I all came on to the stage to have a conversation with the audience. A young woman in the front raised her hand to tell us that she thinks abortion is wrong, but what she learned from the play is that people who decide to have an abortion are trying to make the best possible decision for themselves and their children. She offered what she viewed as the one ethical solution—to have sex only when you're trying to make a baby.

I nodded and thanked her for sharing her viewpoint. I think I started to say something vaguely supportive but noncommittal about the huge diversity of ways that people choose to live their lives. But the great reproductive justice scholar Loretta Ross was also attending this reading (see Ross and Solinger 2017 for more on reproductive justice and her role in the movement). As I am mumbling all my affirmations about this woman's solution, we hear Ross's booming voice from the back: "SEXUAL PLEASURE IS GOOD!" I have to agree with Loretta Ross on this one. Sexual pleasure can be an important part of life, and very few people willingly choose to forgo it. It is not an ideal solution, for most people, to have sex only for procreation.

Given that most people don't have sex only in an effort to make babies, relying on abstinence is not an effective approach to prevent the need for abortion. This leads us to the option favored by my email correspondent.

DURATION OF CONTRACEPTIVE USE

Of course, one can experience sexual pleasure and still protect against pregnancy by using methods of contraception. And this, my email correspondent implies, would reduce the need for abortions. Let me unpack what that means. It means consistently using contraception for potentially more than thirty years—from one's first time having sex to menopause, stopping use only to conceive a few intended pregnancies. Contraception is expensive, and it requires a lot of diligence, forethought, and tolerance of side effects.

Exactly what sort of commitment does it require to prevent pregnancy for a heterosexual woman who begins having sex at age eighteen, starts menopause around age forty-five, and wants to—when she's ready—have two kids? I estimated in my book, *The Turnaway Study* (Foster 2020b), that she would have to take 6,844 contraceptive pills, use condoms every time for 2,350 acts of intercourse, replace her 975 patches or 325 vaginal rings on time, or have four to six intrauterine devices (IUDs) inserted and removed. Most women use more than one method over a lifetime, and most methods are not available over the counter, so she will also have to make regular medical appointments to arrange for the appropriate prescriptions or procedures and make regular trips to the pharmacy to keep up her supplies. And all of this assumes she has consistent access to health insurance and can afford the co-pays.

Even for the woman who uses contraceptives ceaselessly, there would still be significant chances of becoming pregnant. Over a reproductive lifetime, she might still become pregnant as many as two times on the pill, four with condoms, and seven using withdrawal. Indeed, we have the data to see that many people become pregnant despite using contraception. In national data of abortion patients in 2014, over half reported having used contraception in the month they conceived (Jerman, Jones, and Onda 2016). In my Turnaway Study, which was not a random sample of abortion patients but instead intentionally recruited more people seeking abortions later in pregnancy, two-thirds of the participants reported having used a contraceptive method when they became pregnant. Why the difference? In part because when people use contraception, they are slower to recognize that they are indeed pregnant (Foster et al. 2021). But the bigger point is that many people who need abortions were using contraception in the month they conceived that unwanted pregnancy.

It is not that contraception is so flawed that many people become pregnant while using it. Nearly all women of reproductive age (90 percent) have used contraception (Frederiksen et al. 2022). There are so many people who use contraception that even a small percentage of users becoming pregnant creates a significant number of people who are pregnant despite use. Some of these pregnancies are due to failures of the method; fewer than 1 percent of users become pregnant in a year of perfect use of the subdermal implant, sterilization, IUDs, injectables, pill, patch, or ring (Guttmacher Institute 2020)—that's not zero. And most people don't use contraceptives perfectly—never missing a pill, using condoms with every act of intercourse, remembering to place and replace patches and rings. This is what contraceptive effectiveness scientists call "typical use." Typical use contraceptive failure rates are higher than perfect use and, in my opinion, reflect that the world is, indeed, not perfect.

Given the burden of consistently using contraception, it should not be a surprise to learn that most unintended pregnancies in the United States are caused not by contraceptive failure but by gaps in contraceptive use. And by "gaps," I mean not using a method for any period in what could be more than thirty potential childbearing years. When we asked women seeking abortion from six clinics in 2010 about their reasons for not using a method of contraception, two in five reported trouble accessing supplies (Foster et al. 2012). The very next year the Affordable Care Act (aka Obamacare) included a stipulation that employer-covered health insurance include no-co-pay coverage of a wide range of contraceptive methods (U.S. CMS, n.d.). This helped reduce the gaps in coverage for those with private insurance. For those who do not have private insurance, eligibility and program funding for publicly funded family planning services varies tremendously by state.

Yet still, in 2022 one in five uninsured women who participated in a nationwide survey reported that they have at some point stopped using contraception because of the cost (Frederiksen et al. 2022). Access to contraceptives is still far from universal in our country. To circle back to my email correspondent's suggestion about responsibility, we might ask about what role our government plays—and whether it is fulfilling its responsibilities—in meeting the basic health care needs of its citizens.

Meeting Contraceptive Preferences

Besides the hassle and expense of securing a supply of contraception, why else might women not want to use a method? The shockingly simple answer is that most contraceptive methods do not meet everyone's needs (Lessard et al. 2012). They want a method that is highly effective but has few side effects. They want a method that is easy to get and easy to use. Many want control over when and whether to use the method. There are lots of features that users might want in a contraceptive method— one that relieves menstrual symptoms, one that doesn't cause hair loss, one that you can stop using any time without going to a clinic, one that makes female orgasm more likely. (That last one doesn't exist yet, but wouldn't it be wonderful?) My previous studies have found that existing methods of contraception have less than two-thirds of the features that women report are very important to them.

Women of color have somewhat different preferences for contraceptive features than white women, possibly the product of a historically justifiable suspicion of healthcare institutions and providers as well as contraceptive methods (Jackson et al. 2016). The United States has a long history of denying women of color their full humanity and control over reproduction—everything from forced childbearing in the time of slavery to forced sterilization in recent decades. As a result of having stronger preferences, women of color are even less likely to find methods that have their desired features.

Ultimately, what this means is that some women find methods that meet their needs. But for many, preventing unintended pregnancy involves putting up with a host of side effects, regularly going to clinics or pharmacies, and sometimes paying a lot of money out of pocket just to keep using a method they don't like in the hopes of avoiding conception.

Choosing Not to Use Contraception (and Having a Choice)

Finally, we get to the people for whom my correspondent is likely reserving judgment—those who have access to contraception but still don't consistently use it. Are they necessarily being irresponsible?[3] The chance of conception from an act of intercourse is about 3 percent if you don't know where in your menstrual cycle you are. If you are in the six days leading up to ovulation, the risk is about 10 percent (Wilcox et al. 2001). Unfortunately, it isn't easy to know when you are in a six-day window before ovulation. Without careful monitoring of body temperature and cervical mucus, most people can't tell when they are ovulating, much less whether they are in the one-week window before it happens. Many couples, including both those who seek abortions and those who have never had an unwanted pregnancy, have sex without using a method of contraception because sex can be pleasurable and the chance of conception per act is actually quite low (Foster et al. 2012).

And let's take a moment to point out there is an imbalance in both the pleasures and the consequences of heterosexual sex. Sexual intercourse may be more wonderful for the man than for the woman—three-fourths of men report that their last sexual event was quite or extremely pleasurable compared with just under two-thirds of women (Herbenick et al. 2023). If an unintended pregnancy does occur, it will become disproportionately her problem, a burden that she will literally physically carry. Gendered social narratives, purportedly built on the biotechnical aspects of pregnancy and contraception, mean that she bears nearly all the burden of preventing pregnancy as well (Fennell 2011).

This imbalance in the benefits of sex and the burden of its consequences, along with deep-rooted misogyny, contributes to the problem of contraceptive coercion (which is different from coercive sex, as discussed earlier). Contraceptive coercion includes refusing to use a method of contraception (e.g., a condom) or preventing one's partner from using one. We have found that among women who seek abortions, one in five reported that their partner did not want to use birth control; one in twenty reported that their partner forced them to have unprotected sex; and one in 100 reported that their partner messed with their birth control (Foster et al. 2012).

So, although my correspondent pointed out that it was the "responsibility of the woman and man to take the necessary steps to not get pregnant," the woman and man have different motivations and responsibilities and may not be working together toward the same goal.

Could Technology Prevent All Unwanted Pregnancies?

It is tempting to look for easy technological solutions to what seems like an extremely messy personal and social problem. Inherent in the issues of contraceptive development and choice are the complex topics of sex, gender relations, power dynamics, access to health care, the huge range of physiological responses to devices and hormones, the need for control over use, privacy and dependability, and more.

Long-acting reversible methods of contraception ("LARC" methods) have been touted as methods you can just "set and forget" with no room for user error. LARC methods include the contraceptive implant and IUD, the most effective reversible methods of contraception. The idea is that greater use of LARC technologies can bypass the presumed main weak point in effective contraceptive use—users—and thereby reduce unintended pregnancies and abortions. This simplistic and rosy view is often held by people who don't fully acknowledge the pain of insertion for both these methods, the potential for side effects and complications, and the understandable desire for personal control over a method's start and discontinuation—plenty of people do not want to "set and forget" their contraception.

Don't get me wrong: I am a huge personal fan of IUDs. I have had both copper and hormonal IUDs, and they suited me very well. Before menopause, I loved not worrying about pregnancy because of the IUD. And with the hormonal IUD, I loved not getting a menstrual period. However, I know the IUD is not for everyone. When we are talking about a device that is implanted inside one's body, there should be a lot of deference for personal decision-making.

But let's walk through this LARC-first "solution" anyway. In a world possibly preferred by my email correspondent, maybe everyone would get a LARC method before they became sexually active and keep getting them removed and replaced every four years until they decided they were ready to become pregnant. In that world, we would still expect tens of thousands of abortions.[4] It's a large reduction from the hundreds of thousands of abortions we currently have, but it is not a better world. Why? Because such a world would require people using specific contraceptives against their will. I asked 100 scientists and clinicians who research IUDs and implants to estimate the fraction of women who would choose to use an IUD or implant if all barriers to access of these methods were removed (Foster et al. 2015). Their estimate was about a quarter—similar to the levels at the time of LARC use in France and Norway (UN Department of Economic and Social Affairs 2007). In a world of universal LARC use, people would not have autonomy over their own bodies; the majority of people would be using methods against their will. (There would also be no room for people who don't want to plan their pregnancies in advance—those who are happy to live with ambivalence and the possibility of a happy surprise.) In a quest to end unwanted pregnancies, we would be giving up freedom and bodily autonomy.

Sometimes LARC promotion is framed not as a way to reduce abortion but as a way to reduce unintended births or, more grandly, poverty itself. The claim rests on assumptions that poor people are poor because they have too many children, and this leads to an intergenerational cycle of poverty. The assumption is wrong, and as an argument for LARC use, it is troubling. Only a very small percentage of people living below the poverty line are infants or new mothers (Foster 2020a). And although childbirth and a baby's first few years are a time of particular economic vulnerability, it is the lack of paid parental leave, childcare, health care, or assistance to the poor in the United States that is the cause of new parents falling into poverty: a finding that is clear when one compares economic status of new parents across developed countries (Brady, Finnigan, and Hübgen 2017).

In 2020, I published a commentary in the *American Journal of Obstetrics and Gynecology* called "The Problems with a Poverty Argument for Long-Acting Reversible Contraceptive Promotion" where I spelled out why contraceptives cannot prevent poverty and, more to the point, why any reason for promoting this method apart from that it is someone's chosen method will likely backfire (Foster 2020a). Promoting LARC methods for the wrong reasons (e.g., poverty alleviation, population control, environmental concerns, prevention of teenaged childbearing) rather than as the fulfillment of women's own reproductive goals can only have a negative effect on the reputation of these methods. Promotion of family planning for reasons other the woman's own is likely to result in reduced trust, and trust is exactly what is needed to enable women who want a LARC method to use one.

Tying this back to my email correspondent, the point is that contraceptive use is and should be personal. It isn't a means of resolving—or nullifying—social and political debates.

Conclusions

Now I offer one final note to my email correspondent. Implicit in his email is the idea that preventing pregnancy is ethically or morally superior to having an abortion. This moral perspective is not universal. For people who believe that both contraception and abortion are sins, preventing pregnancy means sinning every act, day, or month, which might be worse in their day-to-day life than the possibility of aborting the few unwanted pregnancies that are likely to occur. And, of course, there are people who do not have moral qualms about abortion, who view it as another way, like contraception, to have the number of children you want, when you want them.

You might expect this chapter to end with a final count of how many abortions could be prevented through contraception and the number of pregnancies that should not have been prevented because they were wanted or could not have been prevented because the sex was coerced, the contraception was sabotaged, or the contraceptives failed. In principle, it could be possible to estimate these things, even though all the data are imprecisely measured and the factors are not independent. Some of the youngest women are already counted among the 1 percent who were raped. Some of the wanted pregnancies where poor health led to a desire to terminate were actually conceived as a result of contraceptive failure. Some of the women who did not have a steady supply of contraceptives also had partners who prevented them from using the few packs of pills they had. But the more important point is that, even if contraception were universally available and effective, people would still seek abortions.

The exercise of trying to decide exactly which pregnancies were due to people being irresponsible reminds me of a discussion of the common legal exceptions to abortion bans—for example, those done to save a woman's life or in cases of rape or incest. In the podcast "This Is How We Work Together toward Reproductive Rights" (ACLU of North Carolina 2024), Dr. Beverly Gray, an abortion provider in North Carolina, talks about how trying to define exceptions to bans is like deciding who gets to have a legal abortion—who is in a "sphere of compassion." She says, "There's this lack of understanding of all the other people that live in our community and in our world that need compassion for reasons that aren't in that tight sphere that people who are willing offer exceptions are willing to give." The same exercise is required to decide which pregnant people are worthy of compassion. It is not possible to understand, for somebody else, all the experiences and considerations that go into sex, contraception, and deciding to have an abortion. But we can trust them, as individuals, to be the best judge of their circumstances and how they got there.

The question of whether contraception can avert abortions has gained new significance since the 2022 *Dobbs v. Jackson Women's Heath Organization* Supreme Court decision, which removed the federal protections for abortion rights established under *Roe v. Wade*. If abortion is no longer legal, will people be more likely to prevent unwanted pregnancies? A change in contraceptive use in response to a law change would require many contributing factors, including for people to know that abortion is illegal and therefore more difficult to access or to decide that they are at risk of pregnancy and then have the means to prevent it. I have been skeptical that this cascade of events will occur. Even when abortion was legal, people didn't always know the legal status of abortion until they needed one. Most people have unprotected sex thinking (rightly) that conception is not likely. And people who aren't using contraception have reasons for doing so—either they don't think they are at risk of pregnancy or they don't think that the available methods are good for them (Biggs, Karasek, and Foster 2012).

My skepticism has so far seemed justified given the data that have emerged in the eighteen months after *Dobbs*. The total number of abortions in the United States has actually increased since the Supreme Court allowed abortion state-level bans (Society of Family Planning 2024; see also the chapter by Jenny O'Donnell in this volume). This increase is likely due to reductions in the cost of abortion through telemedicine and online ordering as well as the massive efforts directed toward helping people travel to and pay for in-clinic abortions. However, this increase in abortions suggests that there has not been the drop in demand for abortion that we would have expected had a change in the perception of abortion access inspired people to use contraception more diligently.

My email correspondent and others who would like to see the number of abortions reduced (whatever their position on the legality of abortion) imagine a dynamic and inverse relationship between contraception and abortion wherein "better" use of one can obviate the need for the other. But real people's lives don't work like this. Contraceptive use is motivated by far more than the desire to avoid abortion. Returning to the underlying moral and ethical claim being made about abortion, contraception without abortion is not and can never be enough to achieve reproductive freedom and justice.

NOTES

1. One could say it does not matter, that abortion rights should not be withheld no matter the circumstances of the pregnancy. Otherwise, the outcome is that pregnancy is treated as a punishment for perceived irresponsibility rather than a blessing.

2. Researchers who study clinics and telemedicine count about 1 million abortions per year (Society of Family Planning 2024), which occur to the 65 million women aged fifteen to forty-four in the United States (U.S. Census Bureau, American Community Survey, 2022 1-Year Estimates, S0101: Age and Sex, https://data.census.gov/table/ACSST1Y2022.S0101). We spend thirty years in that age range, so if abortion rates stayed constant, we would average just under 0.5 abortions each.

3. There's an excellent book on this topic by Kristin Luker, *Taking Chances: Abortion and the Decision Not to Contracept* (1975), that examines the topic using in-depth interview data and a sociological perspective.

4. There are 65 million women aged eighteen to forty-four, perhaps half of whom are heterosexually sexually active but not pregnant or seeking pregnancy at any given time. Implants have the lowest failure rate at 0.1 percent per year. So that's 30,000+ unwanted pregnancies. And this does not count all the abortions that would be required for wanted pregnancies gone wrong.

REFERENCES

ACLU of North Carolina. 2024. "Part 2: This Is How We Work Together toward Reproductive Rights." *This Is How . . .* (podcast), March 4, 2024. https://podcasts.apple.com/us /podcast/pt-2-this-is-how-we-work-together-toward-reproductive-rights/id1723863934?i =1000647951201.

Biggs, M. Antonia, Deborah Karasek, and Diana Greene Foster. 2012. "Unprotected Intercourse among Women Wanting to Avoid Pregnancy: Attitudes, Behaviors, and Beliefs." *Women's Health Issues* 22 (3): e311–e318. https://doi.org/10.1016/j.whi.2012.03.003.

Brady, David, Ryan M. Finnigan, and Sabine Hübgen. 2017. "Rethinking the Risks of Poverty: A Framework for Analyzing Prevalences and Penalties." *American Journal of Sociology* 123 (3): 740–786. https://doi.org/10.1086/693678.

Chao, S. 1987. "The Effect of Lactation on Ovulation and Fertility." *Clinics in Perinatology* 14 (1): 39–50.

Coale, A. J. 1965. "Factors Associated with the Development of Low Fertility: An Historic Summary." In: *Proceedings of the World Population Conference. Belgrade, 30 August–10 September 1965.* Vol. 2, *Selected Paper and Summaries: Fertility, Family Planning, Mortality.* Edited by UN Department of Economic and Social Affairs, 205–209. World Population Conference, United Nations.

———. 1971. "Age Patterns of Marriage." *Population Studies* 25 (2): 193–214. https://doi.org/10 .1080/00324728.1971.10405798.

Fennell, Julie Lynn. 2011. "Men Bring Condoms, Women Take Pills: Men's and Women's Roles in Contraceptive Decision Making." *Gender & Society* 25 (4): 496–521. https://doi.org /10.1177/0891243211416113.

Finer, Lawrence B., Lori F. Frohwirth, Lindsay A. Dauphinee, Susheela Singh, and Ann M. Moore. 2005. "Reasons U.S. Women Have Abortions: Quantitative and Qualitative Perspectives." *Perspectives on Sexual and Reproductive Health* 37 (3): 110–118. https://doi.org/10 .1363/psrh.37.110.05.

Foster, Diana Greene. 2020a. "The Problems with a Poverty Argument for Long-Acting Reversible Contraceptive Promotion." *American Journal of Obstetrics and Gynecology* 222 (4S): S861–S863. https://doi.org/10.1016/j.ajog.2020.01.051.

———. 2020b. *The Turnaway Study: Ten Years, a Thousand Women, and the Consequences of Having—or Being Denied—an Abortion.* Scribner.

Foster, Diana Greene, Rana Barar, Heather Gould, Ivette Gomez, Deborah Nguyen, and M. Antonia Biggs. 2015. "Projections and Opinions from 100 Experts in Long-Acting

Reversible Contraception." *Contraception* 92 (6): 543–552. https://doi.org/10.1016/j
.contraception.2015.10.003.

Foster, Diana Greene, Heather Gould, and M. Antonia Biggs. 2021. "Timing of Pregnancy
Discovery among Women Seeking Abortion." *Contraception* 104 (6): 642–647. https://doi
.org/10.1016/j.contraception.2021.07.110.

Foster, Diana Greene, Jenny A. Higgins, Deborah Karasek, Sandi Ma, and Daniel Grossman.
2012. "Attitudes toward Unprotected Intercourse and Risk of Pregnancy among Women
Seeking Abortion." *Women's Health Issues* 22 (2): e149–e155. https://doi.org/10.1016/j.whi
.2011.08.009.

Frederiksen, Brittni, Usha Ranji, Michelle Long, Karen Diep, and Alina Salganicoff. 2022.
"Contraception in the United States: A Closer Look at Experiences, Preferences, and Coverage." KFF: Women's Health Policy. https://www.kff.org/womens-health-policy/report
/contraception-in-the-united-states-a-closer-look-at-experiences-preferences-and-coverage/.

Guttmacher Institute. 2020. "Contraceptive Effectiveness in the United States." *Contraceptive
Use in the United States: Fact Sheet*. https://www.guttmacher.org/fact-sheet/contraceptive
-effectiveness-united-states.

Hamilton, Brady E., Joyce A. Martin, and Michelle J. K. Osterman. 2024. "Births: Provi-
sional Data for 2023." *Vital Statistics Rapid Release*, no. 25. April 2024. https://www.cdc
.gov/nchs/data/vsrr/vsrr035.pdf.

Herbenick, Debby, Tsung-chieh Fu, and Callie Patterson. 2023. "Sexual Repertoire, Duration
of Partnered Sex, Sexual Pleasure, and Orgasm: Findings from a US Nationally Representative Survey of Adults." *Journal of Sex & Marital Therapy* 49 (4): 369–390. https://doi.org/10
.1080/0092623x.2022.2126417.

Jackson, Andrea V., Deborah Karasek, Christine Dehlendorf, and Diana Greene Foster. 2016.
"Racial and Ethnic Differences in Women's Preferences for Features of Contraceptive Methods." *Contraception* 93 (5): 406–411. https://doi.org/10.1016/j.contraception.2015.12.010.

Jerman, Jenna, Rachel K. Jones, and Tsuyoshi Onda. 2016. "Characteristics of U.S. Abortion
Patients in 2014 and Changes Since 2008." Guttmacher Institute. https://www
.guttmacher.org/report/characteristics-us-abortion-patients-2014.

Lessard, Lauren N., Deborah Karasek, Sandi Ma, Philip Darney, Julianna Deardorff, Maureen Lahiff, Dan Grossman, and Diana Greene Foster. 2012. "Contraceptive Features Preferred by Women at High Risk of Unintended Pregnancy." *Perspectives on Sexual and
Reproductive Health* 44 (3): 194–200. https://doi.org/10.1363/4419412.

Luker, Kristin. 1975. *Taking Chances: Abortion and the Decision Not to Contracept*. University of California Press.

National Women's Health Network and SisterSong. 2017. "Long-Acting Reversible Contraception Statement of Principles." Updated February 8, 2017. https://health.usf.edu
/publichealth/chiles/fpqc/larc/~/media/043402D6CF0842DD95DC65E604B07B46.ashx.

Robinson, Warren C. 1986. "Another Look at the Hutterites and Natural Fertility." *Social
Biology* 33 (1–2): 65–76. https://doi.org/10.1080/19485565.1986.9988623.

Ross, Loretta, and Rickie Solinger. 2017. *Reproductive Justice: An Introduction*. University of
California Press.

Sam, Sreya, Sarah Tai-MacArthur, Panicos Shangaris, and Srividhya Sankaran. 2022.
"Trends of Selective Fetal Reduction and Selective Termination in Multiple Pregnancy, in
England and Wales: A Cross-Sectional Study." *Reproductive Sciences* 29 (3): 1020–1027.
https://doi.org/10.1007/s43032-021-00819-5.

Society of Family Planning. 2024. "April 2022 to September 2023." #WeCount Public Report,
February 28, 2024. https://doi.org/10.46621/675707thmfmv.

UN Department of Economic and Social Affairs/Population Division. 2007. "Levels and
Trends of Contraceptive Use as Assessed in 2002." https://www.un.org/development/desa
/pd/sites/www.un.org.development.desa.pd/files/files/documents/2020/Jan/un_2002
_levelsandtrendscontraception.pdf.

Upadhyay, Ushma D., Tracy A. Weitz, Rachel K. Jones, Rana E. Barar, and Diana Greene
Foster. 2014. "Denial of Abortion Because of Provider Gestational Age Limits in the

United States." *American Journal of Public Health* 104 (9): 1687–1694. https://doi.org/10
.2105/AJPH.2013.301378.

U.S. Centers for Medicare & Medicaid Services (CMS). "Health Benefits and Coverage: Birth
Control Benefits." n.d. HealthCare.gov. Accessed September 17, 2024. https://web.archive
.org/web/20240917005309/https://www.healthcare.gov/coverage/birth-control-benefits/.

Wilcox, Allen J., David B. Dunson, Clarice R. Weinberg, James Trussell, and Donna Day
Baird. 2001. "Likelihood of Conception with a Single Act of Intercourse: Providing Bench-
mark Rates for Assessment of Post-Coital Contraceptives." *Contraception* 63 (4): 211–215.
https://doi.org/10.1016/S0010-7824(01)00191-3.

CHAPTER 2

What *Dobbs* Revealed About the Everyday Morality of Abortion

Whitney Arey and Klaira Lerma

Within eighteen months of the Supreme Court's 2022 decision in *Dobbs v. Jackson Women's Health Organization* (*Dobbs*), more than twenty states had implemented abortion restrictions (Center for Reproductive Rights 2024). However, nearly all these laws had one or more exceptions—that is, instances where abortion was legally allowable despite a general prohibition. Broadly, these exceptions fell into four domains: to prevent the death of the pregnant person; to protect the health of the pregnant person; for pregnancies resulting of incest or rape; and in the case of a lethal fetal anomaly (Felix and Sobel 2021).

The concept of exceptions to abortion restrictions is not new. U.S. federal and state-level abortion bans have long distinguished some abortions as exceptions to restrictions. For example, at the federal level, starting in 1977, the Hyde Amendment banned the use of federal funding for abortion while allowing exceptions to pay for terminations in cases of rape or incest or for pregnancies that endanger the life of the pregnant person. Yet in the wake of *Dobbs* and subsequent state-level abortion bans, what is new is clear evidence of how legal exceptions are deeply challenging to implement in practice, leading healthcare workers to fear criminalization and fail to offer the standard of care to obstetric and gynecologic patients (Lift Louisiana et al. 2024; Physicians for Human Rights 2023). Indeed, as the chapter by Danielle Bessett and colleagues in this volume documents, post-*Dobbs*, people have started to pay attention to the failures of abortion "exceptions" to ensure patient health and safety.

Here, we build on this burgeoning awareness to illustrate how abortion exceptions in law are evidence of a much broader social discourse of abortion legitimacy. Extending the term *abortion exceptionalism* to capture how abortion in the United States is—and has been—stratified and regulated in terms of legitimacy, we illustrate the presence and long operation of a social discourse that constructs some abortions as more morally, socially, and politically acceptable than others. In this chapter, drawing on patient and provider accounts of experiences of abortion, we show how this legitimacy rhetoric operates and some of its consequences. Well-established long before the *Dobbs* decision, this discourse of abortion legitimacy influences contemporary understandings of abortion, and understanding this is crucial for making sense of the future of abortion in the United States.

We each bring our individual experiences to this chapter as an abortion worker (K. L.) and as activists and researchers (K. L. and W. A.). For the past decade, we have collectively cared for or interviewed hundreds of people who have considered or had abortions. We draw from reports in the media, peer-reviewed research, and examples from our original research in Texas (K. L. and W. A.) and in North Carolina (W. A.) collected before *Dobbs* (2021–2022 and 2018–2019, respectively).

Abortion Exceptionalism: A Proxy for "Legitimate" Abortions

The term "abortion exceptionalism" was initially coined to describe the legal cases regulating abortion that systematically made abortion less accessible across the United States, enacted in response to the 1973 Supreme Court decision in *Roe v. Wade* that provided constitutional protections for abortion. Put differently, it described the pattern of legislation that treated abortion provision differently from other similar (and sometimes higher risk) kinds of medical care (Borgmann 2014). But the idea that abortion is treated differently and that some abortions are acceptable—and thus exceptions to general bans—extends beyond the law.

Broader social discourse also categorizes abortions in terms of acceptability. For example, abortions for medically complex pregnancy conditions are often referred to in medical practice as "medically indicated" or "therapeutic." Such framing is in contrast to "elective" abortions. However, "elective" here is different from its typical use in medicine as a term for surgeries scheduled for future times; instead, the meaning is that abortions are "voluntary" or lack "legitimate" medical indications (Kimport, Weitz, and Freedman 2016; Smith et al. 2018). In practice, the abortions considered "elective" are valued less and are regulated more strictly.

For example, pre-*Dobbs*, due to state-level restrictions regulating insurance provision for abortion as well as institutional objections to abortion provision (such as the directives at Catholic hospitals), some Texas hospitals only allowed on-site abortions that were deemed "therapeutic" or "indicated" (Merner et al. 2023). As one Texas obstetrician-gynecologist described this policy, "I do medically indicated abortion care. In my organization, we are not allowed to perform elective abortion, or abortion upon request" (Arey et al. 2022). There is not, however, a *clinical* difference: "therapeutic," "indicated," and "elective" abortions all consist of the same medical procedures, and no different skills are required based on the circumstances in which the abortion is chosen. Yet the rules around abortion provision are not the same at every institution (Arey et al. 2023).

Further evidencing the fuzziness of the distinction, treatment for the same conditions has distinctive interpretations in different states, at different hospitals in the same state, and among individual clinicians within the same hospitals. For example, a Texas-based obstetrician-gynecologist described how different hospitals and providers had differing criteria for when an abortion would be considered "medically indicated": "[in] discussions about a patient who received a fetal diagnosis . . . that would eventually result in fetal death, some people see it as non-elective, and some people see it as elective" (Arey et al. 2022). Abortion categorization was surprisingly flexible in practice. This practice of classifying abortions according to exceptions creates a *stratified legitimacy* of abortions, in which people's abortions are valued differently according to interpretations of their circumstances (Kimport et al. 2016). These ideas are not exclusive to the United States and scholars have documented similar practices in a variety of settings (Nandagiri 2019; Leask 2015; Beynon-Jones 2017; Norris et al. 2011).

Many scholars, healthcare providers, and researchers have critiqued categorizing abortions in this way, arguing that separating kinds of abortions based on the reasons for having one amounts to moral judgments on patients and perpetuates abortion stigma. Katie Watson, for example, argues,

> Ultimately, the term *elective abortion* is moral judgment dressed up as medical judgment. Medical versus elective is code for morally justified versus morally unjustified. . . . Every abortion is elective. No pregnant woman with health problems is required to terminate her pregnancy—she can choose to deliver a baby with a disability or a terminal condition, risk her own health to deliver a baby, or decide the risks outweigh the benefits and choose abortion. . . . The distinction between elective and medically indicated abortions is a regressive, destructive conceit. What really distinguishes abortion patients with medical indications is that these pregnant women are presumed to have initially wanted a child—they would not have asked for an abortion if it weren't for this health problem—or, in cases of rape and incest, that they did not consent to sex. The allowance hospitals, private practice groups, and insurers make for medically necessary abortions is not a medical line, it is a sex-discriminatory social line: *We will only care for women who accept the social norms that women are meant to be mothers and that women cannot have sex solely for pleasure instead of for procreation. Mainstream medicine will cast out all others.* (2018, 1176–1177, emphases in original)

It goes beyond medicine. This form of stratified legitimacy in medicine also informs dominant cultural narratives of who is "allowed" to choose an abortion, marking some abortions as legally and medically legitimate. In the case of allowing exceptions for "medically indicated" abortions in some medical spaces, these select abortions are produced as more legitimate than "elective" abortions. This legitimacy rhetoric contributes to cultural stereotypes about who has abortions, often in ways that reflect broader social stereotypes about race and class (Rosenthal and Lobel 2016; Dobbins-Harris 2017) and reinforce stigma toward populations whose abortions are deemed less legitimate (Bommaraju et al. 2016; Caron 2016). These categorizations of abortion and the legitimacy they imply are present in people's moral experiences of their own abortions as well.

EXCEPTIONALISM DISCOURSE IS REPRODUCED IN
AND THROUGH INDIVIDUAL EXPERIENCES

Interviews across research projects have showcased how abortion seekers them-selves can hold negative ideas about the legitimacy of some abortions—and fellow abortion seekers. For example, a patient from North Carolina described her under-standing of abortion morality and how this shifted after she found herself in a situation where she needed an abortion:

> I wasn't really supportive of abortion. I thought that the only people who got abortions were people who were raped or dealing with an incest issue or people who just had too much sex. Like I saw myself—I got into a good college. I have a good paying job. I live a really good life. But living the American Dream post-grad, here I am pregnant by a guy who I know but literally doesn't want any-thing to do with this kid. So, I was like, this can happen to anybody. It doesn't matter who you are, you can get pregnant. But yeah, [my opinion] completely changed. Like I mentioned, there were women who kind of like fell into the cat-egory at the abortion clinic, but when I've been the walking epitome of "you can have a perfect life, and you can still fuck up and get an abortion." So now I guess I'm a part of that group.

In describing other people who "fell into the category," this patient highlighted the ways that stratified legitimacy is repeated and reinterpreted in individual experi-ences. Until she herself faced decision-making around a pregnancy, she relied on stereotypes that often make up dominant U.S. narratives about abortion seekers. More simply put, she had deep assumptions about the type of people who had abor-tions. It took a personal experience of an unintended pregnancy for her to realize that her assumptions were unfounded.

Furthermore, when law, policy, and medicine define some abortions as acceptable, they are marked as culturally legitimate (Leask 2015). This can affect people's understandings of their own abortion experiences. For example, Whit-ney Arey (2021) conducted research at two independent abortion clinics in North Carolina from 2018 to 2019. The first laws that banned abortion after detection of embryonic cardiac activity at approximately six weeks of pregnancy—before the gestational development of a heart—were introduced and passed by four states in 2019 (Georgia, Kentucky, Mississippi, and Ohio) and were referred to as "heart-beat bills" (Pyle et al. 2024). These were the precursors to laws that now have gone into effect in many states after *Dobbs*. Arey found that when these laws were passed in nearby states, patients in North Carolina started discussing their abor-tion using heartbeat language, despite there not being a heartbeat bill in North Carolina, noting in interviews that their abortions would be illegal in other states. For example, a patient who had a medication abortion at approximately six weeks' gestation in North Carolina, soon after the first heartbeat bills had been passed in Georgia in 2019, referenced the laws in thinking about her experience:

The bills that are being passed, it's terrifying. I mean at the point that I had the abortion, the fetus had a heartbeat. I think it's in Georgia and maybe in Ohio I would not have been allowed to have [the abortion]. And that terrifies me, because while I found out ungodly early, I know that a lot of women don't, and to think that someone wouldn't have access to have an abortion. . . . Even in my condition, I have a chronic pain syndrome. I think that contributed to me being so sick during the pregnancy. And to think of someone having to go through the pregnancy in my shoes, not being happy and feeling unsupported, that would just be horrible. And I know that people do, but I couldn't imagine having gone through it. I think that would be very traumatic.

This patient's moral experience of her abortion was shaped in part by imagining how it would have been restricted if she lived in another state. Although she understood her abortion as legitimate, the idea that it would be deemed illegitimate (or, at least, illegal) elsewhere was distressing.

Another patient in North Carolina who had an abortion at about seven weeks' gestation said,

Honestly, with all of these laws, the heartbeat bill being passed, this has really weighed on me a lot recently, but it's all over social media, and it really hurts emotionally because I see people such as my sister and other people that I kinda like grew up with, and they're just like [posting], "you're a murderer and you should kill yourself [for having an abortion]" and blah, blah, blah. And if these people knew that it was their sister and their friends and their schoolmates that had actually went and had an abortion, would they still want me to die? Would they still look at me like a murderer, or did they just have this one biased opinion, and they don't think that, you know, their stepmom, their sister, their best friends are the people that have went and secretly had abortion done and they just don't know about it.

As these quotes illustrate, laws, media coverage, and people's perceptions of them can impact how they think and talk about their own abortion experiences. What was most notable was that no interviews before these bills were passed contained references to heartbeat language, but after the bills were passed patients in North Carolina started using the heartbeat bill language to talk about their own abortions, using the legal gestational limits and the rhetoric about them as a marker for characterizing their own experiences.

So why does this matter for abortion exceptionalism? Laws and policies can create and maintain a distinction between legitimate and nonlegitimate abortions based on categorizations of what abortions are or are not allowed. People then use legitimacy discourse to talk about their own abortions in culturally legible ways, often as exceptional or distinct from the imagined stereotypical abortions. For example, there is high U.S. public support for abortion care in the case of medical emergencies (Schumacher et al. 2024), and in interviews, we saw how framing one's experience as part of this category of abortion was a way to establish rhetorical distance from negative associations with abortion (Braff 2013). In our research in Texas, a woman who had to leave the state to access abortion care due to the gestational limit at the time emphasized in her account the severe fetal health diagnosis she had received:

> Honestly, we didn't even think of it as [an abortion]—I didn't even realize that it would need to be done at an abortion clinic. Because to me, this was an obvious medical issue. My baby's brain was compressed into her skull. She had a hole in her spinal cord. She wasn't going to live. It seemed like this is not—this is a medical condition. It did not seem to me like what you would typically think of someone newly pregnant who doesn't want to be pregnant and wants an abortion.

Not only did a logic of "indicated" shape her understanding of her need for abortion, she deployed it to differentiate herself from the "typical" abortion seeker, whose experience she viewed as different from a medical reason for abortion. Such dual framings and the use of institutionalized exceptionalism language of "indicated" supported her abortion decision as different and legitimate.

In our research and experience, we often have observed that when people are confronted with the realities of abortion experiences or decision-making, they attempt to separate themselves and their experience from negative abortion associations by asserting a moral justification for their abortion. "Othering" is one such discursive response, where people distance themselves from negative constructs of "undeserving" or "illegitimate" abortions by characterizing their abortions as "deserving" or "exceptions" to the norm (Braff 2013; Norris et al. 2011). Exceptionalism discourse is one way to do so. By claiming their abortions were the exception, they could claim moral and cultural acceptability. Frontline abortion clinic staff members in North Carolina described this problem as the belief that "the only moral abortion is my abortion," where abortion stigma often compelled people to justify their reasons for having an abortion as moral and thus different from prevalent abortion stereotypes (Arey 2021).

Along these lines, some people with complex pregnancies did not use the word "abortion" to describe their experience. Instead, they used words like "termination" or "termination for medical reasons" to define their experiences as distinct from other abortions. Another Texan who went to an out-of-state abortion clinic because she was beyond the state's legal gestational limit said, "I wished it wasn't an abortion clinic because it did not feel like an abortion, it felt like . . . I don't know, something about that word just feels like the pregnancy wasn't wanted. I much prefer calling it a termination for medical reasons or compassionate induction." Importantly, this patient's recharacterization of her procedure as different from "abortion" due to a fetal health issue presented her abortion as exceptional even though she failed to meet the criteria for an exception under Texas's (admittedly draconian) law. The frame of exceptionalism persisted even when it was denied by law.

As these examples show, exceptionalism discourse has shaped cultural narratives of what "counts" as an abortion. These findings are consistent with research by Alicia VandeVusse and colleagues (2023), who write, "people do not hold a consistent, shared, biomedically based understanding of abortion, . . . respondents' implicit and explicit views of 'abortion' as a negative and stigmatizing word, outcome or action meant that there was a preference to avoid labeling something an abortion or someone as having an abortion, even when respondents understood the experience to meet the biomedical definition of abortion" (6).

Even as exceptionalism discourse operated to prevent people from initially accepting their experiences as abortions, their experiences of abortion stigma could compel recognition that their experience was, perhaps, not so exceptional. Take this example of a woman with a preexisting health condition who attempted to get an abortion exception under Texas's 2021 heartbeat law:

> Whenever I called [the doctor's office], they sent me to the nurse—for me, I almost felt like my moment of shame, and there was just—I was horrified . . . I tell her, "Hey, can I get something that says that I'm high risk?" She was like, "Oh, do you need something for your job?" I remember feeling like I can't tell her [I want an abortion] because she's gonna judge me, and I just—I don't have the capacity to defend myself right now. There's a lot of shame.

She ultimately traveled out of state and had an abortion, afraid of others' judgment while trying to navigate Texas's law. Even as she identified having a health condition that might have qualified her to receive care as an exception to Texas's law, facing abortion stigma, shame, and having to travel did not feel exceptional. She also discussed how her past stereotypes and stigma toward abortion influenced her own feelings about her abortion.

> I am working through the shame and everything that I associated with the abortion. I think it's just more of an environmental thing. Growing up, there wasn't a lot of education for me [about] abortion, and so as I've gotten older and being blessed enough to be able to attend college and became educated on a lot of different things, I've been able to unlearn those old thoughts and thinking patterns. Be able to develop, I guess, a healthier thought process around abortions. I think the hardest thing through my own process of dealing with abortion was feeling those feelings of shame arise again and having to battle it all over again. I think it's very easy for me to be supportive of other women in this situation. It's very hard for me to be supportive and show myself grace in this situation.

The experience of public understandings of abortion affecting patients' own experiences was a recurring theme. As another Texas patient with a severe fetal health diagnosis said about her experience of abortion stigma,

> Having to travel halfway across the United States, and I think just realizing how much negative connotation just surrounds the word "abortion." It just sucks. Sometimes when we're talking about it with our friends, no one wants to say abortion. It makes me realize how much it's politicized when it shouldn't be, this was—what we had to do was not common, but it's not uncommon. Just—if any-

thing we're supporting [abortion funds], we're sharing our story, and just being open and honest. We have family members who didn't realize we couldn't have this procedure done in Texas, so just not setting an example but "Hey, [the need for abortion] happens to normal people, to very wanted pregnancies, it's not just unwanted pregnancies," so trying to change that stigma surrounding abortions.

This patient's understanding of how the exceptional became unexceptional during the process of seeking an abortion highlights the public misunderstandings surrounding abortion.

Many discussed the general need to expand the public understanding of who has an abortion to include complex pregnancies as a way to combat abortion stigma. For example, a Texan who sought abortion care out-of-state after receiving a serious fetal health diagnosis discussed her and her husband's experience:

I don't feel any shame with what we did. I don't feel that it has to be secret. I feel like what we did was make the most compassionate choice that we could, even though it was the hardest choice for our family. I was actually speaking with the nurse at the clinic about this, and how so many families have to face this kind of situation, but because nobody talks about it, people don't realize—they believe the whole rhetoric around ending a pregnancy as if it's just a simple decision. Even our family members who we have since told, who are very anti-abortion— every single one of them could understand why we made this decision, and none of them expressed any judgment. They were all very supportive, and they were even surprised that this counted as an abortion. I just think there's a lot of misunderstanding about what the law applies to, what constitutes an abortion.

While the decision to have an abortion might be simple or complicated, and depend on individual circumstances, past experiences, and a wide variety of external factors and influences, patients often described situations where they were making the best possible decision for themselves, their families, and their futures. Another Texas patient with a serious fetal health diagnosis likewise described how her understanding of abortion had changed based on her own experience of being denied in-state care: "My understanding of [abortion] really just burst open. I would never have judged someone; I just don't think I understood what went into a decision-making process like that until I was in the middle of a pregnancy and ending it. I think now I'm even more fierce about protecting those rights."

WHY ABORTION EXCEPTIONALISM MATTERS IN A POST-DOBBS REALITY

The *Dobbs* decision, with its effect of increased restrictions across the country, further narrowed the circumstances in which people could access abortion in many states. Most abortion restrictions still have exceptions, and with them persists a public belief that some abortions are legitimate and others less so. We broaden the application of "abortion exceptionalism" to describe how some abortions are perceived as legitimate exceptions while others are not. Further, these discourses of abortion exceptionalism have been institutionalized in laws, media, policy, and medicine. In our research, we have documented how abortion seekers must navigate exceptionalism discourses—such as arbitrary lines drawn by heartbeat bills or prevalent stereotypes about who has abortions and what counts as an abortion—and how people with complex pregnancies used exceptionalism narratives in ways that distance their experiences from negative abortion constructs. This is a form of othering that sometimes reified or contested abortion exceptionalism, as people found that cultural narratives about *who* has abortions and *why* they have abortions did not match their experiences. Many patients we interviewed wanted to share their stories to change the narrative about who is subject to abortion laws and the wide variety of circumstances in which someone might decide to end a pregnancy—catalyzing their experience into advocacy (Lerma et al. 2023).

Understanding how abortion exceptionalism is a proxy for categorization of abortion in terms of legitimacy has potential for broadening the idea of what circumstances constitute a normal, everyday abortion, showing that no abortions are in fact exceptional and all abortions are an integral part of comprehensive reproductive health care. We hope these examples complicate and challenge preconceived notions about abortion. The experiences of patients in our and other research highlight the ways that people are attempting to make the best decisions for themselves and their families in a wide variety of circumstances. Along the way, these efforts are complicated when abortion seekers are forced to confront the dominant social discourses about abortion that insist that only some abortions are legitimate (Doran and Nancarrow 2015; Miller 2023; Tillman, Eagen-Torkko, and Levi 2023).

Ultimately, in their own experiences, the ideas of legitimacy did not serve abortion seekers because most people understand their reasons for having an abortion to be legitimate based on their own lives and circumstances. As we continue to make sense of a post-*Dobbs* United States, attention to and interrogation of this idea of (only) some abortion as legitimate (via law, media, policy, and medicine) will be important. Everyone deserves the right to access abortion care without needing to prove their abortion legitimacy, regardless of their circumstances. As one patient from North Carolina who was a parent of four said about abortion stigma, "You never know what you're gonna do, until your feet cross that bridge. . . . Growing up I always that I would never [have an abortion], until it happened, and I was faced with that decision. So I'll say [stigma] is just through lack of experience and open mindedness."

ACKNOWLEDGMENTS

We would like to acknowledge the people who contributed to the data collection and analysis at the University of Texas at Austin for the research included in this chapter, including Gema Alemán, Gabriela Alvarez Perez, Emma Carpenter, Anna Chatillon, Asha Dane'el, Laura Dixon, Juliette Draper, Ghazaleh Moayedi, Pritika Paramasivam, Lauren Thaxon, Brooke Whitfield, and Kari White. We would also like to acknowledge the people and health care workers who shared their experiences and supported our research, and the abortion facilities we've worked with over the years.

REFERENCES

Arey, Whitney. 2021. "Abortion as Care: Affective and Biosocial Experiences of Abortion Access and Decision Making." PhD. diss., Brown University. https://repository.library .brown.edu/studio/item/bdr:mrtcxb78/.

Arey, Whitney, Klaira Lerma, Anitra Beasley, Lorie Harper, Ghazaleh Moayedi, and Kari White. 2022. "A Preview of the Dangerous Future of Abortion Bans—Texas Senate Bill 8." *New England Journal of Medicine* 387 (5): 388–390. https://doi.org/10.1056/NEJMp2207423.

Arey, Whitney, Klaira Lerma, Emma Carpenter, Ghazaleh Moayedi, Lorie Harper, Anitra Beasley, Tony Ogburn, and Kari White. 2023. "Abortion Access and Medically Complex Pregnancies before and after Texas Senate Bill 8." *Obstetrics & Gynecology* 141 (5): 995–1003. https://doi.org/10.1097/aog.0000000000005153.

Beynon-Jones, Siân M. 2017. "Untroubling Abortion: A Discourse Analysis of Women's Accounts." *Feminism & Psychology* 27 (2): 225–242. https://doi.org/10.1177/0959353517696515.

Bommaraju, Aalap, Megan L. Kavanaugh, Melody Y. Hou, and Danielle Bessett. 2016. "Situating Stigma in Stratified Reproduction: Abortion Stigma and Miscarriage Stigma as Barriers to Reproductive Healthcare." *Sexual & Reproductive Healthcare* 10 (December):62–69. https://doi.org/10.1016/j.srhc.2016.10.008.

Borgmann, Caitlin E. 2014. "Abortion Exceptionalism and Undue Burden Preemption." *Washington and Lee Law Review* 71 (2): 1047–1087. https://scholarlycommons.law.wlu.edu /wlulr/vol71/iss2/13/.

Braff, Lara. 2013. "Somos Muchos (We Are so Many): Population Politics and 'Reproductive Othering' in Mexican Fertility Clinics." *Medical Anthropology Quarterly* 27 (1): 121–138. https://doi.org/10.1111/maq.12019.

Caron, Simone. 2016. Review of *Abortion in the American Imagination: Before Life and Choice, 1880–1940*, by Karen Weingarten. *Journal of American History* 103 (2): 498. https:// doi.org/10.1093/jahist/jaw253.

Center for Reproductive Rights. 2024. "After *Roe* Fell: Abortion Laws by State." https:// reproductiverights.org/maps/abortion-laws-by-state/.

Dobbins-Harris, S. 2017. "The Myth of Abortion as Black Genocide: Reclaiming Our Reproductive Cycle." *National Black Law Journal* 26 (1): 85–127. https://escholarship.org/uc/item /0988p9xp.

Doran, Frances, and Susan Nancarrow. 2015. "Barriers and Facilitators of Access to First-Trimester Abortion Services for Women in the Developed World: A Systematic Review." *Journal of Family Planning and Reproductive Health Care* 41 (3): 170–180. https://doi.org/10 .1136/jfprhc-2013-100862.

Felix, Mabel, and Laurie Sobel. 2023. "A Review of Exceptions in State Abortions Bans: Implications for the Provision of Abortion Services." *KFF* (blog), May 18, 2023. https:// www.kff.org/womens-health-policy/issue-brief/a-review-of-exceptions-in-state-abortions -bans-implications-for-the-provision-of-abortion-services/.

Kimport, Katrina, Tracy A. Weitz, and Lori Freedman. 2016. "The Stratified Legitimacy of Abortions." *Journal of Health and Social Behavior* 57 (4): 503–516. https://doi.org/10.1177 /0022146516669970.

Leask, Marita. 2015. "An Exceptional Choice? How Young New Zealand Women Talk about Abortion." *Australian Feminist Studies* 30 (84): 179–198. https://doi.org/10.1080/08164649 .2015.1046305.

Lerma, Klaira, Whitney Arey, Anna Chatillon, and Kari White. 2023. "Reasons for Participation in Abortion Research in Restrictive Settings." *Contraception* 130: 110324. https://doi .org/10.1016/j.contraception.2023.110324.

Lift Louisiana, Physicians for Human Rights, RH Impact, and Center for Reproductive Rights. 2024 "Criminalized Care How Louisiana's Abortion Bans Endanger Patients and Clinicians." https://phr.org/our-work/resources/louisiana-abortion-bans/.

Merner, Bronwen, Casey M. Haining, Lindy Willmott, Julian Savulescu, and Louise A. Keogh. 2023. "Institutional Objection to Abortion: A Mixed-Methods Narrative Review." *Women's Health* 19: 17455057231152373. https://doi.org/10.1177/17455057231152373.

Miller, Calum. 2023. "The Scourges: Why Abortion Is Even More Morally Serious Than Miscarriage." *Journal of Medicine and Philosophy* 48 (3): 225–242. https://doi.org/10.1093/jmp/jhad014.

Nandagiri, Rishita. 2019. "'Like a Mother-Daughter Relationship': Community Health Intermediaries' Knowledge of and Attitudes to Abortion in Karnataka, India." *Social Science & Medicine (1982)* 239 (October):112525. https://doi.org/10.1016/j.socscimed.2019.112525.

Norris, Alison, Danielle Bessett, Julia R. Steinberg, Megan L. Kavanaugh, Silvia De Zordo, and Davida Becker. 2011. "Abortion Stigma: A Reconceptualization of Constituents, Causes, and Consequences." *Women's Health Issues* 21 (3): S49–S54. https://doi.org/10.1016/j.whi.2011.02.010.

Physicians for Human Rights. 2023. "In Clinicians' Own Words: How Abortion Bans Impede Emergency Medical Treatment for Pregnant Patients in Idaho." https://phr.org/our-work/resources/louisiana-abortion-bans/.

Pyle, Alaina, Shannon Y. Adams, DonnaMaria E. Cortezzo, Jessica T. Fry, Natalia Henner, Naomi Laventhal, Matthew Lin, Kevin Sullivan, and C. Lydia Wraight. 2024. "Navigating the Post-*Dobbs* Landscape: Ethical Considerations from a Perinatal Perspective." *Journal of Perinatology* 44 (5): 628–634. https://doi.org/10.1038/s41372-024-01884-9.

Rosenthal, Lisa, and Marci Lobel. 2016. "Stereotypes of Black American Women Related to Sexuality and Motherhood." *Psychology of Women Quarterly* 40 (3): 414–427. https://doi.org/10.1177/0361684315627459.

Schumacher, Shannon, Ashley Kirzinger, Audrey Kearney, Isabelle Valdes, and Liz Hamel Published. 2024. "KFF Health Tracking Poll March 2024: Abortion in the 2024 Election and Beyond." *KFF* (blog), March 7, 2024. https://www.kff.org/womens-health-policy/poll-finding/kff-health-tracking-poll-march-2024-abortion-in-the-2024-election-and-beyond/.

Smith, Benjamin Elliot Yelnosky, Deborah Bartz, Alisa B. Goldberg, and Elizabeth Janiak. 2018. "'Without Any Indication': Stigma and a Hidden Curriculum within Medical Students' Discussion of Elective Abortion." *Social Science & Medicine* 214 (October): 26–34. https://doi.org/10.1016/j.socscimed.2018.07.014.

Tillman, Stephanie, Meghan Eagen-Torkko, and Amy Levi. 2023. "Ethics, Abortion Access, and Emergency Care Post-*Dobbs*: The Gray Areas." *Journal of Midwifery & Women's Health* 68 (6): 774–779. https://doi.org/10.1111/jmwh.13598.

VandeVusse, Alicia J., Jennifer Mueller, Marielle Kirstein, Joe Strong, and Laura D. Lindberg. 2023. "'Technically an Abortion': Understanding Perceptions and Definitions of Abortion in the United States." *Social Science & Medicine (1982)* 335 (October): 116216. https://doi.org/10.1016/j.socscimed.2023.116216.

Watson, Katie. 2018. "Why We Should Stop Using the Term 'Elective Abortion.'" *AMA Journal of Ethics* 20 (12): E1175–1180. https://doi.org/10.1001/amajethics.2018.1175.

CHAPTER 3

Abortion Restrictions

HOW MUCH HAS ACTUALLY CHANGED

Lindsay Ruhr

Abortion restrictions are not new. At the federal level, probably the most well-known restriction is the Hyde Amendment, which was passed three years after *Roe* and prohibits federal funding from covering abortions in most cases. At the state level, abortion restrictions and bans include waiting periods, parental consent laws, policies limiting or banning insurance coverage from paying for the procedure, restrictions on who can perform an abortion, and limits on how far along in a pregnancy the procedure can be performed. All of these laws can make it difficult for individuals to access abortion care.

Studying pre-*Dobbs* restrictions and their impact on abortion seekers can help us understand and predict some of the impacts of the wave of state-level restrictions implemented after *Dobbs*—and those still to come. In 2015, I conducted research on patients' use and experience of abortion in Missouri after the implementation of a new restriction: a mandatory seventy-two-hour waiting period law. Missouri already had a twenty-four-hour waiting period; this was an extension of that period.

Waiting periods require two visits to the clinic. On the first visit, a pregnant person will typically receive state-mandated counseling (which is not always medically accurate). Then, the clock starts on a required delay until they can have an abortion. Missouri was the third state to enact a seventy-two-hour waiting period, and at the time of my study, four states other than Missouri had a mandatory seventy-two-hour waiting period (Utah, South Dakota, Oklahoma, and North Carolina). As of January 2025, twenty-three states had waiting periods, which were most often twenty-four hours (Guttmacher Institute 2025). As I will show in this chapter, enacting this abortion restriction did not stop abortion or end the demand.

The waiting period was not the first or only abortion restriction in Missouri at the time. In Missouri, only physicians could provide abortions (Guttmacher Institute 2022), excluding other medical professionals such as nurse practitioners. Missouri also had a law requiring the physician performing the abortion to have hospital admitting privileges at a nearby hospital (Guttmacher Institute 2022).

(It is imperative to note that medical procedures far riskier than abortion, such as wisdom teeth extraction, are performed by providers without admitting privileges.) Laws also specified the construction and design requirements for abortion clinic spaces, requirements that do not improve patient safety or outcomes (Roberts et al. 2018). Missouri restricted insurance coverage for the procedure (Guttmacher Institute 2022). Abortions are costly; because the circumstances in which individuals can use their insurance to pay for a procedure are limited, many encountered a substantial financial barrier.

All these restrictions could add up to make the abortion-seeking experience difficult. Before the overturning of *Roe*, the number of abortion providers had steadily decreased in Missouri. By 2017, the vast majority of Missouri counties (97 percent) had no abortion provider, and most Missouri women (78 percent) lived in these counties (Guttmacher Institute 2022). Still, as we will see, many patients successfully overcame these challenges. The remainder of this chapter will use Missouri as a case study to examine one specific abortion restriction: the seventy-two-hour waiting period. As I will show, abortion restrictions are onerous, costly, and have negative impacts, but many abortion seekers nonetheless surmount them. This case study utilizes empirical evidence presented through in-depth research methodology and data tables to draw conclusions about abortion restrictions that are relevant to readers across disciplines.

METHODS

In 2014, when Missouri tripled the mandatory abortion waiting period from twenty-four to seventy-two hours, I was working in sexual and reproductive health care (SRH) in the state. Working in this setting and having a background in social work and public policy, I wanted to evaluate the effects of this change empirically. Before working in SRH, I had heard about various abortion restrictions in the media, but hearing about them and seeing their actual impact on people are two different things. Once I started working in SRH, I saw the people affected by these restrictions, and I heard their stories; the effect of these restrictions became deeply humanized for me. As a researcher, I was interested in how this change to a seventy-two-hour wait affected the patient experience of abortion care—and, indeed, their ability to obtain abortion care. To answer this question, I conducted a study on the effects of the newly tripled waiting period on patients in Missouri beginning in 2015.

At the time the waiting period was extended, Missouri had one clinic that consistently provided abortions. It was located in a metropolitan area near the Missouri–Illinois border on the eastern edge of the state. Given this location, the pregnant persons seeking an abortion who lived in other, often more rural, parts of the state had to travel substantial distances for care, either to this clinic or to another state. For example, if you lived in central Missouri and needed an abortion, you most likely would have had to travel about two hours to reach the sole in-state provider or even farther to access a provider in a neighboring state such as Kansas or Iowa. The mandatory waiting period meant pregnant persons had to make multiple trips to the Missouri abortion provider, which was especially burdensome and expensive for those who lived several hours away. To put it simply, abortion access in Missouri in 2015 was not easy—and this was under *Roe*.

I initially conducted this study to answer one research question: Did switching from a twenty-four-hour to a seventy-two-hour waiting period change abortion rates and patients' experience of seeking abortions in Missouri? Here, I return to these data to consider an additional question that emerged well after my study was complete: How can patients' experiences of a seventy-two-hour waiting period help us anticipate the impact of the *Dobbs* decision in an abortion-restrictive state like Missouri?

Theoretical Framework

My initial hypothesis was that the tripling of the waiting period (from twenty-four hours to seventy-two hours) would prevent a portion of those who wanted an abortion from being able to return for care. I used the theoretical framework of the Integrated Behavioral Model (IBM) to guide the study design. The IBM emerged from two previous theories: the theory of reasoned action (Fishbein and Ajzen 1975) and the theory of planned behavior (Ajzen 1991). The IBM posits that the best predictor of behavior is an individual's intention to perform that behavior. For my research, I focused on several components of this model. I examined *intention*, which in this case means a pregnant person's intention to return to the clinic for an abortion after a seventy-two-hour wait. The *behavior* is obtaining an abortion after the waiting period. And the waiting period itself is an *environmental constraint*. I also explored the roles of attitude toward abortion, perceived norms, and personal agency (perceived control and self-efficacy) in predicting a pregnant person's intention to return to the clinic for an abortion after the waiting period.

Data Sources

To answer my two research questions, I gathered the study data in four formats: (1) retrospective medical records analysis, (2) elicitation interviews, (3) baseline surveys, and (4) follow-up surveys.

- *Retrospective Medical Records Analysis.* The retrospective medical records analysis examined patient medical records at the abortion provider before the law changed, which allowed me to analyze past trends. I analyzed medical records from one year before the seventy-two-hour mandatory waiting period law went into effect (September 2013 to September 2014, when the twenty-four-hour mandatory waiting period was in force) and again one year after (October 2014 to October 2015).
- *Elicitation Interviews.* I conducted twenty semistructured interviews to inform the design of the baseline and follow-up surveys (Fishbein and Ajzen 2010), achieving the recommended target number of fifteen to twenty individuals from the target population (Montaño and Kasprzyk 2015). The

participants for the elicitation interviews were recruited at the clinic from late May through early June 2015. A research team member approached potential participants when they came into the clinic for their first visit, before their seventy-two-hour waiting period began. In a private room, the research team gave each participant an overview of our study, including presenting and explaining the informed consent document. The eligible participants were pregnant, were aged eighteen or older, were seeking an abortion, and could speak and comprehend English without the assistance of a translator. The elicitation interviews consisted of ten questions to measure the various constructs of the IBM, such as intention, attitude, and personal agency. These interviews lasted up to 30 minutes, with the participants' responses recorded by hand. I analyzed these data to inform and revise the study's draft baseline and follow-up surveys.

- *Baseline and Follow-Up Surveys.* I drafted the baseline and follow-up surveys to examine the impact of the seventy-two-hour mandatory waiting period on abortion patients' proceeding to abortion and their experience of seeking abortion care. Constructs of the IBM, such as intention, attitude, perceived norms, personal agency, and environmental constraints, guided the development of several survey questions. Most questions were multiple choice or Likert scale, but some were open-ended. Four experts in SRH and social work research provided feedback on the baseline and follow-up surveys to assess content validity. Recruitment for the baseline survey, similar to the elicitation interviews, took place in the clinic on the day the participants came in for their initial visit to receive counseling and begin the clock on the seventy-two-hour wait. Three weeks after the baseline survey, I conducted the follow-up survey, which could be completed over the phone or online.

Data Analysis

Two independent coders, one of whom was myself, conducted the analysis of the open-ended questions in the baseline and follow-up surveys. We followed a five-step inductive coding process to generate data-driven codes (Boyatzis 1998), letting what we read in the participants' responses guide us in creating the codes.

For the quantitative data, I ran a Mann-Whitney U test in SPSS software to analyze the impact of the tripled waiting period on the number of waited days. I chose a Mann-Whitney U test over a t-test because the data from the days waited in the two retrospective spreadsheets was not normally distributed; more participants were included in the twenty-four-hour waiting period data. I conducted a Firth logistic regression in SAS software using the dichotomous *intention* variable (high intention to return to the clinic after the waiting period versus low intention) as the dependent variable; *attitude, perceived norms, self-efficacy,* and *perceived control* were the independent variables.

Intention to have an abortion was measured in the baseline survey by two statements in which the participants had to rate how strongly they disagreed or agreed on a Likert scale of one (strongly disagree) to seven (strongly agree): "I want to have an abortion" and "After the waiting period, I intend to return to this clinic for an abortion." I found a moderate correlation (n = 131; r = 0.580; P = 0.000) between these two statements. I then created a dichotomous composite variable for intention by combining these two statements. Responses from 1 to 4 were recoded to 0 to represent low intention, and responses from five to seven were recoded to 1 to represent high intention. I used a Firth logistic regression because the intention variable is highly skewed, with 88 percent of the respondents reporting a high level of intention to return after the seventy-two-hour waiting period to have an abortion.

RESULTS

Elicitation Interviews

The analysis of the elicitation interviews found that pregnant persons seeking an abortion were a highly motivated group with a high level of intention to return to the clinic for the procedure after the waiting period. These participants felt confident of their ability to return to the clinic to have an abortion. They felt in control of their reproductive healthcare decision-making. However, the participants did note a few potential barriers to returning for an abortion.

- *Intention to Return after Waiting Period.* The question, "If you want to have an abortion, how certain are you that you can?" measured the IBM construct of *self-efficacy*, which falls under personal agency. Personal agency included perceived control and self-efficacy. Eleven participants said that they were 100 percent certain that if they wanted to have an abortion, they could. Three participants said that they were "very certain" or "really certain." By contrast, three said they were "pretty certain," and one participant said that she was "certain." Only one participant said she did not know if she could return. The final participant said, "Well, I've been talking about it with a lot of people. I've been told that I'm gonna be OK, it's gonna be fine. I'm really early, so it's OK. Two to three months though, that's crazy to have an abortion at that time." From her response, this person seems to believe that because she is "really early" in her pregnancy it is "OK" to get an abortion, but if she had been "two to three months" pregnant the circumstances might have been different.
- *Control Over Whether or Not You Have an Abortion.* The question "How much control do you have over whether or not you have an abortion?" measured the IBM construction of *perceived control*. All twenty participants said that they have "100% control" or "full control" over whether or not they have an abortion. Examples of the responses included "As a woman, I have 100% control" and "complete control, it's my body."
- *Influence of Others on Your Decision to Have an Abortion.* The question "Who might influence your decision about whether or not to have an abortion?" measured the IBM construct of *perceived norms*. Ten participants said that no one else influenced their decision on whether to have an abortion. The

responses included "nobody does, I make decisions for myself" and "it all depends on who you share it with; I don't think anyone can really influence your decision, it's your personal belief, personal situation at that time." Seven participants said that their partner, who in most cases was the person who got them pregnant, can influence their decision. Other responses included the participant's mother, father, and friends.

• *Barriers to Accessing Abortion Services.* The question "If you want to have an abortion, what might stand in your way/prevent you from doing so?" measured the IBM construct of *self-efficacy.* The participants could list as many barriers as they felt applied. Five said that nothing would prevent them from having an abortion if that was what they chose. Five said their financial situation could be a barrier. Other potential roadblocks were emotional barriers, including guilt, fear, and social stigma, transportation to the clinic, an unsupportive partner, clinic protestors, and medical reasons. None of the participants mentioned the seventy-two-hour wait as being a barrier to accessing abortion care.

Baseline and Follow-Up Surveys

A total of 132 pregnant persons completed the baseline survey at the clinic between June and December 2015. Of these 132 participants, 124 (94.0 percent) returned to the clinic after the seventy-two-hour waiting period to have an abortion. Of the eight who did not return, six passed the gestational limit to have an abortion in Missouri during the study period. These six did not follow up with me, so it is possible they either decided against the abortion, traveled to another state for the procedure, or had a miscarriage. Another who did not return for abortion care notified me of a miscarriage that occurred before she could return for an abortion. The last of the eight reported that she had sought abortion services elsewhere. Table 3.1 shows the demographic characteristics of the 132 participants in the baseline survey. The average age of participants was 27.1, and the range was eighteen to forty-four years.

In the baseline survey, I also asked participants what actions they had had to take to get to the clinic for their first visit (see table 3.2). The most common responses were getting time off work (39 participants; 29.5 percent), arranging extra childcare (29 participants; 22 percent), and borrowing money (20 participants; 15.2 percent). Borrowing a car and missing school were each reported by nine people (6.8 percent). Seven participants (5.3 percent) said they had traveled a long distance, and six (4.5 percent) noted they had to take public transportation. Other responses included "lie to people at school," "friend missed class," "children missed school today," and "husband took off work."

The finding that twenty-nine participants arranged for extra childcare is noteworthy because, of the 132 participants, 60.6 percent already had children. More than half of those who had children had more than one child, with one participant reporting that she had nine children.

Of the 132 survey participants, 28 percent lived in rural areas, meaning they had a substantial commute to the clinic. Therefore, it was unsurprising that some

TABLE 3.1

DEMOGRAPHICS OF BASELINE SURVEY PARTICIPANTS

Characteristics	Number and percentage of participants
Race	
White	68 (51.1%)
Black	55 (41.8%)
Other	8 (6.2%)
Missing	1 (0.8%)
Ethnicity	
Not Hispanic or Latina	128 (97.0%)
Hispanic or Latina	4 (3.0%)
Living Area	
Urban	94 (71.2%)
Rural	37 (28.0%)
Missing	1 (0.8%)
Education	
Some high school	8 (6.1%)
High school graduate or GED	36 (27.3%)
Some college or technical school	44 (33.3%)
College graduate (including associates and professional degrees)	42 (31.8%)
Missing	2 (1.5%)
Number of children	
None	49 (37.1%)
1 child	30 (22.7%)
2 children	26 (19.7%)
3 or more children	24 (18.2%)
Missing	3 (2.3%)

participants reported having to borrow a car or travel a long distance. Specifically, some participants stated that they had to "spend 1.5 hours driving one way" and "drive over 130 miles . . . I had to borrow money and a car." Much of the state is rural and lacks adequate access to reliable public transportation, making driving the most feasible mode of transportation for many participants.

TABLE 3.2

REPORTED CHALLENGES OF GETTING TO THE FIRST
CLINIC VISIT

Challenges	Number and percentage of participants
Get time off work	39 (29.5%)
Borrow a car	9 (6.8%)
Borrow money	20 (15.2%)
Arrange childcare	29 (22.0%)
Take public transportation	6 (4.5%)
Miss school or a class	9 (6.8%)
Travel a long distance	7 (5.3%)

Impact on Patient Experience

I used the medical records analysis and survey responses for this question: Did switching from a twenty-four-hour to a seventy-two-hour waiting period change abortion rates and patients' experience of seeking abortions in Missouri? Table 3.3 shows a comparison of the waiting times for pregnant persons based on medical records from the year before the seventy-two-hour waiting period (i.e., during the twenty-four-hour waiting period) and the year after the seventy-two-hour waiting period, alongside the survey results.

For patients who had been subject to the twenty-four-hour waiting period from 2013–2014, the average days waited was 6.1 days with a median of 4.0 days (range: 1–81 days). For the patients during the seventy-two-hour waiting period in 2014–2015, the average number of days waited was 7.6 days with a median of 6.0 days (range: 3–85 days). In other words, under the twenty-four-hour waiting period in Missouri, pregnant persons were already waiting an average of 6.1 days between their first clinic visit to sign an informed consent and their actual procedure date. With the implementation of the seventy-two-hour waiting period, the average wait did increase, but only by 1.5 days. Although this difference was statistically significant ($z = -21.936$; $P = 0.000$), it is not clinically significant. It is not clear whether this 1.5-day difference was meaningful for patients themselves. So, to explore the impact of this difference, I turn to the survey data.

In the baseline survey that I gave to 132 pregnant persons seeking an abortion, I asked the participants whether they had known about the seventy-two-hour waiting period before coming to the clinic for their first of the required two visits. I was surprised by the data, which revealed that thirty-four (25.8 percent) had not known about the waiting period before arriving at the clinic. I will never forget the participant who interrupted me as I read her the informed consent form: "Wait,

TABLE 3.3

COMPARISON OF DAYS WAITED BETWEEN THE REQUIRED TWO CLINIC VISITS

	WAITING PERIOD		Survey participants (N = 132)
	24 Hours	*72 Hours*	
Time period	September 2013– September 2014	October 2014– October 2015	June– December 2015
Number of patients who obtained an abortion after the waiting period	4,978	3,635	124
Days waited between first clinic visit and having an abortion			
Mean	6.1	7.6	6.6
Median (range)	4.0 (1–81)	6.0 (3–85)	6.0 (3–28)

what do you mean I have to wait seventy-two hours? I'm not getting the abortion today?" She then became tearful. Her comment caught me completely off guard: I had included this question in the baseline survey because I had heard anecdotal evidence that some patients did not realize there was a waiting period, but I never expected to encounter such a patient during my data collection. Thirty-four patients reported they had not been aware of the waiting period before their first visit, and thirty of them (88.2 percent) returned later to obtain their abortion.

The follow-up survey asked the participants, "If your abortion appointment was more than three days from your first visit to the clinic, what are the reasons that you waited more than the required 72 hours?" Table 3.4 summarizes these response categories. The findings essentially illustrate that life circumstances such as the patient's job, school schedule, ability to pay for the procedure, or the clinic's hours of operation caused them to wait longer than three days. Their delay was not related to the waiting period law itself.

- *Patient's Schedule.* Many participants had life circumstances that kept them from returning to the clinic after precisely seventy-two hours. For instance, if your only day off work is Tuesdays, you might need to schedule both your first and second clinic visits on Tuesdays, resulting in a seven day wait. The same reasoning can apply to a school schedule or available childcare. "Because I had to work—it was my next available day off, so I had to wait an entire week to have the procedure," wrote one participant, aged twenty-four, who had waited eight days. "I had to wait because I had just started a new job and could not take the time off work," wrote another, aged twenty-five, who waited six days.

TABLE 3.4

REASONS FOR WAITING LONGER THAN 72 HOURS

Reason	Number and percentage of participants
Patient's schedule	11 (25.6%)
Clinic's schedule	5 (11.6%)
Medical reasons	4 (9.3%)
Financial reasons	2 (4.7%)
Unsure of decision	2 (4.7%)
Not applicable	
Did not obtain abortion	3 (7.0%)
Only waited 72 hours	16 (37.2%)

- *Clinic Schedule.* At the time of this survey's data collection in 2015, the clinic only performed abortion procedures four days per week, which meant some pregnant persons had to wait longer than seventy-two hours depending on the day of their first clinic visit. For instance, if your initial clinic visit was on Thursday, the earliest that you could return to have the abortion would be on Tuesday because the clinic was closed on Sundays and did not do procedures on Mondays. This was most likely the situation that this twenty-eight-year-old participant (who had waited four days) described: "It was the weekend, and nothing is done on Mondays; because I had to wait 'til Tuesday because they weren't see[ing] patients or something." Several national holidays also fell during the data collection period, including Independence Day, Labor Day, and Thanksgiving, during which the clinic was closed. This resulted in waits longer than the required seventy-two hours. "My biggest problem is that I have to wait because of the holiday, and now I have to wait until next week . . . because my appointment was canceled last Friday," wrote one participant, aged twenty-two, who had waited seven days.
- *Financial Barriers.* Numerous participants noted the struggle of having to come up with the funds to pay for the abortion or the funds to get to the clinic on two separate occasions. "Coming up with the funds to pay" was cited by one participant, aged thirty-four, who had waited twelve days.
- *Transportation Barriers.* Transportation was a barrier to getting to the clinic because all participants had to make two trips. If they wanted a procedural abortion, they would need someone else to drive them on the day of the procedure if they planned to receive any sedation. "I had to wait for my driver to be available/free to take me," wrote one participant, aged twenty-six, who had waited seven days.

TABLE 3.5

FIRTH LOGISTIC REGRESSION RESULTS FOR IBM
CONSTRUCTS AND INTENTION (N = 120)

Variable	OR (95% CI)
Attitude	2.64 (1.20–5.85)*
Self-efficacy	3.35 (1.46–7.66)**
Race	0.26 (0.04–1.68)
Living location	0.84 (0.15–4.72)
Education	3.10 (0.43–22.30)

CI = confidence interval; IBM = Integrated
Behavioral Model; OR = odds ratio.
*$P < 0.05$.
**$P < 0.01$.

- *Unsure of Decision.* Two participants explained they took extra time between the clinic visits to weigh their decision and be confident about choosing abortion.
- *Not Applicable.* Sixteen participants (37 percent) waited precisely three days, so this question did not apply to them. Also, three of those who completed the follow-up survey did not obtain an abortion, so this question also did not apply to them.

Impact of the Dobbs Decision

To answer the research question How can patients' experiences of a seventy-two-hour waiting period help us anticipate the impact of the *Dobbs* decision in an abortion-restrictive state like Missouri? I examined the association between the dependent variable of intention to return to the clinic after the waiting period and the independent variables of attitude, perceived norms, perceived control, and self-efficacy. I found that 88 percent of the participants expressed a high intention of returning to the clinic after the waiting period.

A Firth logistic regression found that self-efficacy and attitude were statistically significant predictors of intention (table 3.5). Self-efficacy was significantly related to having a high level of intention to return to the clinic for an abortion after the waiting period while holding other variables in the model constant (odds ratio, 3.35; 95% confidence interval, 1.46–7.66; $P = 0.0042$). Attitude toward abortion was also significantly related to having a high level of intention to return to the clinic after seventy-two hours (odds ratio, 2.64, 95% confidence interval, 1.20–5.85; $P = 0.0164$). In other words, pregnant persons who have a more favorable attitude toward abortion and who believe they can return to the clinic after the waiting period have high levels of intention to obtain an abortion. The regression model controlled for race, living location (urban versus rural), and the highest level of education completed. The control variables were all dichotomous. This analysis excluded twelve of the 132 participants due to missing data.

These results related to the theoretical framework indicate the importance of self-efficacy and attitude toward abortion. These two variables were statistically significant predictors of intention to return to the clinic after the mandatory waiting period. These significant findings suggest that looking at and understanding the roles of self-efficacy, attitude toward abortion, and intention to perform a behavior may predict who overcomes the barriers to abortion and who does not.

DISCUSSION

When Missouri tripled its waiting period for abortion, pregnant persons still sought and obtained abortions. Under the twenty-four-hour waiting period, pregnant persons were already waiting nearly a week between their first clinic visit and their actual procedure date. With the implementation of the seventy-two-hour waiting period in 2014, that wait was increased by an average of 1.5 days, still several days longer for many than the law required. These findings show that the extra 1.5 days were not a huge deal for most patients, nor did the duration of their wait stem from the law change. The causes for their delays were straightforward. When asked why they waited longer than seventy-two hours (if they did wait longer than the requirement), the participants reported that schedules—such as the patient's work schedule or the clinic operating schedule—were the most significant factors.

On their first clinic visit, when we asked patients about their intention to return after the waiting period, 88 percent reported a high intention to return. This finding suggests that this group had a high level of self-efficacy and felt a strong sense of control over their reproductive healthcare decision-making. These participants recognized obstacles to making two trips to the clinic, but they planned to overcome these challenges and return after the mandatory wait. Regardless of whether the waiting period was twenty-four or seventy-two hours, all the items the participants had listed as barriers to getting to that first clinic visit—borrowing money or a car, taking public transportation, arranging childcare, or missing school—would remain barriers. Without a waiting period, these challenges would still exist. For example, a patient would most likely still need to arrange for childcare or borrow money even if they could obtain an abortion with a single visit to the clinic and not have to wait at all. However, having to do all of these things twice due to a two-visit requirement can be highly burdensome even when it is doable.

These insights into patients' intentions, self-efficacy, and attitudes toward abortion when abortion was legal can tell us about what we might expect of abortion seekers in the states that, following the overturning of *Roe*, banned abortion. Missouri was one of those states. Its neighbor, Illinois, did not—abortion remained legal in Illinois. Because abortion was already so difficult to obtain in Missouri before *Dobbs*, it is not hard to imagine that banning abortion made little meaningful difference to Missourians. If you could make it to Missouri's lone abortion provider in 2015 (pre-*Dobbs*) and wait a minimum of seventy-two hours, then most likely you could make it directly across the Mississippi River to a clinic in Illinois after Missouri banned abortion. In fact, with its fewer abortion restrictions and more providers, Illinois immediately post-*Dobbs* was a more accessible destination for abortion care than Missouri pre-*Dobbs*. There were clinics in Illinois that were mere miles from the Missouri provider's location. Illinois had no waiting period, so it would most likely require only one trip. Then, more than two years after the *Dobbs* decision, Missouri residents voted to restore abortion rights in the state, changing the status of abortion once again.

There are many new research questions stemming from states' post-*Dobbs* restrictions on abortion and, in the case of Missouri, their undoing. In answering them, it is crucial to build on what we already know about the impact of restrictions, including how they may (or may not) affect the abortion rate.

As a final note, I want to highlight that research on measuring the impact of abortion restrictions is not without challenges and risks. When I was a student gathering these data in 2015, a Missouri politician expressed concerns about my project. This politician thought that my research was using public funds to aid abortion seekers at the clinic. Because I was a student at a state university doing this research as part of my doctoral dissertation and Missouri bans state funds from going toward promoting or encouraging abortion, this was a serious accusation. But he misunderstood my work. My goal was to understand the impact of a new policy, not to promote abortion. Still, this politician's inquiry into my work caused me stress and fear.

I thought this inquiry might significantly delay my graduation or force me to redesign my project completely. The situation also drew the attention of several media outlets, and my partner emailed me one particular story with a note asking me to read the comments. There, I found that someone had posted a link to one of my social media pages, accompanied by some not-so-positive statements. Most of my social media pages were private, but I was still concerned about this particular link because its profile pictures included a photo of myself with my young daughter. I made the decision to temporarily deactivate all my social media accounts, and I no longer include my children in my profile pictures.

Ultimately, I completed my project, graduated, and contributed my findings to the scientific understanding of the impact of abortion restrictions. However, the challenges I faced gave me a long-lasting fear and hesitancy about engaging in abortion research. Nearly ten years later, I have just begun to overcome this fear; I now feel I am in a stable place in my career where it is again safe to engage in the research that I am most passionate about pursuing. For me, the fall of *Roe* at a time when I was living in an abortion-restrictive state in the South was also a motivating factor. I'm glad to be returning to this area of study and to these questions about policy impacts.

While *Roe* may be gone, abortion care and the impacts of current abortion policy are not drastically different from what came before nor completely unknown. Abortion restrictions, such as the tripling of the waiting period in Missouri, worsen the patient's experience. However, as we have seen in Missouri, patients will still strive to overcome these especially onerous restrictions like bans, and many will be successful.

REFERENCES

Ajzen, Icek. 1991. "The Theory of Planned Behavior." *Organizational Behavior and Human Decision Processes* 50 (2): 179–211. https://doi.org/10.1016/0749-5978(91)90020-t.

Boyatzis, Richard E. 1998. *Transforming Qualitative Information: Thematic Analysis and Code Development*. SAGE.

Fishbein, Martin, and Icek Ajzen. 1975. *Belief, Attitude, Intention and Behavior: An Introduction to Theory and Research*. Addison-Wesley.

———. 2010. *Predicting and Changing Behavior: The Reasoned Action Approach*. Psychology Press.

Guttmacher Institute. 2022. "State Facts about Abortion: Missouri." Guttmacher Institute. Accessed March 17, 2024. https://www.guttmacher.org/sites/default/files/factsheet/sfaa-mo.pdf.

———. 2025. "State Laws and Policies as of January 2, 2025: Counseling and Waiting Period Requirements for Abortion." Guttmacher Institute. Accessed April 27, 2025. https://www.guttmacher.org/state-policy/explore/counseling-and-waiting-periods-abortion.

Montaño, Daniel E., and Danuta Kasprzyk. 2015. "Theory of Reasoned Action, Theory of Planned Behavior, and the Integrated Behavioral Model." In *Health Behavior and Health Education: Theory, Research, and Practice*, edited by Karen Glanz, Barbara K. Rimer, and K. Viswanath, 95–124. Jossey-Bass.

Roberts, Sarah C. M., Ushma D. Upadhyay, Guodong Liu, Jennifer L. Kerns, Djibril Ba, Nancy Beam, and Douglas L. Leslie. 2018. "Association of Facility Type with Procedural-Related Morbidities and Adverse Events among Patients Undergoing Induced Abortions." *JAMA* 319 (24): 2497–2506. https://doi.org/10.1001/jama.2018.7675.

CHAPTER 4

Counting Was All We Ever Had

MEASURING CHANGE IN ABORTION
CARE AFTER *DOBBS*

Jenny O'Donnell

THE WRITING ON THE WALL

By the end of 2021, the legal writing was on the wall. A bill introduced in the Texas legislature in the spring of that year, Senate Bill 8 (SB 8), had been signed into law and taken effect on September 1, 2021.[1] The law's structure was novel because it created a right for private citizens to enforce a six-week abortion ban as an attempted workaround for what was otherwise a patently unconstitutional law if enforced by the government. The law also targeted anybody who knowingly "aids or abets" an abortion, which cast a huge chilling effect on patient helpers such as family, friends, abortion funds, and clinic staff.

Although the law was quickly challenged, the U.S. Supreme Court allowed this brazenly unconstitutional law to go into and remain in effect while the case proceeded. That was when it became abundantly clear that the federal right to abortion before viability, codified by *Roe v. Wade* in 1973 and in place for nearly fifty years, was on borrowed time. And indeed, when the Supreme Court ultimately refused to stay the case and allowed SB 8 to go into effect on December 10, 2021, and agreed to hear the challenge to another law from Mississippi that was clearly unconstitutional under *Roe* (*Dobbs v. Jackson Women's Health Organization*), it was a clear signal that *Roe* now had a probable expiration date.

The few months between the SB 8 ruling in December 2021 and the *Dobbs* decision in June 2022 that ultimately overturned *Roe* have been all but washed away in the public's memory. However, those months mattered. On its face and most critically, SB 8 dramatically restricted abortion in one of the most populous states in the nation, reducing the gestational limit from twenty-two weeks to six weeks. Its implementation also afforded a clear picture of what a post-*Roe* America, in which there is no protection for abortion at any gestation, could look like and how patients would be impacted.

Behind the scenes, there was another story that needs to be told. This story started with the oral arguments before the Supreme Court on November 1, 2021. You may ask, in the shadow of the *Dobbs* decision, why do the ninety minutes of oral arguments in the SB 8 case still matter? The answer is because of what it spurred scientists to do.

For me and my colleagues in the scientific community, these oral arguments offered a clear warning shot of the legal terrain ahead, and there was no time to waste. Research can be famously slow (Dennis et al. 2020). Its methodical, systematic, careful nature can be in tension with fast-moving events. It was clear to me and other researchers studying abortion, especially those who had long been tasked with systematically capturing the impact legal machinations have on people seeking to become unpregnant, that we needed a plan for rapid monitoring. Collecting even the most basic numbers would require a major effort—and would be needed with a speed never previously achieved.

This chapter presents the story of the #WeCount project, an effort spurred by the implementation of SB 8 and stood up by the Society of Family Planning in the four months leading up to *Dobbs* in anticipation of a negative outcome. By the time a copy of the draft majority opinion in *Dobbs* was leaked via an unprecedented *Politico* publication on May 2, 2022—over a month before the release of the official Supreme Court ruling—the effort to collect real-time data on abortion provision by all known abortion providers in the United States was underway, led by me and a small team at the Society. But it was far from just us: #WeCount required the collective action of a field of advocates, activists, providers, and researchers. This collective action was in service of getting the count, the number of abortions actually taking place after this massive legal disruption.

Just the Count

At its most basic, the *Dobbs* decision allowed states to ban legal abortion within their borders. And many did. Following the *Dobbs* decision, state legislatures hostile to abortion rights immediately sought to criminalize and ban care. State law enforcement officials hostile to abortion immediately declared their intention to enforce "trigger laws" banning abortion that were already on the books (but unenforceable under *Roe*). Clinics quickly closed, and client appointments were abruptly cancelled. Abortion-providing facilities in neighboring states experienced rapid changes in demand for abortion care, and journalists began reporting about long wait times for appointments. We desperately needed to understand the remaining care landscape and how people were navigating it. For advocates, providers, and researchers alike, decisions on resources—financial and human—hinged on a clear understanding of the fall out, with evidence as an essential check on our projections. But broadly, abortion is a common experience that shifts the trajectories of people's lives, especially as it relates to their health and economic security (Foster 2020). In the wake of this unprecedented disruption, the need for evidence on its impact on people's lives was clear and extremely pressurized.

The number of abortions has always been an important but maddeningly incomplete signal of abortion need, use, and provision. From the perspective of a healthcare provider, the term "volume" is commonly used to refer to the quantity or amount of a particular medical service, procedure, or intervention; procedure, patient, case, or service volume are all indicators that guide the business of providing health care, including abortion services. Volume data are essential for planning, allocating resources, and monitoring the quality of the services provided. Data indicate the demand for services and are carefully monitored in order to make decisions about resource distribution, such as the number of appointments or the staffing needed, to meet need.

In the field of public health, the term "incidence" is used to describe new cases of a specific disease or health condition. Abortion incidence refers to the frequency or rate at which induced abortions occur within a specific population over a defined period. Researchers and public health professionals use abortion incidence data to track trends over time and inform reproductive health policies and interventions. Incidence can also be reflected as a rate (e.g., in 2020, there was an abortion rate of 14.4 abortions per 1,000 women) rather than a count (e.g., in 2020, 930,160 abortions were provided in clinical settings) (Jones et al. 2022). Doing so helps guard against the potential that a higher or lower number of abortions is actually a reflection of changes in the number of people who could potentially become pregnant based on demographic trends. These measures aggregate abortions across the U.S. population, shifting our attention from the level of an individual person's reproductive experience to a population-level indicator.

This frame of incidence can be tricky. The shift from the individual to the population level is necessary but fraught. It is necessary because access to abortion (or lack thereof) can profoundly shape the health and well-being of pregnant people. Understanding these trends at a population level is needed for all efforts related to health and well-being, as well as predictions of demographic changes that underlie plans for system education and for public programs like Social Security.

However, the shift to explore abortion at the population level is fraught because the decision to end a pregnancy is a deeply personal one. One more abortion or one less abortion loses meaning at the aggregate level without the context of a person's reproductive desires. Imagine a single appointment for abortion care, scheduled for a person who at the time of calling the office no longer wishes to be pregnant. If that person does not show up for the appointment, it is impossible to know whether one less abortion is good or bad. For supporters of reproductive justice, if that person decided to continue the pregnancy, the missed appointment is a positive outcome. But if that person did not want to continue the pregnancy and is unable to receive care due to the cost, the logistics, or myriad other factors (Bennett et al. 2023), this is a negative outcome both for the individual and for reproductive justice. Of course, this hypothetical assumes a person's desires related to a given pregnancy are clear and stable. In fact, research shows that people's feelings toward pregnancy can be highly dynamic (Cutler et al. 2018; Strong et al. 2023). Far from existing in a vacuum, these feelings can be influenced not only by a person's own desire or family considerations but also by structural factors such as whether an abortion feels within reach (O'Donnell, Weitz, and Freedman 2011).

So, although we need the count for all the reasons previously discussed, untethering the count from the individual lives tied to each abortion received or not is risky. To evaluate how to interpret a trend in the count—as, say, good or bad—we must always ground the assessment in the meaning of abortion at the individual level. These aggregate numbers represent real people's lives.

UP OR DOWN, GOOD OR BAD?

The meaning of abortion numbers is further complicated by previous efforts to find political "common ground" as abortion became highly polarized in the decades that followed the *Roe* decision. In his 1992 presidential campaign, Bill Clinton popularized the frame of "safe, legal, and rare." During a campaign speech at Pennsylvania State University on April 7, 1992, he said, "Abortion should be safe, legal, and rare. I have never met anyone who is pro-abortion. Being pro-choice is not being pro-abortion." The landmark 1994 International Conference on Population and Development in Cairo, Egypt, codified a similar frame that assumed more abortions to be a negative outcome and less abortions to be a positive outcome: "Every attempt should be made to eliminate the need for abortion" (Berer 2009). This conference marked an essential pivot away from a population control approach, which had been and still is associated with controversial and coercive practices at the individual level and directly or indirectly echoed eugenic language. It marked a shift toward a family planning approach that was a more comprehensive and rights-based framework (Hartmann 1995). However, the assumption underlying both "safe, legal, and rare" and "eliminate the need for abortion" was that abortion is a bad outcome rather than part of a long-standing continuum of tools people have used to control their fertility. This, in turn, prominently reinforced the idea that reducing abortions is a goal upon which people can generally agree.

Filtered through this lens, a decrease in abortion numbers would be viewed as positive, perhaps an indicator that other tools like comprehensive sexual education and contraception are accessible and supporting people to prevent pregnancy. For example, a decline in abortion could be partially driven by the more widespread availability of long-acting and highly effective contraception like intrauterine devices (IUDs) to young people seeking to prevent pregnancy. Research finds, however, that some people who want an abortion are unable to obtain one, problematizing the frame of a decreasing abortion rate as a positive indicator of women's reproductive autonomy (Cohen and Joffe 2020; Foster 2020; Kimport 2021). A decrease in numbers might be a signal of more widespread experiences of barriers to abortion rather than a decreasing need for abortion. And, as can happen in the messy real world, a decrease in abortion numbers could be the effect of both increases in pregnancy prevention *and* barriers to obtaining wanted abortions. All of this underscores the complexity of—and risks inherent in—making sense of abortion numbers.

Worthwhile, but Difficult to Do

In the time between the SB 8 ruling and the *Dobbs* decision that ultimately overturned *Roe*, it was clear that the benefits of counting abortions outweighed the risks. We needed the number to document the effects of this monumental legal change and, for advocates and providers, so every effort could be made to buffer the harm to those losing access to care in their state. But actually doing the work to count is challenging.

Since *Roe*, some states have had a long-standing practice of tracking the number of abortions, though the robustness of these efforts varies from state to state. In some states, healthcare providers are required to report abortion data to the state health department. These reports typically include information on the number of abortions performed, demographic characteristics of individuals seeking abortions, gestational age of the fetus, and other relevant details. Other states collect this information as part of their vital statistics reporting system, which compiles information on births, deaths, marriages, and divorces. Interestingly, states with policies designed to make this care harder to get, such as requiring young people under the age of eighteen to get a parent's consent in order to receive care or imposing a waiting period that mandates a delay between the initial counseling session and the actual abortion, were often the most reliable counters of abortion and the states that protected abortion access produced the least robust data. For example, California has limited data despite many laws designed to support access, such as state funding for care, whereas Mississippi, where the *Dobbs* case originated, has excellent data (Lindbergh et al. 2020).

Building off this reporting at the state level, the Centers for Disease Control and Prevention (CDC) compiles and publishes abortion surveillance reports, which provide national and state-level data on abortions. However, the process is not mandatory at the federal level. This effort relies on aggregated data provided by the states. Some states, such as California, Maryland, and New Hampshire, have declined to participate for years. Further, while the CDC publishes its reports annually, there is often a lag of two to three years from collection to report, making it very difficult to use this evidence to understand the present moment, especially in the midst of rapid changes to state legislation, and even harder to use it to make concrete decisions about where to place resources in service of people's access to care.

Recognizing the obvious limitations of publicly funded efforts both in terms of completeness and timeliness, independent efforts to collect these data have stepped in to fill the gaps. The Guttmacher Institute has served as an essential reporter of the number of abortions in the United States for several decades. Instead of relying on state entities to provide data, its Abortion Provider Census collected data on the availability and provision of abortion services in the United States via a combination of surveys, questionnaires, and direct communication with abortion providers. This effort collected information directly from facilities that provide abortions and shared yearly totals by state and provider type (i.e., standalone clinic, hospital, private practice). However, given the time and effort needed to implement these large-scale, national surveys, these reports were made available on a cadence that was driven by having the private resources in hand to produce them, often every three years prior to the *Dobbs* ruling. State-level restrictions—and the associated impacts on abortion access—began to outpace this cadence of triannual reporting, accelerating in the two decades prior to the *Dobbs* ruling. In the face of the sheer volume and variety of restrictions, the patchwork of these restrictions across each region, and the stop-and-start effect of legal challenges to individual restrictions in the courts in each state, the established habits of monitoring volume were already under pressure; often they were not able to respond to the increasing volatility of the policy environment in a timely way.

Extracting data from public (e.g., Medicaid) and private insurers (e.g., for-profit health insurance companies, which provide plans to individuals accessing insurance via their employment) is another tool for monitoring services used in health care broadly that is often suggested for measuring abortion use. However, once again the ongoing assault of state-level policy renders these approaches ineffective for abortion. Because of common restrictions on the coverage of abortion by public and private insurers, any data extract via these records is severely incomplete. Many states, in addition to prohibiting insurance coverage of abortion via Medicaid at the state level, have also severely restricted insurance coverage of abortion in all private insurance plans written in the state (true of eleven states, as of August 2023; Guttmacher Institute 2023). For the remaining abortion seekers whose insurance will cover abortion care, many people find that the cost of abortion comes in under their deductible (meaning no part of the cost can be absorbed by the insurer), or people avoid using their insurance out of concerns about privacy. Because the majority of abortions are paid for out of pocket, insurance records are an inadequate source for understanding the use of abortion in the United States (Jones and Chiu 2023).

Navigating increasing restrictions on abortion at the state level and the neutralization—likely through successful efforts to other abortion in concrete ways—of typical data sources for counts, researchers studying abortion have been forced to continually innovate. In the lead-up to *Dobbs*, new models for responsive research emerged, such as Resound Research for Reproductive Health. Initially organized as the Texas Policy Evaluation Project (TxPEP) at the University of Texas at Austin in 2011, Resound Research for Reproductive Health conducted timely and rigorous assessments of how policy changes affect people's access to abortion and contraceptive care in and around Texas. Other research endeavors were established in Georgia, Ohio, and Wisconsin to undertake similar data collections and analyses of their states and regions.

As the likely overturning of *Roe* and the removal of federal abortion protections loomed, those of us leading the #WeCount effort knew three things. First, researchers, policymakers, healthcare providers, and advocates, among others, needed and relied on the work of these regional research centers. Second, the existing efforts could not meet the need for rapid monitoring at a national level. Finally, the patchwork of abortion restrictions and the race to create protections and expansions of abortion access would be accelerated and play out across fifty states, making the already complicated project of measurement even more complicated. With an eye toward the domino effect of the anticipated *Dobbs* ruling and building off the expertise and insight of invested researchers, the plan for #WeCount was born.

ENTER #WECOUNT

With no single effort well-positioned to respond, the work to set up a rapid monitoring effort needed a home. With its mission to be the source for abortion and contraception science, the Society of Family Planning provided a critical container for the collective effort that became #WeCount. Founded in 2005, the Society is an academic membership organization for over 1,800 researchers and clinicians contributing to the science and medicine of abortion and contraception as well as serving as the academic home of the Complex Family Planning fellowship, an accredited obstetrics and gynecology subspecialty. At the time of #WeCount's creation and implementation, I served as the senior director of research and evaluation at the Society.

We structured #WeCount to take a census approach; in short, #WeCount aimed to engage all entities providing abortion services rather than using a sample of entities to reflect the whole. With participation entirely voluntary, connecting with and engaging entities providing abortions would demand a large-scale organizing effort. There were over 790 publicly advertising facilities that were open and providing abortion services in 2021. That's a lot of doors to knock on.

Getting Clinics to Answer the Door

At minimum, to reach these facilities and invite them to participate required two things: a complete list of facilities in the United States providing abortions regularly and a method to get in touch with each. Indeed, having a comprehensive list of abortion facilities was itself a research endeavor. Luckily, such a list had already been created by a team at the University of California, San Francisco's Advancing New Standards in Reproductive Health for use by researchers: the Abortion Facility Database. The existence and availability of this list, itself the product of careful scraping of online information, cross-checking with directories, and mystery caller data collection, addressed the first challenge but not the second.

Developing partnerships with facilities providing abortion can be difficult for reasons that mirror the broader context of abortion. For decades, facilities and workers that provide abortion care have been targets of violence and harassment (Joffe 2010). This harassment sometimes uses tactics of espionage: "sting" operations and videos of workers recorded without consent (Pierson 2022). In the face of systematic, highly organized, and constant threats, the facilities and workers that provide abortion care are often—and understandably—wary to partner with people outside their organizations. Facilities' public-facing contact information can be very limited and only offered in service of people seeking abortion care. In some cases, finding any contact information for a facility is a challenge, and having a general email address is a far-cry from a conversation with the person who is positioned to commit to the organization's participation in an effort like #WeCount.

Membership organizations for abortion facilities, such as the National Abortion Federation and the Abortion Care Network, have policies that forbid sharing the contact information of individuals working in member facilities. This compounded the difficulties of connecting with facilities. Activating preexisting relationships, state by state and facility by facility, was key. Networked facilities that provided abortions joined in bulk, fueling the project's momentum. Existing data collection efforts, such as those led by state-based research groups, buoyed the effort from the outset, doubling back to facilities already reporting to regional centers to ensure each consented to pass along their count to this national effort.

The professional reputation of the Society helped somewhat in this task. As a hub for scientists doing research on and clinicians providing contraception and abortion, the Society was known as a trusted organization to many (but far from all) who own, manage, or work in facilities that provide abortion services. This name recognition assured contacts at abortion facilities that #WeCount researchers were genuine and not intending the harass or otherwise harm them. This removed a critical barrier for the project's implementation, but it did not obviate the need for a huge recruitment effort. It got #WeCount in the door, but it would only be successful if abortion clinics and other organizations providing abortion services decided to participate. Members of the Society of Family Planning emailed, texted, and called colleagues in their networks to urge them to participate. Clinician members were especially critical to the effort, advocating within their own institutions to execute data-sharing agreements and reaching out to former coworkers and employers on the project's behalf.

Right-Sizing the "Ask"

In April 2022, a mere two months before an expected Supreme Court decision, #WeCount publicly launched and began seeking the participation of the hundreds of facilities providing abortion care. We needed to document the "before" to enable better understanding of what would come after *Dobbs*. Initially, we hoped to collect information from each facility including monthly counts of number of abortions, number of abortions by type (procedural or medication), number of abortions by gestation, number of abortions by state of residence of patient, number of adolescent patients, and number of complex cases (e.g., people seeking care who have medical conditions that make abortion more clinically or socially complex to provide). Still on the table at that time was the possibility of collecting additional data, specifically, patient race and ethnicity data, data on public versus private insurance eligibility, or other demographic data that would help monitor not just the care provided but to whom.

This list, enticing in its potential to support fieldwide insights, was gutted almost immediately after conversations with experts at the Abortion Care Network and in clinic settings. The number of abortions was within reach, exportable from administrative records of sites providing abortions, tucked in their billing data. Any information that was related to the "who" of the patient or the "what" of the care, though, was held in medical records, which meant for us a complex electronic health records system at best or a mound of paper files held under lock and key at worst.

At the wise counsel of leaders of the Abortion Care Network, we anchored #WeCount around the smallest ask that would make a research contribution: we said to ourselves, against the backdrop of the fall of *Roe*, that "the least we can ask is the most we can ask." The project, after all, was poised to ask for time and effort from facilities that were bracing for and then experienced massive upheaval driven by the overturning of nearly fifty years of legal precedent. The project had a greater chance of success if it reduced its ask.

Abortion Care Network leaders also helped us understand the importance of differentiating between information held in a healthcare organization's billing records from that held in patient records. Because the number of abortions is held in billing records, they can be extracted by a range of workers. By contrast, the information held in patient records is not always easy to extract and aggregate. An unshakeable (and HIPAA-required[2]) commitment to patient confidentiality ensures that these records are only accessible to workers who rely on their use to provide care. Like the entirety of health care, facilities that provide abortions are at various stages of adopting electronic medical records (Evans 2016). Even if all facilities had electronic medical records, querying them effectively for the wish list of information in #WeCount's early imagination would have required a level of consistency across different entities that was virtually impossible in practice.

We scaled back. At the moment of launch, it was just the count. Recruitment began in earnest.

Recruiting Against the Clock

This was not simply door knocking: some entities providing abortion care had no physical door. Separate from the *Dobbs* ruling, abortion care was in transition. #WeCount's recruitment efforts took place against the backdrop of an expansion of how abortion could be and was provided via telehealth. As the chapter from Tracy Weitz in this volume details further, the emergency measures put into place to protect public health during the early years of the COVID-19 pandemic had accelerated this transition, as it did for telehealth across health care. Notably, the U.S. Food and Drug Administration's 2021 revision of the rules guiding mifepristone's use had opened up the possibility for telehealth across the sector of abortion provision, and virtual-only entities providing abortion care were newly coming online. It was essential for #WeCount to include these entities, not only because their participation in abortion provision had yet to be captured by previous reporting efforts but also because we suspected these providers were a growing part of abortion provision.

It was a race against the clock to engage all entities providing abortion care in time to capture the fallout of the *Dobbs* decision. Years of monitoring abortion policy meant the field anticipated some states would immediately ban or severely restrict abortion. For the facilities in states guaranteed or very likely to immediately ban or severely restrict abortion, their likely post-*Dobbs* closure would make it much more difficult to get their pre-*Dobbs* numbers in hand. On May 2, 2022, *Politico* published a copy of the draft majority opinion in *Dobbs*. Many facilities had already agreed to participate in #WeCount, but concrete evidence of what would become the final Supreme Court decision in the case was sobering and prompted many others to sign on.

The day that the *Dobbs* decision came down in June 2022 was eerily quiet for the people working on #WeCount. The months prior had felt urgent and high-stakes to reach the facilities most likely to close—before their ability to share pre-*Dobbs* counts was lost. Now the work was to ensure enough participation of the facilities that remained open for the data to be usable. The weeks that followed the ruling offered an immediate proof of research concept: reporters and the public already wanted and needed the data #WeCount produced.

The pressure was high. Reporters were calling frequently, insistently requesting early findings. Some suggested they might be able to get the information faster via their own efforts, a clear indication of their naivety about the complexity of this effort (as previously described) and of their possible hubris. Here, the value of collaborative research shown through. It was only because of the partnership between abortion providers and scholars and their collective time and effort that we could produce accurate numbers. Put simply, it would be impossible for individual journalists and advocates to do this. Faced with excellent but not complete participation from all providers, the application of research expertise was essential to get the best count.

With a first release of data planned for October 2022, the timing was tight. The main contributors of data could only promise numbers six weeks after the close of the month of service. This would mean that, to capture the numbers in the first two months after the *Dobbs* decision (July and August 2022), large portions of data would only be available in early October, leaving precious few weeks to conduct the analysis, aggregate the report, and impute the numbers from the few facilities that had not signed on to share their counts with us.

We did it anyway. On October 28, 2022, #WeCount publicly released its first report and provided a first look at the number of abortions after *Dobbs*—and how that compared to pre-*Dobbs* counts.

EARLY FINDINGS

In the first and subsequent data releases, #WeCount hit home the value of observed numbers over predicted numbers generated from thoughtful, scientific models. The models forecasting what would happen when *Roe* fell were excellent, predicting geographical effects of the fall of *Roe*. Yet still, they were not always right; abortion seekers—and some state legislatures, voters, and judges—operated differently than predicted. Real numbers helped correct and revise our predictions.

Because the state bans were implemented (and sometimes enjoined) at various dates rather than all at once, the maps reflecting the numbers fluctuated. Abortion rate decreases in a given state and increases in another created a call-and-response effect that would shift from month to month. Which states would receive out-of-state travelers seeking abortion care? What impact would gestational limits have in the states that severely restricted but did not outright ban abortion? What would the *Dobbs* decision do to the total number of abortions in the country? How would telehealth play out in the post-*Dobbs* world? The data did not always show what many expected and often challenged the entrenched narratives from various actors within and outside the abortion service delivery world about what *Dobbs* would mean for abortion.

Take, for example, which states would receive out-of-state travelers seeking abortion care. Prior to *Dobbs* and to prepare the infrastructure of abortion provision, researchers and others completed modeling efforts to forecast the impact of the fall of *Roe*. None of these reports were made available to the public at the time; often they were not even shared widely within the networks of professionals who do concrete work to support abortion services (Myers 2024). These forecasts were built on differing underlying assumptions, and they reflected differing narratives of how people make decisions as they navigate to care, yielding distinct but largely complementary predictions.

One informed assumption related to transportation. Research capturing the effect of the SB 8 six-week ban in place in Texas for the ten months before the *Dobbs* ruling showed that people unable to obtain in-state care drove to present for services out of state (White et al. 2022). When paired with the experiences of people seeking care and those supporting them, this made sense. People seeking abortion care are more likely to have limited resources, and many live below the poverty line (Jones and Chiu 2023). Air travel is a luxury; even with outside financial support, out-of-state clinics may be beyond the reach for a person seeking care, introducing many unknowns to an already stressful path to care. Further, travel by car means a support person could accompany the person seeking care without additional cost.

Scaled to thinking about the travel patterns of post-*Dobbs* patients, this should have meant that the states likely to receive an influx of people seeking abortion care were those that bordered or were geographically close to the states with bans (e.g., Kansas), not the states farther afield that perhaps had more robust infrastructure or resources to provide care (e.g., Washington). In the early #WeCount findings, however, these informed assumptions did not fully pan out. There were surprise and hidden "surges" in states such as Minnesota and North Carolina, which did not fit the expected criteria for receiving out-of-state abortion seekers because of their relative distance from the states that immediately banned abortion after *Dobbs*. This sent a clear message to us as researchers that many people preferred to spend what amounted to days in the car to go to a relatively small facility rather than hours in a plane to reach a large facility or waiting longer for an appointment at a facility (of any size) that was a shorter driving distance away.

Another example is the impact of gestational bans. Again, research capturing the impact of SB 8 showed the number of in-state abortions was approximately halved, surprising many who had characterized such bans as functionally equivalent to a complete ban. #WeCount also found a similar pattern wherein strict gestational bans substantially reduced but did not eliminate in-state abortions.

Finally, #WeCount was the first effort to capture the number of abortions on a monthly basis, and, by design, it did so during a time of extreme legal volatility and instability that had not been seen since *Roe* first established the right to abortion in 1973. At the state level, the numbers were intuitive: an abortion ban going into effect effectively brought the number of abortions in that state to almost zero (with the occasional abortion because of a medical emergency allowed). Many states bordering the states with bans experienced large increases in the number of abortions obtained, both in terms of absolute numbers and as a percentage increase when compared with the previous monthly volume.

But once we applied a national lens, the findings were surprising. There was a significant deficit in abortions in the first two months after *Dobbs* (July and August 2022) as compared with the two months collected to serve as a baseline (April and May 2022), with comparable numbers over the course of the nine months after. Reflecting on a year of data after the *Dobbs* ruling, however, a surprising finding emerged: there were more abortions obtained in the first year after the elimination of the federal right to abortion than a census of abortions in 2020 had recorded (Society of Family Planning 2024). These findings suggested that the number of abortions provided in and by abortion facilities was actually increasing, after it had declined for decades. And this increase did not even account for the thousands of abortions taking place by international telehealth and outside formal healthcare settings (Aiken et al. 2022, 2024).

A LEGACY OF QUESTIONS

What drives people to choose to get care in certain states? What makes abortion still obtainable when severely restricted, limited to under six weeks' gestation? How has *Dobbs* changed the distribution of gestations when people obtain care? Why were there more abortions in the year after the *Dobbs* ruling? Notably, and perhaps most critically, #WeCount numbers have prompted questions about the *who*. In a highly racialized and deeply unequal health system, it is very likely that the "who" matters (Dehlendorf, Harris, and Weitz 2013). Who are the people who could (and could not) successfully obtain care out of state? Who are the people self-managing their abortion at home? Who are the people forced to continue a pregnancy?

The #WeCount data in hand is not able to answer these questions. The project's very design is simply to describe volume, not to explain it. Tracking the number of abortions is the floor, not the ceiling, of what is needed to understand the present moment and what brought us to this point. Even so, these are questions that could not have been formulated without the #WeCount data. Beyond being a story of collective effort, working against the clock and producing data that was of service in a moment of crisis, this may be the effort's more lasting legacy. With its simple counts, #WeCount has spurred new, relevant, and timely questions that we will be answering decades into the future.

ACKNOWLEDGMENTS

I hold deep gratitude for the many people who made #WeCount possible through their careful work, especially Drs. Ushma Upadhyay, Alison Norris, and Amanda Dennis, and close colleagues Claire Yuan and Vanessa Arenas, as well as all those who have participated or encouraged participation in this collective effort. A heartfelt thanks as well to my wife.

NOTES

1. Texas Senate Bill 8 (Texas Heartbeat Act of 2021), https://capitol.texas.gov/tlodocs/87R/billtext/pdf/SB00008F.pdf; Tex. Health & Safety Code Ann. §§ 171.201–171.212 (West 2021).

2. The Health Insurance Portability and Accountability Act of 1996 (HIPAA) and its subsequent amendments protect the confidentiality, integrity, and availability of individually identifiable healthcare data from improper uses and disclosures, including data stored and transmitted electronically. See the Department of Health and Human Services pages "HIPAA for Individuals" (https://www.hhs.gov/hipaa/for-individuals/index.html) and "HIPAA for Professionals" (https://www.hhs.gov/hipaa/for-professionals/index.html).

REFERENCES

Aiken, Abigail R., Jennifer E. Starling, James G. Scott, and Rebecca Gomperts. 2022. "Requests for Self-Managed Medication Abortion Provided Using Online Telemedicine in 30 US States Before and After the *Dobbs v. Jackson Women's Health Organization* Decision." *JAMA* 328 (17): 1768–1770.

Aiken, Abigail R., Elizabeth S. Wells, Rebecca Gomperts, and James G. Scott. 2024. "Provision of Medications for Self-Managed Abortion Before and After the *Dobbs v. Jackson Women's Health Organization* Decision." *JAMA* 331 (18):1558–1564.

Bennett, Amber H., Catherine Marshall, Katrina Kimport, Julie Deardorff, and Anu M. Gómez. 2023. "'Have You Ever Wanted or Needed an Abortion You Did Not Get?' Data from a 2022 Nationally Representative Online Survey in the United States." *Contraception* 123: 110007.

Berer, Marge. 2009. "The Cairo 'Compromise' on Abortion and Its Consequences for Making Abortion Safe and Legal." In *Reproductive Health and Human Rights: The Way Forward*, edited by Laura Reichenbach and Mindy Jane Roseman, 152–164. University of Pennsylvania Press.

Cohen, David S., and Carole Joffe. 2020. *Obstacle Course: The Everyday Struggle to Get an Abortion in America*. University of California Press.

Cutler, Alice, Bailey McNamara, Natasha Qasba, Holly P. Kennedy, Lori Lundsberg, and Annabelle Gariepy. 2018. "'I Just Don't Know': An Exploration of Women's Ambivalence about a New Pregnancy." *Women's Health Issues* 28 (1): 75–81.

Dehlendorf, Christine, Lisa H. Harris, and Tracy A. Weitz. 2013. "Disparities in Abortion Rates: A Public Health Approach." *American Journal of Public Health* 103 (10): 1772–1779.

Dennis, Amanda, Rebecca Manski, and Jenny O'Donnell. 2020. "Assessing Research Impact: A Framework and an Evaluation of the Society of Family Planning Research Fund's Grantmaking (2007–2017)." *Contraception* 101 (4): 213–219.

Evans, R. Scott. 2016. "Electronic Health Records: Then, Now, and in the Future." *Yearbook of Medical Informatics* 25 (Supplement 1): S48-S61.

Foster, Diana E. 2020. *The Turnaway Study: Ten Years, a Thousand Women, and the Consequences of Having—or Being Denied—an Abortion*. Scribner.

Guttmacher Institute. 2023. "Regulating Insurance Coverage for Abortion." Guttmacher Institute, August 31, 2023. https://www.guttmacher.org/state-policy/explore/regulating -insurance-coverage-abortion.

Hartmann, Betsy. 1995. *Reproductive Rights and Wrongs: The Global Politics of Population Control*. Rev. ed. South End Press.

Joffe, Carole E. 2010. *Dispatches from the Abortion Wars: The Costs of Fanaticism to Doctors, Patients, and the Rest of Us*. Beacon Press.

Jones, Rachel K., and Diana W. Chiu. 2023. "Characteristics of Abortion Patients in Protected and Restricted States Accessing Clinic-Based Care 12 Months Prior to the Elimination of the Federal Constitutional Right to Abortion in the United States." *Perspectives on Sexual and Reproductive Health* 55 (2): 80–85.

Jones, Rachel K., Mia Kirstein, and Jessica Philbin. 2022. "Abortion Incidence and Service Availability in the United States, 2020." *Perspectives on Sexual and Reproductive Health* 54 (4): 128–141.

Kimport, Katrina. 2021. *No Real Choice: How Culture and Politics Matter for Reproductive Autonomy*. Rutgers University Press.

Lindberg, Laura, Kathryn Kost, Isaac Maddow-Zimet, Shannon Desai, and Mia Zolna. 2020. "Abortion Reporting in the United States: An Assessment of Three National Fertility Surveys." *Demography* 57 (3): 899–925.

Myers, Caitlin. 2024. "Forecasts for a Post-*Roe* America: The Effects of Increased Travel Distance on Abortions and Births." *Journal of Policy Analysis and Management* 43 (1): 39–62.

O'Donnell, Jenny, Tracy A. Weitz, and Lori R. Freedman. 2011. "Resistance and Vulnerability to Stigmatization in Abortion Work." *Social Science & Medicine* 73 (9): 1357–1364.

Pierson, Brendan. 2022. "Abortion Foes Largely Lose $2.4 Mln Appeal over Planned Parenthood Videos." Reuters, October 21, 2022. https://www.reuters.com/legal/litigation /abortion-foes-largely-lose-24-mln-appeal-over-planned-parenthood-videos-2022-10-21/.

Politico Staff. 2022. "Read Justice Alito's Initial Draft Abortion Opinion Which Would Overturn Roe v. Wade." *Politico*, May 2, 2022. https://www.politico.com/news/2022/05/02 /read-justice-alito-initial-abortion-opinion-overturn-roe-v-wade-pdf-00029504.

Society of Family Planning. 2024. "April 2022 to September 2023." *#WeCount Public Report*, February 28, 2024. https://doi.org/10.46621/675707thmfmv.

Strong, Jenny, Ernestina Coast, Emily Freeman, Ann M. Moore, Alison H. Norris, Oluwaseyi Owolabi, and Chloe H. Rocca. 2023. "Pregnancy Recognition Trajectories: A Needed Framework." *Sexual and Reproductive Health Matters* 31 (1): 2167552.

White, Kari, Gabriela Sierra, Krystal Lerma, Alexis Beasley, Lisa G. Hofler, Kristina Tocce, Vinita Goyal, Tony Ogburn, Joseph E. Potter, Samuel L. Dickman. 2022. "Association of Texas' 2021 Ban on Abortion in Early Pregnancy with the Number of Facility-Based Abortions in Texas and Surrounding States." *JAMA* 328 (20): 2048–2055.

Toward a Unified Conceptualization of Abortion Access

Jane W. Seymour and Jenny Higgins

THE IMPORTANCE OF CONCEPTUALIZING ACCESS

Both before and after *Dobbs*, scholars have endeavored to document changes to the U.S. abortion landscape and seekers' challenges in obtaining abortions, using the term "abortion access" to describe the object of their studies. To this end, researchers often call factors that prevent people from obtaining abortions "barriers to abortion access," and public health scholars have focused on interventions that could help people obtain wanted abortions—that is, ensure "abortion access." But what if not everyone is using this term the same way? What does the field of abortion research really mean by "abortion access?"

While there is likely agreement that abortion access refers to the ability of abortion seekers[1] to obtain wanted abortions, there is significant heterogeneity in how scholars operationalize abortion access, ranging from distance to services to the cost of an abortion. This inconsistency leaves the literature fragmented and has real-world consequences. Given that no unifying conceptualization exists, the literature fails to, among other things, systematically identify barriers to obtaining wanted abortions and thus take advantage of opportunities to develop interventions that most effectively improve health and well-being. Moreover, when the literature fails to capture "access" consistently, we miss the opportunity to understand factors that constrain or expand abortion services, interest in abortion, and interest in providing abortion care. A unified conceptualization of abortion access can clarify abortion scholarship, making the literature easier to interpret, synthesize, and act upon, as well as showing gaps in the existing research on the subject.

In this chapter, we call on the public health literature, specifically work by Roy Penchansky and J. William Thomas (1981) as expanded upon by Emily Saurman (2016), to address this need. We propose that abortion access is an umbrella concept constituted by six subdomains. In their foundational conceptualization,

Penchansky and Thomas specify five subdomains that collectively make up healthcare access: availability, accessibility, accommodation, affordability, and acceptability. Subsequently, Saurman updated the conceptualization to include a sixth subdomain: awareness.[2]

We aim to orient the field toward a unified conceptualization of abortion access by defining each of the six subdomains that together constitute abortion access. We examine research on how each subdomain is associated with facilitating or constraining abortion seekers' ability to obtain abortions, and then we draw on the Wisconsin context for further illustration. We primarily focus on examples where abortion seekers were entirely unable to obtain abortions; however, it is important to note that our framing captures how abortion access can also be limited or nonexistent for abortion seekers who obtain an abortion but not as they wanted. After defining and contextualizing each subdomain (summarized in table 5.1), we offer thoughts about their interconnectedness and why meeting abortion seekers' wants and preferences is foundational to defining abortion access. We conclude by offering suggestions for how scholars and those using research to advance health and well-being might use our conceptualization.

Abortion Access in Wisconsin

Wisconsin was once considered supportive of abortion access. But in 2010 a sea-change gerrymandered election resulted in an anti-abortion majority in state government that passed a host of abortion restrictions, including a twenty-four-hour waiting period; a ban on the use of telehealth to provide abortions; prohibitions on insurance coverage for state employees that meant state workers had to pay out of pocket for abortions; and a twenty-week gestational duration ban, which meant that anyone seeking an abortion later in pregnancy had to travel out of state or forgo abortion altogether (Williamson, Ufot, and Higgins 2023). Combined with the state's existing Medicaid ban, which meant that people who relied on public insurance had to pay out of pocket for abortions, these changes led the Guttmacher Institute, a research institute that studies abortion and abortion policy, to designate Wisconsin as "extremely hostile" to abortion rights by 2014.

In June 2022, abortion services were only available at stand-alone abortion-providing facilities, where most abortions take place across the United States, in three Wisconsin counties: Dane (one clinic), Sheboygan (one clinic), and Milwaukee (two clinics) (see figure 5.1). At that time, nearly 70 percent of people of reproductive age in Wisconsin lived in a county with no abortion clinic (WISH 2014).

June 2022 brought more changes to the Wisconsin abortion-provision landscape. When the *Dobbs* decision was released, all abortion providers in the state—in clinics, hospitals, and private practices—stopped offering abortions. In overturning the federal right to abortion, the *Dobbs* decision allowed an 1849 Wisconsin law that some interpreted as criminalizing abortion to go (back) into effect. Initially, there was an open question as to whether the law was enforceable. Over a year later, a state circuit court ruled that the 1849 law did not prohibit voluntary abortions. In September 2023, Planned Parenthood of Wisconsin resumed

TABLE 5.1

SUMMARY OF ABORTION ACCESS SUBDOMAIN CONCEPTUALIZATIONS AND EXAMPLES FROM THE WISCONSIN CONTEXT

Abortion access subdomain	Conceptualization	Examples from the Wisconsin context
Availability	Relationship between presence/absence, volume, and type of abortion offered and the demand for abortion overall as well as for the specific types of abortion among abortion seekers	Between June 2022 and September 2023, an 1849 law was interpreted as an abortion ban, so no services were available in the state.
Proximity	Relationship between where abortion services are located and where abortion seekers live	Forty percent of Wisconsin's abortion clinics closed between 2010 and 2017. Increased driving distances to care were associated with decreases in county-level abortion rates and increases in county-level birth rates.
Accommodation	Relationship between how abortion services are organized and abortion seekers' ability to utilize that abortion service	The 20-week gestational duration ban means that abortion seekers later in pregnancy must leave the state or forego abortion altogether.
Affordability	Relationship between the cost of abortion and abortion seekers' ability to pay those costs, including through insurance coverage	The law prohibits abortion care coverage for enrollees in Medicaid (BadgerCare), plans offered on the state's Health Insurance Marketplace, and insurance plans for state employees, meaning most residents must pay out of pocket for abortion.
Acceptability	Relationship between abortion seekers' expectations of what abortion services and providers "should" be and what services and providers are; whether abortion seekers believe it is acceptable to have an abortion	Laws require healthcare practices discordant with evidence-based practice: 24+ hours before the abortion, the abortion seeker must obtain an ultrasound and the provider must display and explain the images.
Awareness	Abortion seekers' knowledge of correct information about abortion services and their ability to use that knowledge to obtain abortions	Abortion care churn has sowed confusion among Wisconsinites about abortion legality and availability.

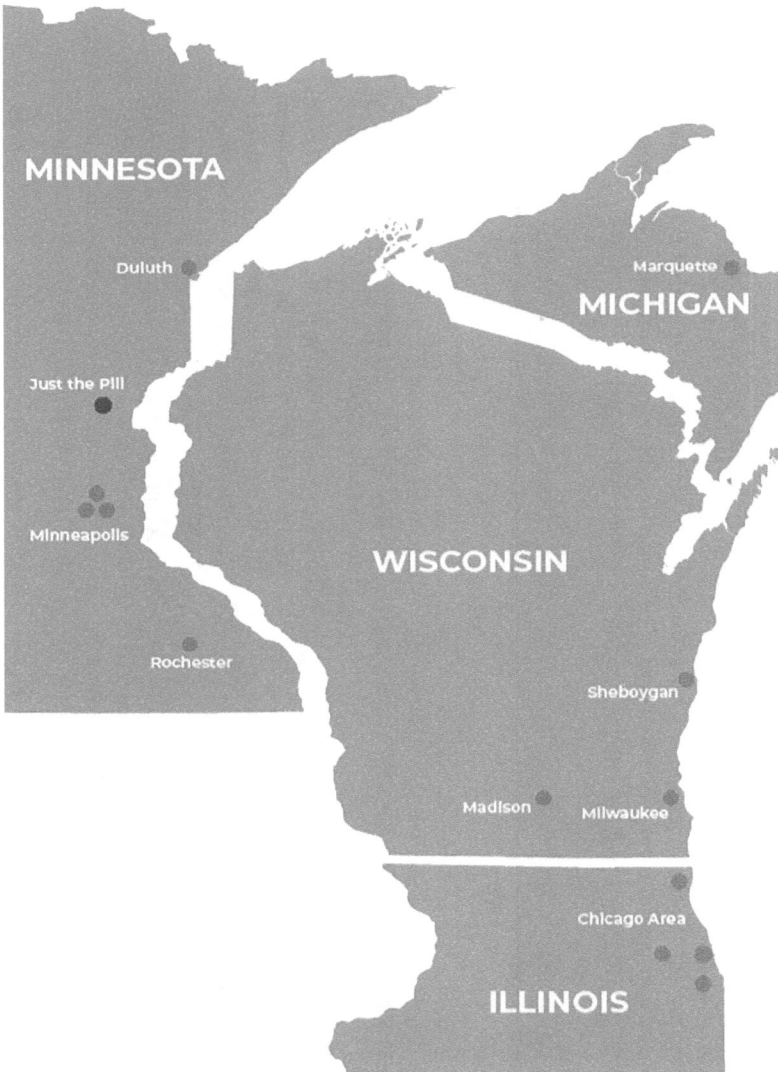

Figure 5.1. Map of abortion clinics in Wisconsin and the neighboring states of Minnesota, Michigan, and Illinois immediately before the *Dobbs* decision in June 2022. Clinic locations are noted by grey dots.

abortion services at two locations. The other two pre-*Dobbs* abortion clinics—another Planned Parenthood location and independent provider Affiliated Medical Services—began offering services again in December 2023 and March 2024, respectively. Given Wisconsin's hostility to abortion rights and the significant abortion landscape changes over time, it is an apt setting to illustrate the various subdomains of access and how they can be constrained.

A CONCEPTUALIZATION OF ABORTION ACCESS

Abortion Availability

In the context of abortion access, we define availability as the relationship between the presence/absence, volume, and type of abortion offered and the demand for abortion overall as well as for specific types of abortion. Abortion types vary both by method (i.e., medication or procedural abortion) and model of care delivery (e.g., in-clinic, via telehealth, self-managed). When we consider abortion availability, we ask, "Are there sufficient numbers of each type of abortion to meet the demands of those who seek abortion?" (Readers might wonder how geography relates to access, but we will discuss that issue in the "proximity" subdomain.) Abortion availability could be operationalized as whether any medication abortion appointments are available at a given clinic or what the average wait time is for an appointment in each U.S. state.

We know from existing evidence that lack of abortion availability can prevent abortion seekers from obtaining wanted abortions. Put simply, abortion availability is central to "access." For example, Heidi Moseson and colleagues (2022) reported findings from a study of individuals recruited online who considered abortion. The participants reported that scarcity of abortion services affected their ability to obtain abortions. This finding echoes Katrina Kimport's (2021) study of prenatal care patients who reported having considered abortion, some of whom noted that lack of local providers deterred them from obtaining an abortion.

Availability of abortion type is consequential as well. Moseson and colleagues (2022) found that some participants did not obtain an abortion because they desired a medication, rather than procedural, abortion, but medication abortion was not available. In other words, these individuals' preference for medication abortion was so strong that when they were unable to obtain that method, they did not obtain an abortion at all.

The work by Moseson's group also indicates that people's perceptions of whether abortion is available are important in determining whether they have access to abortion. Deep and widespread abortion stigma, both at healthcare and community levels, affects these perceptions. For example, abortion stigma and what scholars call "abortion exceptionalism" (Joffe and Schroeder 2021)—that is, treating abortion differently from other healthcare—mean that abortion care has been divorced from other standard reproductive healthcare. As a result, abortion is largely provided in stand-alone, siloed clinics. In other words, people cannot rely on their general gynecologic or primary care providers for abortion care. This may contribute to them miscalculating its availability. Community-level abortion stigma also means that conversations about abortion and its availability are not common, even among close friends or family members (Cowan 2014).

In Wisconsin, abortion availability is constrained (in some cases to the point of unavailability) both directly and indirectly. As a direct constraint, between June 2022 (i.e., *Dobbs*) and September 2023, Wisconsin had *no* formal abortion availability while the state's 1849 law was being considered by Wisconsin courts. After the clinics began to reopen in September 2023, one offered only medication abortion, constraining abortion type choice. Even after their reopening, as was the case pre-*Dobbs*, the clinics are only located in Dane, Sheboygan, and Milwaukee counties, leaving the northern parts of the state without abortion clinic availability.

Other restrictions indirectly affect availability by constraining who is eligible to be an abortion provider in the state. Wisconsin's physician-only restriction prohibits advanced practice clinicians, including nurse practitioners and physicians' assistants, from providing abortion, even as other states allow it and evidence shows they can safely and effectively provide medication and procedural abortion (Porsch et al. 2020). This restriction reduces the number of potential abortion providers, which can negatively impact availability.

Other policies and practices indirectly constrain the number of abortion providers and thus abortion availability. Many Wisconsin physicians trained as abortion providers are prohibited from offering abortions by their employers. The high proportion of Catholic healthcare systems in the state plays a key role. In addition to limiting abortion access, as detailed by Lori Freedman's chapter in this volume, many religiously affiliated healthcare systems prohibit their physicians from moonlighting as abortion providers (Higgins, Schmuhl, et al. 2021). Similarly, secular healthcare systems exhibited conservatism in their interpretation of the 1849 law, and after *Dobbs* they were less willing to allow their physician-employees to work part time at Planned Parenthood. For example, physicians at UW Health (the University of Wisconsin health system) faced institutional barriers to resuming off-campus abortion care shifts after the state court's determination that the 1849 law does not prohibit voluntary abortion. By constraining the number of abortion providers both indirectly and directly, Wisconsin laws and practices constrain abortion availability.

Abortion Proximity

Within the field of abortion research, we define abortion proximity as the relationship between where abortion services are located and where abortion seekers live. When we consider proximity, we ask, "Are abortion services close enough to those who seek abortion?" Abortion proximity could be operationalized as the proportion of the U.S. population with the capacity for pregnancy living within a given drive time of an abortion-providing facility or as the number of miles a patient must travel to get to the nearest clinic.

It is well documented that proximity, frequently operationalized as distance or drive time to abortion care, affects abortion seekers' ability to obtain abortions. Most common in the literature is evidence that as abortion proximity decreases, abortion rates decrease, and birth rates increase. In one study by Kirsten Thompson and colleagues (2021), they calculated 2015 county-level abortion rates and found a dose–response relationship between a county's distance from the closest abortion provider and the rate of abortion among people living in that county; as distance from care increased, the abortion rate decreased. More recent findings, published by Caitlin Myers in 2024, indicated that an increase in county-level distance to care decreased the county-level abortion rate and increased the county-level birth rate. Given that there is no evidence to suggest that desire for abortion varies significantly by geography, these studies, which show people living in counties with poorer abortion proximity reported both fewer abortions and more births compared with those living in counties with better abortion proximity, indicate that proximity matters for abortion access.

As expected, we see the same findings in Wisconsin. Between 2010 and 2017, 40 percent of the state's abortion clinics closed, dramatically impacting abortion proximity for large swaths of the state's residents. Joanna Venator and Jason Fletcher (2021) found that increases in county-level driving distances to abortion clinics because of these closures were associated with decreases in county-level abortion rates and increases in county-level birth rates. Given the absence of other factors that could explain changes in the abortion and/or birth rates in the study period, abortion clinic closures and resulting decreases in abortion proximity appear to be associated with people carrying pregnancies to term that they would have terminated if abortion care were more proximal.

Abortion Accommodation

We define accommodation as the relationship between how abortion services are organized and abortion seekers' ability to utilize those services. When we consider accommodation, we ask, "Are abortion services offered in such a way that abortion seekers can utilize those services?" Abortion accommodation could be operationalized as whether an abortion seeker can find services open during hours they are not at work or whether there is a legally mandated prerequisite to obtaining abortion care (e.g., a required waiting period between abortion counseling and care provision) that can make it more difficult for at least some abortion seekers to obtain abortions.

Evidence unequivocally documents that unaccommodating services prevent people from having wanted abortions. One example is state- and clinic-level gestational duration limits. Studies of people who considered or sought abortion but did not end up obtaining an abortion report that gestational duration limits imposed by states and/or enacted by clinics obstructed them from obtaining wanted abortions (Bennett et al. 2023; Kimport 2021; Moseson et al. 2022; Upadhyay et al. 2014).

As another example, in their study of people seeking abortion information online, Moseson and colleagues (2022) found that a clinic's refusal to disclose the cost of an abortion before a clinic visit and a state-imposed waiting period—which in effect meant two clinic visits were required to obtain abortion care—made abortion impossible to obtain for some participants. Sarah Roberts and colleagues (2020) similarly reported that a two-visit requirement was a reason that some abortion seekers who participated in their study did not obtain wanted abortions.

In Wisconsin, a twenty-week gestational duration ban has been in place since 2015. That is, people who need abortion later in pregnancy are unaccommodated in the state. Wisconsin law, like the state laws faced by participants in the Moseson study, also requires two appointments to obtain an abortion as well as a twenty-four-hour waiting period between those appointments, even though abortion patients could safely and effectively obtain procedural abortion in one visit or obtain medication abortions by telehealth or through self-management, never setting foot in a physical clinic. By forcing people to spend more time traveling to and engaging with care, when only one visit (or fewer) is medically indicated, this restriction undermines accommodation.

Finally, parental consent laws are unaccommodating for young Wisconsinites. Wisconsin is one of thirty-six states that compels minors to receive written consent for an abortion from at least one parent, adult family member, guardian, or legal custodian, unless they are legally emancipated (Alvarez and Williamson 2023). The only alternative is for the young abortion seeker to petition the court to waive the parental consent requirement through the judicial bypass process. However, this process can be difficult if not impossible for young people to navigate, so it severely constricts abortion accommodation for affected abortion seekers. If young people were truly accommodated, they would be able to obtain abortions without the need to comply with such bureaucratic procedures.

Abortion Affordability

We define affordability as the subdomain that examines the relationship between the cost of abortion and abortion seekers' ability to pay those costs, including through insurance coverage. Perhaps obviously, when we consider affordability, we ask, "Can abortion seekers cover the cost of abortion services?" Abortion affordability may be operationalized as the average cost of medication abortion in the state or the total of out-of-pocket expenses a patient pays for the abortion, including travel costs.

The abortion literature contains many examples of how the unaffordability of abortion prevents abortion seekers from obtaining wanted abortions. Many studies have found that the cost of abortion was a reason that abortion seekers did not obtain an abortion (Bennett et al. 2023; Higgins, Lands, et al. 2021; Moseson et al. 2022; Roberts et al. 2019; Roberts, Berglas, and Kimport 2020; Upadhyay et al. 2014, 2021). This body of research describes lack of insurance coverage, including as a result of insurance coverage bans; travel costs; out-of-pocket costs broadly; and constrained economic conditions as influencing participants' inability to access abortions. Kimport (2021) highlights the ways in which lack of insurance coverage, a structural enforcement of abortion unaffordability, interacts with other existing financial vulnerabilities to make abortion yet more unaffordable to the extent that it prevents people from obtaining wanted abortions.

In Wisconsin, state law prohibits three major groups of insurers—Medicaid (BadgerCare), plans offered on the state's Health Insurance Marketplace, and insurance plans for state employees—from offering abortion care coverage. The bulk of Wisconsinites are covered by these insurers, so they are forced to pay for abortion out of pocket. Abortion care typically costs between $500 and $1,000 (though the costs may exceed $3,000) (Roberts et al. 2014; Upadhyay et al. 2022; McCann 2022).

This cost is unattainable for many; upward of 40 percent of U.S. people could not cover an unexpected $400 expense. At least 10 percent of Wisconsinites currently experience poverty (U.S. Census Bureau, n.d.), and as many in one in four (24 percent) experience food insecurity (Bergmans et al. 2019). In other words, for many Wisconsin abortion seekers, who are disproportionately likely to live under the federal poverty level (i.e., less than $20,000 a year for a single parent and child; Jerman, Jones, and Onda 2016) and face financial scarcity, the cost of abortion care would be "catastrophic" (Zuniga, Thompson, and Blanchard 2020).

Abortion Acceptability

In the context of abortion access research, acceptability has two components. First, acceptability measures the relationship between abortion seekers' expectations of what abortion services and providers should be and what the services and providers are. When we consider abortion acceptability from this angle, we ask, "Are the abortion services and providers acceptable to abortion seekers?" Abortion acceptability could be operationalized as whether the clinic offers evidence-based care or whether abortion patients perceive their care to be high quality.

The second component of abortion acceptability is whether an abortion seeker believes it is acceptable to have an abortion. This component of our abortion access conceptualization expands on Penchansky and Thomas's work, which did not specifically consider stigmatized healthcare services. In the context of abortion, acceptability encompasses abortion seekers' internalized feelings about the (un)acceptability of having an abortion. From this angle, we consider abortion acceptability and ask, "Is it acceptable to the abortion seeker to have an abortion?" In this case, abortion acceptability could be operationalized as whether abortion seekers experience interpersonal pressure to remain pregnant or whether abortion seekers perceive that their community holds anti-abortion beliefs.

Perhaps due to a more dominant focus on the subdomains of proximity and affordability, the field is ripe for more research on the first component of abortion acceptability: whether existing services and providers are acceptable to abortion seekers, and the effect of (non)acceptability of services and providers on whether abortion seekers obtain abortions. For example, researchers may wish to consider documenting how legal and financial constraints on abortion contribute to abortion seekers considering existing services to be unacceptable. One can imagine that the presence of protestors outside a clinic, long waits, and relative lack of privacy could affect the acceptability of abortion (Aiken et al. 2018; Arey 2023; Kimport 2021).

What is clear from the existing evidence is that the second component of abortion acceptability—internalized beliefs about the acceptability of having an abortion—has an impact on abortion seekers. When community and societal perceptions of abortion acceptability are poor, some abortion seekers internalize the unacceptability of abortion and cannot obtain the abortion that they want. For example, the literature abounds with examples of how abortion stigma affects those who consider and seek abortion. Moseson and colleagues' (2022) study found that perceived abortion stigma from partners, families, communities, and healthcare providers were all reasons that abortion seekers failed to obtain abortions. Similarly, Kimport's (2021) work identifies how anti-abortion narratives made abortion "unchooseable" for participants. Additionally, "influence" or "pressure" from others deterred abortion seekers from obtaining abortions in Ariana Bennett and colleagues' (2023) national survey, indicating the role that the second component of abortion acceptability can play in preventing people from obtaining abortions.

While the first component of abortion acceptability—whether services and providers are acceptable to abortion seekers—has not been a focus of the abortion literature, the Wisconsin context has examples of how deviations from evidence-based care could result in poor abortion acceptability. For example, Wisconsin law requires that at least twenty-four hours before the abortion, the abortion seeker must obtain an ultrasound, and the provider must display and explain the images and provide a means to visualize any cardiac activity. This policy, too, runs counter to medical evidence; routine ultrasound is not medically necessary for first trimester abortion, and a patient's viewing of an ultrasound image is irrelevant to their care. Research by Ushma Upadhyay and colleagues (2017) found that the mandatory ultrasound law had a negligible effect on pregnancy continuation at one Wisconsin clinic; however, in-depth interviews with some patients who viewed their ultrasound images revealed that viewing could compel complex emotions, both negative and positive. While ultrasound viewing may be acceptable to some abortion seekers, it was not acceptable to all. As Upadhyay and colleagues write, "laws about whether to force women to view their ultrasounds are not a question of quality of care but instead are a question of values regarding whether the state should use legislation to attempt to influence women's abortion decisions" (21). Research should investigate the impact of these policies on abortion seekers' impressions of abortion acceptability and in turn their ability to obtain wanted abortions.

Abortion Awareness

Finally, awareness refers to abortion seekers' knowledge of accurate information about abortion services and their ability to use that knowledge to obtain abortions. When we consider abortion awareness, we ask, "Do abortion seekers know what they need to about abortion services, and can they act on that knowledge to obtain abortions?" Awareness could be operationalized as the proportion of abortion seekers with a correct understanding of how abortion laws impact their abortion seeking or whether an abortion seeker knows of an abortion clinic.

Lack of abortion knowledge directly connects to constrained abortion access. In the study of online abortion seekers by Moseson and colleagues (2022), many participants described not having received all the abortion-related information they needed, including whether abortion was legal in their state, whether there were gestational duration limits, what was the cost of care, what to expect from an abortion, and how to find an appointment. Moreover, many people hold misperceptions about abortion's safety and sequelae, so the abortion seekers in this study also reported desiring information about abortion's long-term effects (or lack thereof) on fertility and other health outcomes. In all these cases, the participants identified that diminished abortion awareness contributed to their not obtaining wanted abortions. Similarly, Sarah Roberts, Nancy Berglas, and Katrina Kimport (2020) note that few prenatal care clinic patients who considered and did not obtain an abortion had accurate knowledge of the abortion process, evidencing how awareness is consequential to obtaining an abortion.

In Wisconsin, particularly since the *Dobbs* decision, an ever-shifting interpretation of abortion policies has sown confusion among abortion seekers, hindering awareness. For example, while the 1849 law was being considered by the courts, all abortion clinics in the state stopped offering services, resuming (as described earlier) more than a year later. Such abortion care churn—the chronic uncertainty about the potential for clinic closures or other service delivery changes (McGowan, Norris, and Bessett 2020)—has led to a lack of awareness among abortion seekers in states such as Ohio. We expect similar undermining of awareness in Wisconsin following the uncertainty of abortion legality post-*Dobbs*. Indeed, in October 2022, anywhere from 34 to 67 percent of Wisconsinites were unsure about the legality of various aspects of reproductive healthcare, including whether abortion was legal at any point during a pregnancy.[3]

Furthermore, in interviews we conducted with Wisconsinites who reported considering abortion in the post-*Dobbs* landscape, abortion seekers have expressed confusion about abortion availability, legality, and access (findings not yet published). Even when interviewees knew that they could not obtain abortion in Wisconsin, they worried that they might be breaking the law if they left the state to obtain abortion in a neighboring state. Others expressed lack of clarity about the state's gestational duration limit and whether they were still eligible for care. Although studies have not examined whether this lack of awareness has led to Wisconsinites not obtaining wanted abortions, evidence does indicate a similar lack of awareness as consequential to abortion seekers in other studies of barriers to access.

Interrelated Nature of Abortion Access Subdomains

For the purposes of elaborating our conceptualization, we have defined abortion access as whether an abortion seeker obtains any abortion. In turn, we illustrated how each of six subdomains contribute to that ability to obtain an abortion, positing abortion access as dependent on all six. Now we highlight three points about the importance of considering these subdomains in relation to one another.

First, key to our conceptualization of abortion access is the need to meet the conditions for abortion availability, proximity, accommodation, affordability, acceptability, *and* awareness. If just one of these subdomains is constrained or absent (for one or more abortion seekers), comprehensive abortion access is not present. Let's take a Wisconsinite living on a low income who knows they live a few blocks from the Water Street Planned Parenthood clinic in Milwaukee, where appointments are available, the clinic's services accommodate their needs, and those services are acceptable to them. Even with these subdomains of access met (i.e., availability, proximity, accommodation, awareness, and acceptability), because this person has BadgerCare insurance and the state bans abortion coverage through this insurer, they would need to pay for care out of pocket. If this person cannot afford to pay out of pocket and cannot obtain funding through other sources, abortion is not affordable, and they do not have abortion access. A determination of abortion access depends on meeting the conditions for all six subdomains for a given abortion seeker.

Second, essential to our conceptualization is that whether each subdomain of access is met varies between individuals, even those living close to one another. Following from the last example, if that Wisconsinite's neighbor was the same in every regard except for the fact that they had sufficient resources to pay for the cost of abortion (i.e., abortion was affordable), that person would have abortion access. Population-level abortion access, in turn, may vary by focal population, with some meeting the conditions of all subdomains of access (e.g., Wisconsinites like our second individual) and others not (e.g., Wisconsinites like our first individual). Measuring population-level abortion access is crucial for informing interventions to better serve abortion seekers and address oppressive structures, but any population-level measure of abortion access or any one of its subdomains can suffer from the ecological fallacy. That is, the experience of the population (i.e., a population-level measure) cannot stand in for the experience of the individual (i.e., an individual-level measure).

Third, the six abortion access subdomains are highly interrelated. For example, our Wisconsin examples illustrate an overlap between abortion acceptability, availability, and proximity. Before the *Dobbs* decision, 69 counties in Wisconsin did not have an abortion provider, and upward of 17 percent of all Wisconsin abortion patients traveled out of state for care. From June 2022 to September 2023, all abortion seekers had to leave the state for abortion care within the formal healthcare system unless they were facing a life-threatening situation. Research by Katrina Kimport and Maryani Rasidjan (2023) documents that being forced to leave one's state for an abortion can cause significant emotional burdens in the form of stress, anxiety, and shame. These emotional costs can be exacerbated by forced disclosure of abortion due to travel or by stigmatization in the process of an in-state denial of care, potentially reducing the acceptability of abortion. In other words, subdomains of access—in this case, proximity and availability or lack thereof—are consequential not only for their individual contributions to abortion access but also for their impact on each other.

Finally, we reiterate a caveat first noted at the start of the chapter: we have primarily focused on the curtailing of abortion access for those who were unable to obtain any abortion. But abortion seekers may also not have abortion access when they obtain an abortion that is different from the abortion that they wanted. This relates to acceptability. For example, patients who seek procedural abortion but are only able to obtain medication abortion lack access to the abortion they wanted. Similarly, if a person is unable to pay for an abortion out of pocket or through insurance and faces delays as they navigate obtaining financial support from an abortion fund, they do not have access to the abortion they wanted.

To ensure that we center abortion seekers, researchers must not assume that these individuals wish only to be not pregnant. Abortion seekers have many desires that are informed by a variety of factors, including structural and medical racism. For example, prior negative encounters with the healthcare system may lead Black abortion seekers to be more likely to prefer self-managed abortion over other forms compared with white abortion seekers because this delivery model requires less interaction with the formal healthcare system (Ralph et al. 2020). To ignore individual desires and assume that all people who want an abortion and get one have had the abortion they want does a disservice to efforts to ensure high-quality abortion experiences for all. Attending to the multiple elements of acceptability helps capture this aspect of evaluating abortion access.

MOVING TOWARD ABORTION ACCESS

To assess people's ability to obtain wanted abortions, and along the way consider the breadth of the organizational and cultural structures that enable or constrain that access, we must consider this abortion access conceptualization in totality—that is, all or nothing. For people committed to ensuring abortion access, we recognize that, given the constraints on each subdomain of access, the need for conditions of all to be met, and their interrelated nature, achieving full abortion access for all abortion seekers may feel out of reach. We suggest approaching the concept of abortion access similarly to the concept of social justice; although true justice cannot exist until all people experience equitable conditions for life and liberty, we can take individual steps toward justice, ensuring that more people live with those conditions, even in the absence of full liberation for all. In the case of abortion, individual improvements in the conditions of the six subdomains move us toward abortion access, even when abortion access is not achieved. For example, ensuring abortion affordability alone does not guarantee abortion access, but abortion affordability contributes to abortion access.

Although theories and frameworks are often relegated to classrooms and academic discourse, we imagine a public life for this conceptualization of abortion access. Moving forward, we propose that researchers and scholars explicitly consider this conceptualization when evaluating existing literature on "abortion access" and when developing research questions, study designs, analyses, and dissemination on the topic. Our conceptualization is based in a public health tradition, but we believe it holds benefits for sociology, including medical sociology. By explicitly aligning abortion access–related research with this conceptualization, the field can make clearer the assumptions and limitations of existing and future work. In turn, those who put research findings to use, including policymakers, healthcare funders and practitioners, and advocates, will be more able to identify points of intervention and areas where more information is needed to understand constraints and facilitators for all subdomains of access. Ultimately, by more accurately and precisely conceptualizing and evaluating abortion access, the field will be better equipped to advance health and well-being effectively and efficiently.

ACKNOWLEDGMENTS

The authors thank the anonymous family foundation that supports the work of the University of Wisconsin—Madison Collaborative for Reproductive Equity (UW CORE).

NOTES

1. We use the term "abortion seekers" to refer to individuals who consider, desire, search for, and/or ultimately obtain care. Our language is inclusive of those who desire an abortion but never take formal steps to seek or obtain one.

2. A common criticism of Penchansky and Thomas's original conceptualization is that laypeople often use accessibility interchangeably with access and making accessibility a subdomain of access is confusing. Although the "5 As" may be easy to remember, we believe that "proximity" is more easily understood by a lay audience, so we use this term for our conceptualization.

3. Michael W. Wagner, "2022 CCCR-CORE Reproductive Rights Survey of Georgia, Ohio, Texas, and Wisconsin," email to authors, 2022.

REFERENCES

Aiken, Abigail R. A., Kathleen Broussard, Dana M. Johnson, and Elisa Padron. 2018. "Motivations and Experiences of People Seeking Medication Abortion Online in the United States." *Perspectives on Sexual and Reproductive Health* 50 (4): 157–163. https://doi.org/10.1363/psrh.12073.

Alvarez, B., and A. Williamson. 2024. "Abortion Care for Minors in a Post-*Roe* Wisconsin." *CORE Brief*, January. University of Wisconsin Collaborative for Reproductive Equity. https://core.wisc.edu/documents/abortion-care-for-minors-in-a-post-roe-wisconsin/.

Arey, Whitney. 2023. "Experiences with Small and Large Numbers of Protesters at Abortion Clinics in North Carolina." *Contraception* 120 (April): 109919. https://doi.org/10.1016/j.contraception.2022.109919.

Bennett, Ariana H., Cassondra Marshall, Katrina Kimport, Julianna Deardorff, and Anu Manchikanti Gómez. 2023. "'Have You Ever Wanted or Needed an Abortion You Did Not Get?' Data from a 2022 Nationally Representative Online Survey in the United States." *Contraception* 123 (July): 110007. https://doi.org/10.1016/j.contraception.2023.110007.

Bergmans, Rachel S., Lara Coughlin, Tomorrow Wilson, and Kristen Malecki. 2019. "Cross-Sectional Associations of Food Insecurity with Smoking Cigarettes and Heavy Alcohol Use in a Population-Based Sample of Adults." *Drug and Alcohol Dependence* 205 (December): 107646. https://doi.org/10.1016/j.drugalcdep.2019.107646.

Cowan, Sarah K. 2014. "Secrets and Misperceptions: The Creation of Self-Fulfilling Illusions." *Sociological Science* 1 (November):466–492. https://doi.org/10.15195/v1.a26.

Higgins, Jenny A., Madison Lands, Taryn M. Valley, Emma Carpenter, and Laura Jacques. 2021. "Real-Time Effects of Payer Restrictions on Reproductive Healthcare: A Qualitative Analysis of Cost-Related Barriers and Their Consequences among U.S. Abortion Seekers on Reddit." *International Journal of Environmental Research and Public Health* 18 (17): 9013. https://doi.org/10.3390/ijerph18179013.

Higgins, Jenny A., Nicholas B. Schmuhl, Cynthie K. Wautlet, and Laurel W. Rice. 2021. "The Importance of Physician Concern and Expertise in Increasing Abortion Health Care Access in Local Contexts." *American Journal of Public Health* 111 (1): 33–36. https://doi.org/10.2105/AJPH.2020.305997.

Jerman, Jenna, Rachel K. Jones, and Tsuyoshi Onda. "Characteristics of U.S. Abortion Patients in 2014 and Changes Since 2008." Guttmacher Institute, May 2016. https://www.guttmacher.org/report/characteristics-us-abortion-patients-2014.

Joffe, Carole, and Rosalyn Schroeder. 2021. "COVID-19, Health Care, and Abortion Exceptionalism in the United States." *Perspectives on Sexual and Reproductive Health* 53 (1–2): 5–12. https://doi.org/10.1363/psrh.12182.

Kimport, Katrina. 2021. *No Real Choice: How Culture and Politics Matter for Reproductive Autonomy.* Rutgers University Press.

Kimport, Katrina, and Maryani Palupy Rasidjan. 2023. "Exploring the Emotional Costs of Abortion Travel in the United States Due to Legal Restriction." *Contraception* 120 (April): 109956. https://doi.org/10.1016/j.contraception.2023.109956.

McCann, Allison. 2022. "What It Costs to Get an Abortion Now." *New York Times*, September 28, 2022. https://www.nytimes.com/interactive/2022/09/28/us/abortion-costs-funds.html.

McGowan, Michelle L., Alison H. Norris, and Danielle Bessett. 2020. "Care Churn—Why Keeping Clinic Doors Open Isn't Enough to Ensure Access to Abortion." *New England Journal of Medicine* 383 (6): 508–510. https://doi.org/10.1056/NEJMp2013466.

Moseson, Heidi, Jane W. Seymour, Carmela Zuniga, Alexandra Wollum, Anna Katz, Terri-Ann Thompson, and Caitlin Gerdts. 2022. "'It Just Seemed like a Perfect Storm': A Multi-Methods Feasibility Study on the Use of Facebook, Google Ads, and Reddit to Collect Data on Abortion-Seeking Experiences from People Who Considered but Did Not Obtain Abortion Care in the United States." *PLoS One* 17 (3): e0264748. https://doi.org/10.1371/journal.pone.0264748.

Myers, Caitlin. 2024. "Forecasts for a Post-*Roe* America: The Effects of Increased Travel Distance on Abortions and Births." *Journal of Policy Analysis and Management* 43 (1): 39–62. https://doi.org/10.1002/pam.22524.

Penchansky, Roy, and J. William Thomas. 1981. "The Concept of Access: Definition and Relationship to Consumer Satisfaction." *Medical Care* 19 (2): 127–140. https://doi.org/10.1097/00005650-198102000-00001.

Porsch, L., M. Dragoman, H. Jones, K. Steinle, and I. Dayananda. 2020. "Advanced Practice Clinicians and Medication Abortion Safety: A 10-Year Retrospective Review." *Contraception* 101 (5): 357. https://doi.org/10.1016/j.contraception.2020.03.016.

Ralph, Lauren, Diana G. Foster, Sarah Raifman, M. Antonia Biggs, Goleen Samari, Ushma Upadhyay, Caitlin Gerdts, and Daniel Grossman. 2020. "Prevalence of Self-Managed Abortion Among Women of Reproductive Age in the United States." *JAMA Network Open* 3 (12): e2029245. https://doi.org/10.1001/jamanetworkopen.2020.29245.

Roberts, Sarah C. M., Nancy F. Berglas, and Katrina Kimport. 2020. "Complex Situations: Economic Insecurity, Mental Health, and Substance Use among Pregnant Women Who Consider—but Do Not Have—Abortions." *PLoS One* 15 (1): e0226004. https://doi.org/10.1371/journal.pone.0226004.

Roberts, Sarah C. M., Heather Gould, Katrina Kimport, Tracy A. Weitz, and Diana Greene Foster. 2014. "Out-of-Pocket Costs and Insurance Coverage for Abortion in the United States." *Women's Health Issues* 24 (2): e211–e218. https://doi.org/10.1016/j.whi.2014.01.003.

Roberts, Sarah C. M., Katrina Kimport, Rebecca Kriz, Jennifer Holl, Katrina Mark, and Valerie Williams. 2019. "Consideration of and Reasons for Not Obtaining Abortion among Women Entering Prenatal Care in Southern Louisiana and Baltimore, Maryland." *Sexuality Research and Social Policy* 16 (4): 476–487. https://doi.org/10.1007/s13178-018-0359-4.

Saurman, Emily. 2016. "Improving Access: Modifying Penchansky and Thomas's Theory of Access." *Journal of Health Services Research & Policy* 21 (1): 36–39. https://doi.org/10.1177/1355819615600001.

Thompson, Kirsten M. J., Hugh J. W. Sturrock, Diana Greene Foster, and Ushma D. Upadhyay. 2021. "Association of Travel Distance to Nearest Abortion Facility with Rates of Abortion." *JAMA Network Open* 4 (7): e2115530. https://doi.org/10.1001/jamanetworkopen.2021.15530.

Upadhyay, Ushma D., Chris Ahlbach, Shelly Kaller, Clara Cook, and Isabel Muñoz. 2022. "Trends in Self-Pay Charges and Insurance Acceptance for Abortion in the United States, 2017–20." *Health Affairs* 41 (4): 507–515. https://doi.org/10.1377/hlthaff.2021.01528.

Upadhyay, Ushma D., Katrina Kimport, Elise K. O. Belusa, Nicole E. Johns, Douglas W. Laube, and Sarah C. M. Roberts. 2017. "Evaluating the Impact of a Mandatory Pre-Abortion

Ultrasound Viewing Law: A Mixed Methods Study." *PLoS One* 12 (7): e0178871. https://doi
.org/10.1371/journal.pone.0178871.
Upadhyay, Ushma D., Ashley A. McCook, Ariana H. Bennett, Alice F. Cartwright, and
Sarah C. M. Roberts. 2021. "State Abortion Policies and Medicaid Coverage of Abortion
Are Associated with Pregnancy Outcomes among Individuals Seeking Abortion Recruited
Using Google Ads: A National Cohort Study." *Social Science & Medicine* 274 (April): 113747.
https://doi.org/10.1016/j.socscimed.2021.113747.
Upadhyay, Ushma D., Tracy A. Weitz, Rachel K. Jones, Rana E. Barar, and Diana Greene
Foster. 2014. "Denial of Abortion Because of Provider Gestational Age Limits in the
United States." *American Journal of Public Health* 104 (9): 1687–1694. https://doi.org/10
.2105/AJPH.2013.301378.
U.S. Census Bureau. n.d. "U.S. Census Bureau QuickFacts: Wisconsin." Accessed Febru-
ary 13, 2024. https://www.census.gov/quickfacts/fact/table/WI/PST045223.
Venator, Joanna, and Jason Fletcher. 2021. "Undue Burden beyond Texas: An Analysis of
Abortion Clinic Closures, Births, and Abortions in Wisconsin." *Journal of Policy Analysis
and Management* 40 (3): 774–813. https://doi.org/10.1002/pam.22263.
Williamson, A., M. I. Ufot, and J. A. Higgins. 2023. "Wisconsin State Laws Impacting Abortion
Access." *CORE Brief*, revised September 2023. University of Wisconsin Collaborative for
Reproductive Equity. https://core.wisc.edu/documents/wisconsin-state-laws-impacting
-abortion-access/.
Wisconsin Department of Health Services (WISH). 2014. Wisconsin Interactive Statistics on
Health Query System. Wisconsin Department of Health Services. Accessed October 9, 2014.
https://www.dhs.wisconsin.gov/wish/index.htm.
Zuniga, Carmela, Terri-Ann Thompson, and Kelly Blanchard. 2020. "Abortion as a Catastrophic Health Expenditure in the United States." *Women's Health Issues* 30 (6): 416–425.
https://doi.org/10.1016/j.whi.2020.07.001.

PART II

What the Fall of *Roe* Revealed About Abortion Provision

CHAPTER 6

Shift Work

ABORTION CARE IN AN EVER-CHANGING LANDSCAPE

Kelly Marie Ward and Barbara A. Alvarez

Since the late 1800s, due largely to changing social, legal, and cultural contexts, abortion work in the United States has experienced shifts to and from professionalized medicine. By "professionalized medicine," we mean health-related care that occurs within the context of formal medical institutions (e.g., hospitals and clinics) by credentialed healthcare workers (e.g., doctors and nurses). Indeed, the push and pull between mainstream health care and nonprofessional, radical, and/or community-based care has been a driving force in shaping the abortion workforce for over a century. And changes to abortion work will surely continue in a post-*Dobbs* landscape. In this chapter, we introduce three factors that have shaped the abortion workforce over time; situate abortion work within larger healthcare structures of the twenty-first century; take stock of the abortion workforce at the time of this writing; and then finally discuss what this may mean for the future of abortion work and research on abortion workers in a post-*Dobbs* America. Throughout, we pay particular attention to medical assistants, using their experiences and changing role as a window into major historical and anticipated shifts in the abortion workforce.

CRIMINALIZATION OF ABORTION

For most of the twentieth century, abortion was criminalized in the United States. Given *Roe*'s nearly fifty-year tenure of protecting the right to abortion, this can be hard to imagine, but *Roe* was not decided until 1973. It can also be hard to imagine another fact about the history of abortion in the United States: the criminalization of abortion in the United States in the twentieth century was not about the morality of abortion. Rather, it was a byproduct of the emergence of professionalized medicine.

Prior to the twentieth century, when women knew they were pregnant and wanted to terminate the pregnancy, they used abortifacients (medicinal plants and herbs) or engaged in activities thought to induce a miscarriage, such as strenuous physical exercise, trauma to the abdomen, or hot baths, with varying success (Devereux 1954; Gordon 2002; Himes 1936). These practices were passed down by community healers and midwives. In the United States, enslaved women and eventually free Black women and immigrants primarily held these reproductive health knowledges. In addition to serving their communities, they were sought out by white and upper-class folks for a range of reproductive needs, including preventing pregnancy, delivering babies, and providing abortions (Bonaparte 2023). This means of acquiring an abortion was largely unchanged for centuries, from the earliest days of pregnancy termination until the late nineteenth century.

It was then, in the late 1800s, that quasi-professionals entered the abortion workforce and became another option for people looking to terminate pregnancies. These workers were not the midwives of centuries prior. Instead, they were mostly white men who dealt with a wide range of health conditions and advertised their services in local newspapers (Beisel and Kay 2004). Also called homeopaths, they advertised remedies for "uterine" dysfunction or retained menses. These advertisements stated the medicine was not for "married women," which served as a coded message that these remedies would terminate pregnancies (Reagan 1997). Pregnancy outcomes of these practitioners' interventions were varied and sometimes very poor.

Meanwhile, members of the emerging medical field—physicians—sought to serve these same patients, but not with so-called remedies or with the expertise of generations of midwives. Instead, they claimed the mantle of medicine. Over a period of years in the late nineteenth century, physicians sought to distinguish themselves from homeopaths (labeling them quacks) and midwives as a way to claim patients and their own expertise and to build business. Central to this effort was laying claim to expertise over pregnancy and its outcomes, arguing that only doctors should be allowed to facilitate pregnancy termination. To make their case, they marshalled anti-abortion rhetoric and deployed a claim of authority based in science—and it worked. By distancing themselves from and disparaging other abortion practitioners and, indeed, undercutting the legitimacy of abortion all together, physicians secured a space for themselves as a skilled and exclusive professional group. Their professional success rested on having wrested the provision of abortion from midwives and homeopaths, and, in conjunction with new state-based anti-abortion legislation, they obtained a monopoly on the procedure. By the turn of the century, only licensed physicians could perform abortions.

Just as important, in addition to asserting authority over the procedure itself, physicians also claimed authority over whether a woman could *have* an abortion. This was a major shift. Rather than a personal decision about a non-medical issue that a woman could privately handle on her own, pregnancy termination was now legally controlled by the medical profession. By 1910, all states except Kentucky had adopted legislation to criminalize abortion outside of the supervision of a doctor (Lewis and Shimabukuro 2001). And doctors were far less inclined to support women's desire for abortions than prior abortion practitioners. This meant that a woman could not legally obtain an abortion through the medical system except under rare circumstances.

In these ways, the criminalization of abortion outside of doctor supervision did several things. For one, it medicalized abortion. Now a doctor had to be involved in what had previously been understood as a non-medical event. For two—and central to our focus here—it created a professionalized version of abortion care. This was a shift from midwives, traditional healers, and "quacks" to a professionalized and "scientific" abortion workforce of mostly educated and credentialed white men.

Now located in the purview of medicine, abortion availability—for whom and when—was, in turn, subject to more shifts as health care changed. As health care became less individualized and private and more hospital-based over the course of the twentieth century, abortion became more regulated within medicine. Early twentieth century advances in medicine meant that some of the few health conditions that had traditionally been considered contraindications for pregnancy (e.g., tuberculosis, cardiovascular disease, etc.), and thus a justification for abortion, were less common, further limiting the circumstances in which abortion was allowable. Other medicalized frameworks grew the circumstances in which abortion was allowable: by the mid-twentieth century, doctors increasingly cited mental health or "psychiatric" reasons for providing abortions (Luker 1984). Even with these changes in what was considered an indication for abortion, however, the assessment of a doctor remained central to the determination of whether a woman could have one.

As more medical care was consolidated in hospitals, abortion decisions became administrative. Hospitals convened therapeutic abortion boards, or panels of doctors to approve or reject applications for abortions. Therapeutic abortion boards were designed to make sure that doctors were strictly adhering to the approved reasons for abortion and not overprescribing abortions. Physicians would present their recommendation to this board, which was a committee of other doctors (usually obstetrician-gynecologists and psychiatrists), and the board would approve or deny the abortion. In effect, therapeutic abortion boards limited access to abortion. Importantly, these boards did not exist for patient benefit; they were a sort of protection for the hospital. As such, their primary concern was that a patient did not qualify for an abortion, not that a doctor had failed to provide the desired abortion care to a patient. Thus, for the middle decades of the twentieth century, pregnant people seeking a legal abortion had to convince a doctor and then a hospital board that pregnancy termination was necessary for their own health and safety.

For various reasons, including the onerousness of this process, some abortion seekers circumvented this system all together. They sought out illegal abortions and got information about where to get abortions through their social networks (Kaplan 2019). Alongside a highly regulated and medicalized hospital-based abortion workforce was an underground and illicit abortion workforce.

STAND-ALONE CLINICS: A POST-*ROE* RESPONSE
TO SHIFTS IN ABORTION CARE

The 1973 decision on *Roe v. Wade*, which legalized abortion in all U.S. states and territories, led to significant changes in abortion work and a shift of abortion care from hospitals to clinics. These stand-alone clinics, which often provided a range of sexual and reproductive healthcare services, could be private or not-for-profit and were not affiliated with any hospitals. With the *Roe* decision, pregnant people no longer needed permission from doctors and therapeutic abortion boards. They could decide for themselves to have an abortion in a stand-alone clinic.

Despite the messaging of abortion as a choice "between a woman and her doctor," abortion clinics largely took doctors (and hospitals) out of a gatekeeping role. This change was also liberating for pro-choice doctors who now could provide abortion care without being overly surveilled by hospital administrators (Luker 1984). Feminist reproductive health advocates wanted healthcare settings structured according to the ideals of women's autonomy, reproductive freedom, and egalitarian practices (Hume 2023; Nelson 2015). In other words, abortion clinics were purposefully set apart from traditional medical settings as (at the time) a radical alternative.

Within ten years of *Roe*, most abortions were performed in free-standing clinics, which included large, affiliated groups of nonprofit clinics such as Planned Parenthood, independent clinics, and private clinics (Jones and Jerman 2017). Relevant to the focus in this chapter, this move from hospitals to clinics changed not only where abortions were happening but also what abortion work looked like and who participated in abortion work.

Some of these changes could arguably be characterized as a sort of demedicalization of abortion work as non-medical professionals were integrated into clinics (Halfmann 2011). This new space for abortion created new occupations and types of abortion workers. Doctors worked in these clinics, but the clinics were not driven by a purely medical mission (Halfmann 2011). Some clinics incorporated progressive ideologies emphasizing egalitarian relationships among the staff and recognition of power imbalances based on race and gender (Simonds 1996). This made it possible for new lay (non-medical) staff to participate in abortion care, and the abortion counselor emerged as a new occupation (Joffe 2013). Some abortion counselors were trained as social workers, but they were not medical professionals. The abortion counselor's job, in addition to getting informed consent and explaining the details of the procedure, was to provide time and space for the abortion seeker to process the decision and to offer resources and support either in groups or in one-on-one sessions (Joffe 2013). This expansion of the abortion workforce to include non-medical workers was a small shift away from physician dominance in abortion care.

MANAGED CARE AND ABORTION WORK

Stand-alone abortion clinics were a new organizational structure—and it quickly became a popular one. Clinics had to rapidly develop structures and processes to provide abortion care to high volumes of patients. This meant using space, personnel, and time efficiently. Physician-only laws, prohibiting non-physicians from performing abortions, remained in place in most states, which meant that doctors were needed legally for their credentials and expertise. But other non-medical staff were equally important in the clinics (Halfmann 2011; Simonds 1996).

Concurrent with the move to stand-alone clinics were broader shifts in health-care provision spurred by the demands of large managed care insurance compa-nies and reimbursement structures (Scott et al. 2000). Though free-standing abortion clinics were not part of big managed care systems, these clinics were influ-enced by the ideals and practices of managed care. Both contexts sometimes con-tract with doctors and other specialists (rather than hiring them as staff), both seek to streamline care to reduce inefficiencies and maximize productivity, and both have to navigate complicated insurance reimbursement structures (Kavanaugh, Jones, and Finer 2011; Scott et al. 2000). One of the consequences of this new arrangement of health care was the growth of allied health occupations, a cate-gory of health workers who are not doctors or nurses but are increasingly integral to healthcare provision, including in abortion clinics.

This type of work includes medical assistants (MAs), workers who are cross-trained in administrative and some clinical duties. They have less education and training than doctors and nurses, are paid less, and hold the least status in the healthcare hierarchy. Depending on where they work, they may perform only administrative tasks and have little interaction with patients, or they may do clin-ical work such as taking vital signs and assisting doctors. During the first two decades of the twenty-first century to the present, MAs have been instrumental in many clinical settings that offer reproductive health care.

MAs are on the list of fastest-growing fields (U.S. Bureau of Labor Statistics, n.d.), and they represent a new demographic of healthcare worker. Unlike doctors who tend to be white, highly educated, and affluent, MAs more closely reflect the racial, ethnic, and socioeconomic demographics of the communities in which they work (Chapman, Marks, and Dower 2015). From an organizational perspective, MAs are a relatively cheap yet valuable source of labor—particularly useful for clin-ics striving to maximize revenue and reduce costs. The nineteenth century move to medicalize abortion resulted in highly educated white men as the primary abor-tion worker, but the *Roe* decision and the demands of managed care opened the door for a more diverse abortion workforce.

Prior research documenting the arrangement and allocation of work in abor-tion clinics has found that MAs are engaged in some of the most stigmatizing aspects of abortion work, with little access to the more valorizing parts of the job (Ward 2021). Here, we look at the role of MAs in abortion work and what their participation tells us about broader conceptualizations of abortion work and healthcare work in general. Specifically, we put forth that MAs offer a useful point of analysis to understand the dynamic push/pull to and from professionalized med-icine in abortion work.

Medical Assistants: A New Type of Abortion Worker

To investigate patterns and shifts in abortion work in the last few decades, we now turn to a brief discussion of MAs in abortion work using ethnographic and interview data collected in a stand-alone abortion clinic in California. The first author collected data over eighteen months during 2016–2017. As a supportive social and legal context for abortion (then and now), California presented an opportunity to understand abortion work that is relatively unfettered by state-level anti-abortion legislation. For instance, by 2017 California was one of a few states that allowed some advanced practice clinicians (namely, nurse practitioners, certified nurse-midwives, and physician assistants) to perform abortions. By examining the unique position of MAs in abortion clinics, we can better understand the tensions between professionalized and comparatively new unskilled labor in abortion work.

The study site was a busy comprehensive sexual and reproductive health clinic. In addition to abortion, the clinic offered preventive health screenings (e.g., pap smears), tested for sexually transmitted infections, treated infections and disorders, dispensed contraception, and performed some advanced gynecological procedures such as colposcopies. The clinic saw patients seven days a week. Procedural abortions were provided two to three days a week; on those days, upward of twenty patients were on the schedule for an abortion. (Most patients seeking medication abortions were sent to a nearby affiliated clinic that specialized in medication abortion.) Of the staff of about thirty people, about a quarter were MAs. The MAs were all women of color, mostly Latina, and they had worked there anywhere from a few months to over twenty years.

Despite what many may assume about abortion workers, the MAs in the clinic under study did not get their MA certification with the goal of providing abortion care or even reproductive health care. The typical trajectory to them working at the clinic was as follows: they were interested in working in the medical field, they got their medical assisting certification, and then they found their way to the clinic either through social networks or just saw the clinic was hiring and applied. Working at the clinic was a step forward in putting their education and credentials to use—and it was a paying job. Some of the MAs wanted to continue their education and get a nursing degree, which would advance them in the medical profession; others were satisfied with their current job and had no immediate plans for further education or training. Ideologically, although some MAs did think of themselves as "pro-choice" before working at the clinic, none of them sought out work at the clinic *because* of the clinic's mission or their own beliefs about reproductive rights. Abortion work was aligned with their career goals, not because they wanted paid work that contributed to access to abortion but because they wanted to work in health care.

For the most part, the MAs enjoyed their jobs at the clinic; they liked assisting doctors with procedures, they liked that they did not have to do front desk duties (which was a common task for MAs employed in other settings), and they liked the feeling of helping people. Comparing their experiences working in other types of healthcare settings, the MAs found working in the abortion clinic to be more satisfying. They had more diverse clinical duties and gained advanced skills such as ultrasound guidance and procedure assisting.

Three of the MAs in the study—Chloe, Alex, and Sam[1]—talked about being fascinated by the biological aspects of their work, and they noted that procedural abortion allowed them to see things they otherwise would not have. For example, they enjoyed being able to see different stages of fetal development. Sam acknowledged that what may be off-putting to others about their role is what fascinated her about the work, noting that "it may be weird, because [the fetal remains] looks really gory and everything, but it still amazes me." The opportunities contributed to their job satisfaction.

This clinic had relatively high numbers of procedural abortions, compared with some neighboring clinics that only provided medication abortions. Sam and Nicole both explained that they preferred to do the more advanced clinical work (associated with procedural abortions) rather than the more administrative work associated with medication abortion. For medication abortion, MAs typically collected a urine sample and entered basic information (e.g., blood pressure, heart rate, weight) into the patient's electronic chart. Procedural abortion also allowed MAs to work directly with physicians whereas with medication abortion they could be working with nurse practitioners. In addition to abortions, one of the MAs, Chloe, described how much she enjoyed helping the doctors with more advanced gynecologic procedures, including colposcopies, cervical biopsies, and sterilization procedures. One of the doctors quipped that Chloe was so skilled that she could probably do an abortion procedure herself. Chloe viewed these supportive roles as the most important part of her job because she was "there for the doctors if they need anything."

MA positions are located in a vast array of healthcare settings. Depending on the job, one may have very little patient interaction and have a lot of paperwork and computer work. One MA at the study site, Nicole, briefly left to work in another healthcare setting. But she was unhappy there, and eventually she came back to the abortion clinic. She explained that she was unhappy with the amount of administrative office work that she was required to do at the other job: "I didn't go to school to do front office stuff. . . . And I missed the surgical, like I missed all that." Nicole got her medical assisting credential with the goal of doing hands-on health care with patients, and working an abortion clinic allowed her to realize this goal.

Not all MAs were excited about assisting with procedural abortions. Juliana, for example, felt abortion work was important, but she found some aspects of the work distasteful. She liked that she was helping people. At the same time, she explained she was "uncomfortable" assisting with second-trimester abortions, although she did not elaborate further on the reasons for that discomfort. Despite her own feelings about participating in some abortion care, she defended her work—and her involvement in abortion care—to friends and family.

In addition to the medical aspects of their work, MAs saw themselves as providing essential care to patients in the form of emotional support and to the larger clinic as they facilitated smooth operations. Because they are the first clinical staff to meet patients, MAs are often the first to provide emotional care to patients. Alex described this role as like being an "emotional sponge" for people with a variety of life stories and experiences. She said that, of the range of patient experiences she had encountered, it was the most difficult to be with patients "who have been sexually abused and have been pregnant because of result of it." Alex shared that as she prepared them for the abortion she would "just [try] to hold their hand and tell them everything is going to be okay. Well, you don't know everything's going to be okay with them after they leave, but at least for this little part everything will be fine." Juliana also discussed the difficulty and emotional toll of the "hard cases," which she did not think she was adequately trained to handle: "I don't think we're trained emotionally, they kind of just throw us [in]." Juliana's reflection identifies emotional labor as an underdeveloped area in MAs general training and in specialized training at the clinic.

Alex approached this role as an opportunity to be the "glue" of the clinic. Alex noted that being an MA required one to "make sure that the RNs [registered nurses] are happy, that the doctors are happy, and the recovery nurse is happy, and the manager is happy, and the patient flow is going just right because you are the one kind of transporting everyone everywhere they need to go . . . if it weren't for this position, it would be really hard. Operations would be more difficult." Other MAs shared Alex's assessment of juggling different tasks and supporting different people in the clinic and recognized how essential their position was to the functioning of the clinic.

Like other occupations in abortion work that navigate social disapproval, stigma, and judgment, MAs described a job that can be socially isolating. MAs talked about navigating how to explain to friends, family, and even strangers about their job title and the reality of their work. This could lead to awkward and uncomfortable situations. For instance, Chloe described her in-laws as religious people who stopped talking to her for a while when they learned she worked at an abortion clinic. Even her husband did not like to hear about her workdays. She said, "When I talk about the abortions and stuff. He doesn't like to hear it." Others reported they had lost friends because of their chosen job. Juliana said that someone had refused to maintain a friendship with her because her abortion clinic work conflicted with the friend's religious beliefs. In other cases, after initial disapproval, friends and family were accepting of their work in abortion, if not necessarily supportive. For instance, some MAs' parents accepted their work despite opposition to abortion, reasoning that the pay and benefits outweighed the moral conflict. MAs learned strategies to avoid uncomfortable conversations, especially with strangers. They described feeling out whether the other person would be receptive to their profession. For instance, Alex explained that she gave a "generic response" when people ask what she does for a job: "If they keep asking, it's like, well, it's a surgical site, and we do very specific specialized cases, and, yeah, [I] usually stop there."

The pull of MAs into the abortion workforce over the last several decades extended the category of abortion worker beyond the highly trained and professionalized physicians and nurses of abortion care before and immediately after *Roe*, while also cementing abortion work as highly medicalized and reflecting the norms and practices of larger healthcare systems. This brief examination of MAs in abortion work provides some insight into the effects of larger healthcare structures on abortion work. The integration of lower-status, less-skilled workers into abortion care meant a change in who can be categorized as an abortion worker. No longer only those who are responsible for actively terminating the pregnancy, auxiliary clinic staff are now doing the work of abortion.

The Ever-Changing Abortion Workforce

With this context of how abortion work in the United States has been organized over time and some of the factors that have contributed to changes in the abortion workforce, we can start to anticipate the state of abortion work in the post-*Dobbs* era. What do the legal changes for abortion mean for abortion work and workers? And how does this help us understand the arrangement of healthcare work at large? With *Dobbs v. Jackson Women's Health Organization* in 2022, the Supreme Court ended the federal protections guaranteed by *Roe v. Wade* and *Planned Parenthood of Southeastern Pennsylvania v. Casey*, and abortion became an issue decided by individual states.

Because of laws already on the books to be "triggered" by the end of *Roe*, abortion became illegal in some states overnight. Other states moved swiftly to ban abortion within their borders. Clinic closures were immediate, instigating another shift on the abortion workforce. In the first 100 days after the *Dobbs* decision, sixty-six clinics in fifteen different states stopped providing abortion services; in the thirteen states that had abortion bans, all clinics stopped providing abortions. Additionally, twenty-six clinics shut down completely, while forty were still in operation by providing services other than abortion (Kirstein, Dreweke, and Jones 2022).

Medical professionals at these locations either lost their jobs or, in the case of clinics that stayed open for other services, had a significant change in their duties. For the MAs who lost their jobs with the abortion clinic closures, there are open questions about the ease with which they were able to find work in other healthcare settings. Do the skills they developed in procedural abortion afford them some advantage when looking for a new job? There are also open questions about the extent to which they will find alternative employment satisfying, especially if it lacks the opportunity for advanced clinical work.

Of course, the effects of clinic closures on abortion workers are not restricted to the states where clinics have closed. To be clear, clinic closures are not a new phenomenon. Prior to *Dobbs*, anti-abortion state-level legislation targeting abortion providers and clinics had reduced the number of clinics in the United States providing abortions. For example, between 2012 and 2022, the number of abortion clinics decreased by 35 percent (Abortion Care Network 2022). And those closures can affect the clinics that remained open. Clinic closures in one state can increase demand in other states. Immediately following *Dobbs*, the states that neighbored or were surrounded by states that banned abortion experienced the largest surge in abortion patients (Society of Family Planning 2022).

The increase in patients means that some clinic workers may find that their job duties are reallocated, even if they are in a state where abortion remains legal. Clinics that previously provided comprehensive reproductive care might shift to primarily providing abortion care, for instance, to meet the increased patient demand. This means clinic workers' job duties also shift. It remains to be seen how permanent a shift this would represent—that is, will clinics adjust to increased demand and grow to return to their pre-*Dobbs* practices, or will this represent the latest iteration in the organization of abortion care, with clinics more commonly specializing in abortion? Thinking about the mobility of the abortion workforce, will MAs who worked in abortion care in states that now ban abortion relocate to the states where their skills are in demand? Given the relatively lower socioeconomic status of MAs and their associated lower mobility, this option is more likely for doctors and nurses.

TELEHEALTH AND SELF-MANAGED ABORTION

For example, with the move away from in-person care, MAs like those described earlier may be less necessary. Their previous role in medication abortion included tasks that are no longer considered necessary for safe care (e.g., taking vitals or urine samples), pointing to the latest shift in the abortion workforce. MAs may still be used for entering medical data in charts and other administrative tasks, but these tasks may not be satisfying, as evident in the comments from the MAs interviewed earlier. Additionally, the rise of telehealth and self-managed abortion (wherein a person manages their own abortion, usually with medication abortion pills outside the formal healthcare setting; see also the chapter by Tracy Weitz in this volume) could mean that MAs may have fewer interactions with patients or opportunities to provide the emotional labor that some MAs value. They may have fewer opportunities the for hands-on, "scientific" medical care they characterized as meaningful interactions with patients and working closely with doctors. It is also possible that the changing landscape of abortion care could increase the opportunities for MAs to be involved in patient care. Because abortion bans contribute to delays in obtaining care—and medication abortion is not available in the United States to abortion seekers after eleven weeks' gestation—there may be an increased number of patients needing abortions later in pregnancy, which could represent more opportunities for MAs to be involved in clinical care.

The rise of telehealth and self-managed abortion may also usher in new types of abortion workers. Abortion seekers may need to rely on lay knowledges and community-based networks (perhaps including the internet) to navigate these options and may look to a new type of abortion worker for guidance and support in their experience of abortion. These "workers" may be more akin to abortion accompaniers or doulas, roles that have been developed by activists and advocates to support aborting people and do not require formal medical training. We should be asking who or what makes up the "abortion workforce" in self-managed abortion? Is this a turn to the complete deprofessionalization of abortion care? What of the people who are responsible for the websites that sell and ship the pills? Is this a new category of abortion worker?

Although these workers are dissimilar to the homeopaths of the mid- to late 1800s in that the products they sell are safe and effective, there are similarities in the ability for abortion seekers to privately use market-based solutions for pregnancy termination. This emerging context may be not only a de-skilling of abortion work but also a step toward further de-centering physicians in abortion care.

Conclusion

Understanding the changes and features of abortion work can help illuminate central processes and practices of health care and medicine. Thinking about medicalization, looking at the abortion workforce illustrates that the push/pull to and from medicalization is dynamic and multifaceted. Where health care and medicine happen (e.g., at home or in hospitals) depends on many things: politics, culture, scientific advances, and even patient preferences. Who is involved in providing health care also changes with social contexts, creating ebbs and flows in de/professionalization. When we consider medical dominance (or medicalization), abortion demonstrates how messy and nonlinear this process can be (Halfmann 2011). This is not unique to abortion care and abortion work. Other areas of health care that are highly politicized, such as gender-affirming care and prepregnancy care (the "zero-trimester"), also have to contend with complex contexts and competing interests involving physicians, a wide variety of experts, politics, and a shifting legal environment (shuster 2021). Analyzing these healthcare contexts from the perspective of the work involved in providing this care is a fruitful area for inquiry into how social and cultural contexts shape the healthcare workforce.

Additionally, as health care of all kinds moves toward more virtual care, the options for private, market-based care increase. Abortion work can serve as an example for what is to come in other sectors. Take, for example, hormone replacement therapy (HRT) for menopause. The online market for HRT has been steadily increasing and is projected to continue increasing over the next decade (Strategic Market Research 2022). Through these pathways, people seeking these treatments do not need to make appointments with their primary care physicians or even interface with the providers within their managed care networks. They can search for for-profit companies online who have doctors on staff to prescribe the medications and have them shipped directly to people's homes. Like telehealth for abortion, this form of health care is direct-to-consumer and reduces the need for auxiliary workers trained in health care, instead largely relying on workers who can manage data online and process and ship orders. This work does not require taking medical histories or assessing vital signs, nor does it require the worker to have medical knowledge. This pathway to accessing what has historically been exclusively under the purview of medicine signals not only a deprofessionalization of healthcare work but a potential demedicalization of treatments like HRT.

Abortion care has a long history of responding to shifting political, legal, and cultural climates—and the post-*Dobbs* landscape is the latest catalyst for change. From community-based midwives to professionalized physicians and from therapeutic abortion boards to stand-alone clinic staffers, telehealth, and self-managed abortion facilitators, as abortion work has changed, so too has the profile of abortion workers. In the contemporary moment, alongside attention to what *Dobbs* means for the legality of abortion across the United States, the evolving history of abortion work suggests that we also ought to pay attention to how abortion work and abortion workers respond. Such consideration will offer insights into abortion work: how abortion workers navigate the once-again-shifting bounds of politics, law, and culture and indeed how broader patterns of healthcare delivery and ongoing struggles relate to the (de)medicalization and (de)professionalization of health care.

NOTE

1. All participant names used here are pseudonyms.

REFERENCES

Abortion Care Network. 2022. "Communities Need Clinics: The New Landscape of Independent Abortion Clinics in the United States." https://abortioncarenetwork.org/wp-content/uploads/2022/12/communities-need-clinics-2022.pdf.

Beisel, Nicola, and Tamara Kay. "Abortion, Race, and Gender in Nineteenth-Century America." *American Sociological Review* 69, no. 4 (2004): 498–518.

Bonaparte, Alicia D. "Regulating Childbirth: Physicians and Granny Midwives in South Carolina." In *Birthing Justice: Black Women, Pregnancy, and Childbirth*, edited by Julia Chinyere Oparah and Alicia D. Bonaparte, 30–42. Routledge, 2023.

Chapman, Susan A., Angela Marks, and Catherine Dower. "Positioning Medical Assistants for a Greater Role in the Era of Health Reform." *Academic Medicine* 90 no. 10 (2015):1347–1352.

Devereux, George. 1954. "A Typological Study of Abortion in 350 Primitive, Ancient and Preindustrial Societies." In *Therapeutic Abortion: Medical, Psychiatric, Anthropological, and Religious Considerations*, edited by Harold Rosen, 97–152. Julian Press.

Gordon, Linda. 2002. *The Moral Property of Women: A History of Birth Control Politics in America*. University of Illinois Press.

Halfmann, Drew. 2011. "Recognizing Medicalization and Demedicalization: Discourses, Practices, and Identities." *Article Health* 16 (2): 186–207.

Himes, Norman E. 1936. "Medical History of Contraception." *New England Journal of Medicine* 210: 576–581.

Hume, Angela. 2023. *Deep Care*. AK Press.

Joffe, Carole. 2013. "The Politicization of Abortion and the Evolution of Abortion Counseling." *American Journal of Public Health* 103 (1): 57–65.

Jones, Rachel K., and Jenna Jerman. 2017. "Abortion Incidence and Service Availability in the United States, 2014." *Perspectives on Sexual and Reproductive Health* 49 (1):17–27.

Kaplan, Laura. 2019. *The Story of Jane: The Legendary Underground Feminist Abortion Service*. University of Chicago Press.

Kavanaugh, Megan L., Jones, R. K., and Finer, L. B. 2011. "Perceived and Insurance-Related Barriers to the Provision of Contraceptive Services in US Abortion Care Settings." *Women's Health Issues* 21 (3): S26-S31.

Kirstein, Marielle, Joerg Dreweke, and Rachel K. Jones. 2022. "100 Days Post-*Roe*: At Least 66 Clinics across 15 US States Have Stopped Offering Abortion Care." Guttmacher Institute, October 3, 2022. https://www.guttmacher.org/2022/10/100-days-post-Roe-least-66 -clinics-across15-us-states-have-stopped-offering-abortion-care.

Lewis, Karen J., and Jon O. Shimabukuro. 2001. *Report for Congress, Abortion Law Development: A Brief Overview*. Congressional Research Services.

Luker, Kristin. 1984. *Abortion and the Politics of Motherhood*. University of California Press.

Nelson, Jennifer. 2015. *More Than Medicine: A History of the Feminist Women's Health Movement*. New York University Press.

Reagan. Leslie J. 1997. *When Abortion Was a Crime: Women, Medicine, and Law in the United States, 1867–1973*. University of California Press.

Scott, W. Richard, Martin Ruef, Peter J. Mendel, and Carol A. Caronna. 2000. *Institutional Change and Healthcare Organizations: From Professional Dominance to Managed Care*. University of Chicago Press.

shuster, stef M. 2021. *Trans Medicine: The Emergence and Practice of Treating Gender*. New York University Press.

Simonds, Wendy. 1996. *Abortion at Work: Ideology and Practice in a Feminist Clinic*. Rutgers University Press.

Society of Family Planning. 2022. "April 2022 to August 2022." *#WeCount Report*, October 28, 2022. https://societyfp.org/wp-content/uploads/2022/10/SFPWeCountReport_Aprto Aug2022_ReleaseOct2022-1.pdf

Strategic Market Research. 2022. "Hormone Replacement Therapy Market by Therapy Type (Thyroid Hormone Replacement Therapy, Estrogen Replacement Therapy, Human Growth Hormone Replacement Therapy, Progestogen Hormone Replacement Therapy, Testosterone Replacement Therapy), Route of Administration (Parenteral, Oral, Others)" Report ID: 67307763. https://web.archive.org/web/20221116180037/https://www.strategicmarketresearch .com/market-report/hormone-replacement-therapy-market.

U.S. Bureau of Labor Statistics. n.d. "Occupational Outlook Handbook, Medical Assistants." U.S. Department of Labor, updated August 29, 2024. https://www.bls.gov/ooh/healthcare /medical-assistants.htm.

Ward, Kelly M. 2021. "Dirty Work and Intimacy: Creating an Abortion Worker." *Journal of Health and Social Behavior* 62 (4): 512–525.

CHAPTER 7

The Great Fallacy That American Catholic Hospitals Practice Medicine Without Abortion

Lori Freedman

AAPLOG [the American Association of Pro-Life Obstetrician Gynecologists], the movement's leading medical organization, argues that "direct abortion is not medically necessary to save the life of a woman." The organization suggests that doctors may separate "a mother and her unborn child for the purposes of saving a mother's life," but not with the intention *of taking a fetal life. (Zeigler 2022, emphasis in original)*

In 2008, my colleagues and I published six disconcerting clinical stories in an article entitled, "When There's a Heartbeat: Miscarriage Management in Catholic-owned Hospitals," in the *American Journal of Public Health* (Freedman, Landy, and Steinauer 2008). The stories showed how, in U.S. Catholic health care institutions, abortion prohibitions required that physicians deny medical treatment or delay it until miscarrying patients became sick enough that their life was threatened or the fetus died, whichever came first. How exactly religious restrictions impacted miscarriage treatment had little documentation in the peer reviewed health literature at the time. Patients likely did not know that in other medical settings they would be offered treatments sooner. Sometimes, perhaps due to vague branding, the patients didn't even know they were in a Catholic hospital (Guiahi et al. 2014; Hafner 2018; Wascher et al. 2018). In fact, before this moment, few who did not work in Catholic obstetric services understood that patient safety and well-being was routinely compromised when pregnancy termination became necessary (Freedman et al. 2018; Freedman and Stulberg 2013; Wingo et al. 2020). It seemed as if my co-authors and I had stumbled upon an antiquated corner of medicine that strangely failed to advance along with women's rights. From my vantage now, after the constitutional right to abortion has been overturned, I see it differently: these hospitals are a model for state abortion bans post-*Dobbs*.

After that first article, my co-authors and I learned that Catholic health care is no small corner of medicine. Americans have little awareness of how numerous and influential Catholic healthcare institutions really are (Guiahi, Sheeder, and Teal 2014; Stulberg et al. 2019; Wascher et al. 2018). Catholic hospitals are run by large health systems around the United States with names that may not signal to all their religious affiliation, such as Common Spirit and Ascension. Founded more than a century ago by orders of nuns and priests under the authority of a local diocese with a mission to care for the poor, Catholic hospitals have modernized, proliferated, and consolidated into large Church-affiliated health systems with few clergy present anymore and a solidly corporate mission standard in U.S. health care (Gabow and Berwick 2023; Kutney-Lee et al. 2014; Lown Institute 2024). Although they maintain a reputation for caring for the poor today, in reality they provide less than average charity care or Medicaid services (Solomon et al. 2020).

Religious policies still govern care, however. Operating as a Catholic hospital means following a set of mandatory directives written by the U.S. Conference of Catholic Bishops (an organization of male clergy and theologians) that, among other things, prohibit abortion and various reproductive services within Catholic hospitals (U.S. Conference of Catholic Bishops 2018). Although the Catholic Church does not fund the care, it essentially owns the land and the buildings. Today, the reach of Catholic health care—and, thus, the Directives—is large. Altogether, as of 2020, about one in six U.S. hospital patients finds themselves being treated in a facility governed by the religious policies of the Catholic bishops (Solomon et al. 2020). In these facilities, doctors must routinely tell patients they are not allowed to offer abortion and related care, including for obstetric complications. That said, the Catholic hospitals have never really existed without abortion.

Post-*Dobbs*—and even in the run-up to *Dobbs*—antiabortion advocates, antiabortion professional medical associations including some obstetrician-gynecologists, and vocal legislators claimed that abortion is never necessary (Bopp 2022; Catholic News Agency 2022; Surana 2022; Ziegler 2022). Some made dubious medical claims, but others offered what, at its surface, seemed factual. They pointed to Catholic hospitals, whose Directives prohibit abortion, and said patients were fine there without abortion care. In so doing, they aimed to negate the claims of public health and reproductive health experts—including the American College of Obstetricians and Gynecologists, the primary professional association of physicians specializing in women's reproductive health, who warned that banning abortion would compromise people's health, including people experiencing miscarriage. In response, an author on the conservative news site the *National Review* called such safety concerns disingenuous: "Never mind that for decades now, Catholic hospitals, which don't perform elective abortions, have somehow managed to treat pregnant women with ectopic pregnancies or miscarriages" (Desanctis 2022).

But the idea that abortion is never necessary in Catholic hospitals is a fallacy. Catholic hospital patient outcomes have been adequate only because abortion care was available nearby—and sometimes even within these "abortion-prohibitive" spaces.

WHAT ARE THE DIRECTIVES?

The Directives, officially entitled the "Ethical and Religious Directives for Catholic Healthcare Services," are a set of seventy-seven policies that the U.S. Bishops require hospitals to abide to be officially deemed Catholic. Codified in the mid-twentieth century, the Directives have been revised by the bishops about every other decade as new conflicts in care surfaced. The policies address many things, including financial arrangements and governing structures, but over one-third of the Directives restrict sexual and reproductive care. Specifically, the Directives allow for only medical practices that support the Catholic hierarchy's views of marriage and personhood.

In relation to marriage, the Directives stick to the Catholic religious doctrine that sex should only occur for the purpose of procreation between a married man and woman; no other sexual or procreative pathway is acceptable. Because sex just for pleasure is unacceptable, Directives 52 and 53 prohibit contraceptives and sterilization procedures, male or female. In vitro fertilization is also prohibited; as Directive 41 states, "it separates procreation from the marital act in its unitive significance." Likewise, the use of donated sperm or eggs is not allowed because, as Directive 40 states, "it is contrary to the covenant of marriage, the unity of the spouses, and the dignity proper to parents and the child." Basically, there's only one way to make a baby: heterosexual married sex. And all sex must try to make a baby. Importantly, the Directives apply to all patient care in Catholic hospitals whether you subscribe to those beliefs or not.

In relation to the personhood of the fetus or embryo, the Directives oppose abortion under any circumstance. As Directive 45 states, "abortion (that is, the directly intended termination of pregnancy before viability or the directly intended destruction of a viable fetus) is never permitted. Every procedure whose sole immediate effect is the termination of pregnancy before viability is an abortion, which, in its moral context, includes the interval between conception and implantation of the embryo." Because of Directive 45, Catholic hospitals will not offer abortion services for any fetal indication. Even if the fetus has no brain or has a disease ensuring it will die in its first days, weeks, or months, no procedure that hastens its demise is allowed. When a fatal fetal diagnosis is made early in pregnancy, Catholic hospital policy compels the pregnant person to continue to gestate the pregnancy another five or six more months even though abortion would be safer. (Given the cruelty of this policy, patients in this situation often then seek out an abortion provider elsewhere.)

However, there is one critical directive that allows physicians to perform an abortion, though not in so many words. Directive 47 applies to obstetric emergencies, allowing abortion to save a pregnant patient's life. It states, "Operations, treatments, and medications that have as their direct purpose the cure of a proportionately serious pathological condition of a pregnant woman are permitted when they cannot be safely postponed until the unborn child is viable, even if they will result in the death of the unborn child." This is the "medical exemptions" clause, so to speak, and it is, in practice, critical for patient safety.

Within a Catholic hospital, if a patient is experiencing some type of pregnancy complication that threatens her life (excessive bleeding or infection, for example), the Directives permit the doctor to treat that threat through use of a theological justification: the principle of "double effect." Double effect, when applied to obstetric complications, holds that a clinician cannot *intentionally* end the life of the fetus because within Catholicism this is considered "evil." However, clinicians are permitted to *directly* intervene with intention of doing "good." To give an example, if a pregnant woman arrives feverish and cramping, a clinician might examine her and find that the pregnancy is doomed—whether the fetus is still alive or not—because she has an infection in her uterus. Directive 47 means in this context that the clinician can save the pregnant woman's life by treating her infection, which entails emptying her infected uterus. Of course, the treatment will kill the fetus in the process. This is *expected*, but it is not *intended*, an important theological clarification.

Only the saving of the pregnant patient's life is *intentional*, and fetal death along the way is the *unintentional* effect. Sound familiar? This language of intentionality has permeated antiabortion rhetoric about whether and how to include exemptions to state abortion bans for the "life or health of the mother" (AAPLOG 2013; Steupert 2023; Ziegler 2022). It is religious, not medical language.

THE DIRECTIVES VERSUS STANDARD MISCARRIAGE MANAGEMENT

Although the Directives are clear, clinicians do not always follow them to the letter. Miscarriage happens in about one in ten recognized pregnancies, and it is likely even more common if including instances where individuals don't yet know they are pregnant (ACOG 2018). Only a small portion of those become obstetric emergencies that occur while a fetus still has a heartbeat even after the pregnancy is otherwise seriously compromised. The American College of Obstetricians and Gynecologists (ACOG) advises that when an obstetric complication arises too early for the fetus to survive after delivery, the standard of care is for doctors to first determine whether they can save the pregnancy. They may not be able to save it because, for example, the amniotic sac has completely ruptured, leaving the patient and fetus vulnerable to infection, or because the patient already has an infection, or because the patient is bleeding and her cervix is opening up. Though only about 10 percent of identified pregnancies miscarry annually, there are many ways for pregnancy loss to occur, some more clinically complicated than others. If the loss is inevitable, ACOG advises physicians to offer the patient three standard options about how to proceed: (1) watch and wait, (2) give medication to induce labor, or (3) do a procedure to evacuate the uterus (ACOG 2018).

The six doctors in our 2008 "heartbeat" publication explained they that they had to seek permission from their Catholic hospital's ethics committee before being able to offer patients the latter two choices because both treatments can cause an abortion. Catholic hospitals have ethics committees made up of a mix of health professionals and lawyers, usually led by a clergyperson. They serve as gatekeepers to the prohibited reproductive care in this context. To get permission to treat, doctors have to persuade the clergyperson on the hospital's ethics committee that intervention is medically necessary to save the pregnant patient's life (Hamel 2014). Physicians have reported that even after they determined that pregnancy loss was inevitable, their hospital's ethics committee required them to wait for a fever to set in to prove infection threatened the patient's life. Some were not willing to take that risk and to practice below the standard of care, so they worked around the Directives in a variety of ways or left the job.

After the "heartbeat" publication drew considerable attention and concern from advocates, scholars, and some news outlets, my colleagues and I began new research to look more deeply and broadly at how the Directives work in practice. We also wanted to gain a more detailed understanding of physicians' experiences in managing previable pregnancy loss (i.e., miscarriage) in Catholic hospitals. How consistently was the principle of double effect applied? What did this look like for patients, and how did physicians navigate the process of arriving at a theological justification to intervene?

The Directives in Practice

After interviewing about fifty more physicians throughout the country, in as many different Catholic hospitals, we learned that the way they navigated around the prohibition varied (Freedman 2023; Freedman and Stulberg 2013). For example, even though the Directives prohibit direct referrals to abortion providers, the most common and uncomplicated workaround physicians used involved sending patients to abortion clinics nearby for care, in some cases judiciously avoiding a paper trail. One physician told me, "So mainly the workaround is that . . . I can verbally tell them. I can say, 'You go to Planned Parenthood.'" In other cases, doctors made direct referrals to abortion clinics in nearby cities. For example, another doctor said, "If we have a patient who has a known anencephalic baby . . . we refer them to [a large Southern city]." Following *Dobbs*, the state that city is in has a total ban on abortion.

Related to miscarriage management, some Catholic hospital ethics committees permitted abortion procedures to be performed early in the pregnancy loss process when a patient's temperature elevated slightly, some only later when she was quite sick. Some physicians endeavored to get permission from the ethics committee to intervene by massaging the language, sometimes by exaggerating the signs of infection, as one doctor explained while comparing and contrasting the experiences of working in Catholic and non-Catholic hospitals: "And in the Catholic hospital you had to wait till they get sick, which was kind of foolish when you knew the prognosis was so poor. So you have to wait till they got an infection . . . we would cut corners, and so if they got to [a temperature of] 99 [degrees], we would call it a

fever. And we would induce them. Because we were protecting their life and trying to salvage their uterus, so they didn't get a serious infection that they needed
a hysterectomy."

Some doctors offered to transfer patients quickly to abortion providers nearby
so their patients would not have to get sick at all. And still other doctors avoided
the whole treatment/referral problem by communicating early to their patient to
go to a non-Catholic hospital if miscarrying. Yet across all these workarounds,
there was one very important consistency: physicians relied heavily on abortion
care to keep their patients safe.

So while antiabortion advocates have argued that abortion is never necessary
and that Catholic health care serves as a proven model of how medicine could function safely under abortion bans, the assertion is simply untrue. In these obstetric
complications, it was not a matter of *if*, but rather *how*, *when*, and *where* to get abortion care.

Who the Directives Have Failed

Workarounds serve as an *escape valve* for Catholic hospitals stuck in a quandary
where religious leadership prohibits abortion but the physicians working there
know abortion is often necessary for patients' health and well-being. Historians
studying Catholic health care in other times and places corroborate this pattern
(Joyce 2002; Martucci 2023; Wall 2011). Without workarounds, more patients in
Catholic hospitals in need of abortion would have become sick or suffered neglect—
what I call *doctrinal iatrogenesis* (Freedman 2023). It is the extra efforts of physicians employing workarounds that has kept patients in Catholic hospitals safe.

But the workarounds do not work consistently, as evidenced by several lawsuits
Catholic hospitals have faced in the past decade. For example, the American Civil
Liberties Union represented both Tamesha Means and Mindy Swank in lawsuits
against Catholic hospitals (Kaye et al. 2016). Ms. Means, a Black woman who was
eighteen weeks pregnant, lived in a city where her only options for care were Catholic hospitals. Ms. Swank, a white woman who was twenty weeks pregnant, had
planned to have her delivery in a Catholic hospital. Both were repeatedly refused
emergency abortion care when they began to miscarry. In Ms. Means case, she had
signs of infection and began to pass the pregnancy in the lobby of the Catholic hospital during her third attempt to get care. Ms. Swank was finally admitted to her
hospital when she was twenty-seven weeks pregnant and hemorrhaging. Neither
of these women received the standard of care for managing their miscarriage—
because the institutions where they sought care were governed by the Directives.

The survival of patients with obstetric complications in Catholic hospitals often
depends on alternative access to abortion care, but these pathways have vanished
with the abortion bans. In states that have banned or severely restricted abortion,
a miscarrying patient can no longer be driven to a nearby non-Catholic hospital
or an abortion clinic for a procedure, not unless they live close to the border of a
state with no ban. Doctors can no longer stretch the truth about how bad a patient's

symptoms are or seek an ethics committee's permission to do an abortion based on the doctrine of double effect. Even if an ethics committee in a Catholic hospital did approve an abortion procedure, they could not protect physicians from criminal liability for violating state law.

Some state abortion bans have made workarounds unavailable or questionably legal, despite concerns voiced even by the current president and CEO of the Catholic Health Association. Quoted in a Catholic publication, CEO Sister Haddad said, "The E.R.D.s [Ethical and Religious Directives] aren't restrictive. They're allowing things to happen that some states are prohibiting right now. And that's going to be an issue for all of us" (Clarke 2022). That is, leaders like Sister Haddad want the public to know Catholic health care institutions have a means of "making exceptions" to keep patients safe when *they* deem abortion medically and theologically justifiable. State abortion bans actually strip Catholic hospital ethics committees of this authority, which their physicians have depended on to get around the Directives' abortion prohibitions.

Indeed, Sister Haddad is right: minus Directive 47 and the commonly used workarounds or escape valves, many patients in Catholic hospitals would have died, just as Savita Halapannavar died in Ireland in 2012 when abortion was fully banned. Halapannavar, a dentist and Indian immigrant, came to a hospital in her second trimester complaining of severe back pain (a sign of infection) and, aware she was losing the pregnancy, begged for them to help her, to give her an abortion. They refused: they admitted her but told her they could only "watch and wait," given the nation's abortion law. She died because, by the time they finally intervened, she had a full-body infection. This tragedy prompted broad public outrage and ultimately the lifting of Ireland's abortion ban.

Revelations, Post-*Dobbs*

One revelation since *Dobbs* has been the insight that in states with abortion bans *all hospitals will function like Catholic hospitals but without their routinely used escape valves.* That is, these state policies look as strict as the Directives on paper but without Directive 47, the principle of double effect, an ethics committee to approve qualifying abortions, or the commonly used referral pathways to abortion providers nearby. I hold Catholic hospitals, Catholic health systems, and professional groups such as the Catholic Health Association responsible for having made medicine without abortion look possible when it really is not. It was a sneaky and harmful obfuscation.

The second revelation has been that it is increasingly evident that *state abortion bans draw heavily on the language and rationales used in Catholic doctrine,* betraying the close collaboration between religious antiabortion actors and state policy makers. This is to say, these policies are theological, not medical. They are a deliberate—and to date successful—comingling of church and state to the detriment of women's health and obstetric practice throughout states with bans (Bendix 2022).

CONCLUSION

Catholic hospitals were never abortion free, and the concept was a mirage. State legislators and antiabortion advocates have incorrectly presumed that Catholic hospitals successfully practiced medicine without abortion; this has and will continue to have negative consequences for those experiencing obstetric complications. In states with abortion bans, where saving patients' lives and protecting their future fertility has become precarious, some doctors are leaving, and those who stay must navigate this precarity at the cost of their patients' well-being.

Abortion has always been an important treatment for certain obstetric complications both in and out of Catholic hospitals. At minimum, more transparency from leaders in Catholic health care is required to dispel this fallacy—perhaps a more explicit version of that modeled by the Catholic Health Association's CEO Sister Haddad—so that our laws leave room for lifesaving obstetric care, for god's sake.

ACKNOWLEDGMENTS

This chapter draws on data and analysis published in Lori Freedman, *Bishops and Bodies: Reproductive Care in American Catholic Hospitals* (2023). Thank you to Rutgers University Press and to Debra Stulberg for the many ways you have shaped the book and earlier, related publications.

REFERENCES

American Association of Pro-Life Obstetricians and Gynecologists (AAPLOG). 2013. "Premature Delivery Is Not Induced Abortion." December 4, 2013. https://aaplog.org/premature -delivery-is-not-induced-abortion/.

American College of Obstetricians and Gynecologists (ACOG). 2018. "ACOG Practice Bulletin No. 200: Early Pregnancy Loss." *Obstetrics & Gynecology* 132 (5): e197–e207.

Bendix, Aria. 2022. "What Overturning of Roe v. Wade Means for Life-Threatening Pregnancies That May Be Exceptions to Abortion Bans." *NBC News*, June 30, 2022. https://www .nbcnews.com/health/health-news/abortion-ban-exceptions-life-threatening-pregnancy -rcna36026.

Bopp, James, Jr. 2022. "National Right to Life Committee Proposes Legislation to Protect the Unborn Post-Roe." Bopp Law Firm (blog), June 16, 2022. https://www.bopplaw.com /national-right-to-life-committee-proposes-legislation-to-protect-the-unborn-post-roe.

Catholic News Agency. 2022. "Ectopic Pregnancies, Miscarriage: Abortion Is 'Never Necessary,' These Doctors Say." *Detroit Catholic*, August 8, 2022. https://www.detroitcatholic.com /news/ectopic-pregnancies-miscarriage-abortion-is-never-necessary-these-doctors-say.

Clarke, Kevin. 2022. "Providers Push Back on Abortion Criticism: 'This Country Would Be in Dire Straits without Catholic Health Care.'" *America Magazine*, October 12, 2022. https://www.americamagazine.org/politics-society/2022/10/12/catholic-hospitals -abortion-243931.

Desanctis, Alexandra. 2022. "The Disingenuous Debate over Ectopic Pregnancy and Miscarriage." *National Review*, June 27, 2022. https://www.nationalreview.com/corner/the -disingenuous-debate-over-ectopic-pregnancy-and-miscarriage/.

Freedman, Lori. 2023. *Bishops and Bodies: Reproductive Care in American Catholic Hospitals*. Rutgers University Press.

Freedman, Lori R., Luciana E. Hebert, Molly F. Battistelli, and Debra B. Stulberg. 2018. "Religious Hospital Policies on Reproductive Care: What Do Patients Want to Know?" *American Journal of Obstetrics and Gynecology* 218 (2): 251.e1–251.e9.

Freedman, Lori R., Uta Landy, and Jody Steinauer. 2008. "When There's a Heartbeat: Miscarriage Management in Catholic-Owned Hospitals." *American Journal of Public Health* 98 (10): 1774–1778.

Freedman, Lori R., and Debra B. Stulberg. 2013. "Conflicts in Care for Obstetric Complications in Catholic Hospitals." *AJOB Primary Research* 4 (4): 1–10.

Gabow, Patricia A., and Donald M. Berwick. 2023. *The Catholic Church and Its Hospitals: A Marriage Made in Heaven?* American Association for Physician Leadership.

Guiahi, M., J. Sheeder, and S. Teal. 2014. "Are Women Aware of Religious Restrictions on Reproductive Health at Catholic Hospitals? A Survey of Women's Expectations and Preferences for Family Planning Care." *Contraception* 90 (4): 429–434.

Hafner, Katie. 2018. "As Catholic Hospitals Expand, So Do Limits on Some Procedures." *New York Times*, August 10, 2018. https://www.nytimes.com/2018/08/10/health/catholic-hospitals-procedures.html.

Hamel, R. 2014. "Early Pregnancy Complications and the Ethical and Religious Directives." *Health Progress* 95 (3): 48–56. https://www.chausa.org/publications/health-progress/archive/article/may-june-2014/early-pregnancy-complications-and-the-ethical-and-religious-directives.

Joyce, Kathleen M. 2002. "The Evil of Abortion and the Greater Good of the Faith: Negotiating Catholic Survival in the Twentieth-Century American Health Care System." *Religion and American Culture* 12 (1): 91–121.

Kaye, Julia, Brigitte Amiri, Louise Melling, and Jennifer Dalven. 2016. "Health Care Denied." American Civil Liberties Union, May 2016. https://www.aclu.org/issues/reproductive-freedom/religion-and-reproductive-rights/health-care-denied.

Kutney-Lee, Ann, G. J. Melendez-Torres, Matthew D. McHugh, and Barbra Mann Wall. 2014. "Distinct Enough? A National Examination of Catholic Hospital Affiliation and Patient Perceptions of Care." *Health Care Management Review* 39 (2): 134–144.

Lown Institute. 2024. "Nonprofit Hospitals Receive Billions More in Tax Breaks Than They Invest in Their Communities." *Lown Institute Hospital Index*, March 26, 2024. https://lownhospitalsindex.org/hospital-fair-share-spending-2024/.

Martucci, Jessica. 2023. "'It Gives the Mother the Best Chance for Her Life': U.S. Catholic Health Care and the Treatment of Ectopic Pregnancy." *Bulletin of the History of Medicine* 97 (1): 48–56.

Solomon, Tess, Lois Uttley, Patty HasBrouck, and Yoolim Jung. 2020. "Bigger and Bigger: The Growth of Catholic Health Systems." Community Catalyst, February 8, 2020. https://communitycatalyst.org/resource/bigger-and-bigger-the-growth-of-catholic-health-systems/.

Steupert, Mia. 2023. "Pro-Life Laws Protect Mom and Baby: Pregnant Women's Lives Are Protected in All States." *Lozier Institute*, September 11, 2023. https://lozierinstitute.org/pro-life-laws-protect-mom-and-baby-pregnant-womens-lives-are-protected-in-all-states/.

Stulberg, Debra B., Maryam Guiahi, Luciana E. Hebert, and Lori R. Freedman. 2019. "Women's Expectation of Receiving Reproductive Health Care at Catholic and non-Catholic Hospitals." *Perspectives on Sexual and Reproductive Health* 51 (3): 135–142.

Surana, Kavitha. 2022. "'We Need to Defend This Law': Inside an Anti-Abortion Meeting with Tennessee's GOP Lawmakers." *ProPublica*, November 15, 2022. https://www.propublica.org/article/inside-anti-abortion-meeting-with-tennessee-republican-lawmakers.

U.S. Conference of Catholic Bishops. 2018. "The Ethical and Religious Directives for Catholic Healthcare Services." United States Conference of Catholic Bishops. http://www.usccb.org/about/doctrine/ethical-and-religious-directives/upload/ethical-religious-directives-catholic-health-service-sixth-edition-2016-06.pdf.

Wall, Barbra Mann. 2011. *American Catholic Hospitals: A Century of Changing Markets and Missions*. Rutgers University Press.

Wascher, Jocelyn M., Luciana E. Hebert, Lori R. Freedman, and Debra B. Stulberg. 2018. "Do Women Know Whether Their Hospital Is Catholic? Results from a National Survey." *Contraception* 98 (6): 498–503.

Wingo, Erin E., Jocelyn M. Wascher, Debra B. Stulberg, and Lori R. Freedman. 2020. "Antici-
patory Counseling about Miscarriage Management in Catholic Hospitals: A Qualitative
Exploration of Women's Preferences." *Perspectives on Sexual and Reproductive Health* 52 (3):
171–179.
Ziegler, Mary. 2022. "Why Exceptions for the Life of the Mother Have Disappeared." *The
Atlantic*, July 25, 2022. https://www.theatlantic.com/ideas/archive/2022/07/abortion-ban
-life-of-the-mother-exception/670582/.

CHAPTER 8

Dobbs Reinvigorated the Potential of Mifepristone to "Change Everything"

Tracy A. Weitz

In the early 1990s, American abortion rights activists touted the potential of the French abortion pill RU-486 to "change everything" about abortion in the United States by making abortion more accessible and less socially controversial. In this chapter, I trace whether and how the abortion pill (known by its compound name mifepristone) realized that potential. Unsurprisingly, "changing everything" is easier said than done. As I will detail, from the outset the potential of the abortion pill in the U.S. market was eroded by a complex regulatory regime that limited the drug's diffusion outside established abortion clinics. Abortion advocates, in turn, failed to effectively challenge these constraints; indeed, they leaned into limiting medication abortion to the existing network of providers because protecting abortion rights was conflated with protecting abortion clinics. In its first twenty years, medication abortion did not change much of anything about accessing abortion in the United States, but ironically mifepristone's potential was reinvigorated by both the COVID-19 pandemic and the 2022 U.S. Supreme Court decision overturning *Roe v. Wade* in the *Dobbs v. Jackson Women's Health Organization* decision.

Mifepristone works by blocking the hormone progesterone, which is essential for sustaining a pregnancy. It disrupts the pregnancy's development and eventually causes the uterus to shed its lining; it is used in combination with a prostaglandin, which causes the uterus to contract and expel the products of conception.[1] In the United States, mifepristone is used in combination with the prostaglandin misoprostol to perform a medication abortion. Although medication abortions can be performed using only misoprostol, the scientific evidence for this practice was not fully established in 2000 when the U.S. Food and Drug Administration (FDA) approved mifepristone for distribution. Today, scientific evidence supports the safe use of misoprostol alone for abortions. However, because it has a slightly higher failure rate and is associated with greater cramping and discomfort (Raymond et al. 2023), almost all medication abortions in the United States are done with the mifepristone/misoprostol regimen (Jones, Kirstein, and Philbin 2022). In the United States, mifepristone/misoprostol is used for abortions through eleven weeks of pregnancy although globally the drugs are used for abortions throughout pregnancy, with differing amounts of medications and timing of dosages (WHO 2022a; Wu et al. 2021).

The means of offering medication abortion remained stagnant after the 2000 approval, with cumbersome in-person clinical requirements and limited sites of provision until 2020 when the COVID-19 pandemic forced all healthcare providers to reevaluate the need for face-to-face contact to obtain medical care, especially for care that involved simply taking medication. New clinical guidelines supported medication abortion provision without a physical examination, which allowed for care delivery via telemedicine. Consequently, new telemedicine providers that offered only medication abortions quickly entered the market. Ultimately these changes were more incremental than transformative because they continued to affirm the medicalized model for abortion care.

Perhaps counter to the anti-abortion underpinnings of the 2022 Supreme Court decision in *Dobbs*, the majority decision catalyzed a reckoning with the limitations of the extant model of dispensing medication abortion. Indeed, *Dobbs* catapulted the need for and safety of self-managed abortion (SMA) into national attention, igniting a conversation that had been long stymied by abortion rights supporters' overinvestment in medicalization as the means for protecting and securing abortion rights. This chapter explores how *Dobbs* reinvigorated the potential of medication abortion to radically reconfigure abortion meaning and access in the United States, illustrating how *Dobbs* fostered a reimagining of practices in ways that more fully serve the diverse preferences and needs of abortion seekers.

FDA Approval and the Immediate Blunting of the Promise of the Abortion Pill

A *Time* magazine cover in June 1993 showed a woman holding up a pill that it boldly declared to be "The Pill That Changes Everything" (Heisler 1993). The pill in question, RU-486, was made by the French pharmaceutical company Roussel Uclaf, and it had been approved in France in 1988 as an abortifacient for pregnancies up through forty-nine days (seven weeks). After the drug company succumbed to U.S.-based anti-abortion intimidation and announced that it would not manufacture the drug, the French health minister declared RU-486 to be the "moral property of women" (Charo 1991) and threatened to seize the drug's patent if Roussel Uclaf refused to produce it. The company reversed its position and agreed to manufacture the drug but only for French women.

Across the Atlantic, with the prospect of abortion by pill, U.S. abortion rights activists envisioned a way to resolve the abortion culture wars wherein anti-abortion activists had been directly, violently targeting the facilities that offered abortion care and the doctors who were known to perform abortions (Blanchard 1994; Wilson 2013). By the mid 1990s, nationally there were fewer than 900 outpatient clinics offering abortion care, and over 90 percent of all U.S. abortions were performed in those facilities (Henshaw 1998). Lawrence Lader, the founding chair of NARAL, the nation's largest abortion-related social movement organization,[2] declared the importance of the drug in the title of his 1991 book: *RU 486: The Pill That Could End the Abortion Wars and Why American Women Don't Have It*. Feminists advocating for the drug's approval lauded its potential to be dispensed by any women's health care provider, thus allowing women to avoid abortion clinics and to use the drug discreetly (Joffe and Weitz 2003).

Because the drug was used early in pregnancy, advocates for its widespread availability further argued that it would defang the anti-abortion movement's focus on graphic images of fetuses (typically depicting pregnancies at more advanced gestational ages) and even potentially blur the distinction between abortion and contraception (Jackman 2002; Lader 1995). Supporters of RU-486 hoped that abortions could move out of abortion clinics, and the public nature of the abortion conflict would be eliminated as a result (Talbot 1999).

Perhaps because they understood the potential of a pill to end a pregnancy, or simply because they opposed all efforts to expand abortion options, anti-abortion activists vehemently opposed FDA approval of the drug. Using their influence over the federal executive branch under President George H. W. Bush, anti-abortion advocates secured an importation ban on the drug (Haussman 2013). It would take the election of a pro-choice president (Bill Clinton in 1992) and the transfer of the U.S. patent rights from Roussel Uclaf to a nonprofit organization, the Population Council, to officially move the FDA to consider the drug's approval under the compound name mifepristone.

However, many roadblocks to FDA approval of mifepristone remained, including the need for U.S.-specific clinical trials. Based on those studies, the FDA gave tentative approval to mifepristone in September 1996, finding the drug safe and effective. Because the FDA had already approved misoprostol for other nonabortion uses, only mifepristone needed to be specifically approved for medication abortion to become available. The remaining steps to approval of mifepristone centered around "manufacturing and labeling issues," but overcoming these last hurdles would take four years and require feats unusual for pharmaceutical trajectories (Joffe and Weitz 2003). First, although the Population Council retained the rights to the drug patent, they still needed to secure a pharmaceutical company that would agree to manufacture the drug. Fearing anti-abortion targeting, no existing U.S. companies were willing. Eventually a new company, Danco Inc., was created to produce and market mifepristone in the United States. Establishing a manufacturing site, creating and testing labels, and completing all the final steps eventually yielded final approval by the FDA in September 2000.

The result of this ten-year battle was unsatisfying to both sides. Abortion opponents were unhappy with the approval. Abortion supporters were unhappy with constraints on mifepristone's approved use that created meaningful barriers to mainstream adoption of the drug. Of the many restrictions, the most inhibiting was the requirement that physicians register as certified prescribers and dispense the medication directly to patients—so it could not be dispensed via pharmacies (Joffe and Weitz 2003). Thus, for the first twenty years of its use in the United States, medication abortion was only offered within the confines of the very structure—the stand-alone abortion-providing clinic—the early advocates had hoped the drug would make irrelevant.

THE MOMENTUM TO KEEP DIFFUSION CONTAINED

Abortion care is a business, and a tough one to keep financially solvent. At the time of mifepristone's approval in 2000, the majority of abortion patients were low-income (Jones, Darroch, and Henshaw 2002), and federal law prohibited these individuals from using their public insurance (Medicaid) to pay for abortion care (Fried 2007). Research had demonstrated that the inability to pay for an abortion due to Medicaid restrictions significantly impacted abortion seekers' ability to obtain a desired abortion (Cook et al. 1999). Further, although some states did use state funds to cover abortions for residents using public insurance, the reimbursement rates for care were significantly lower than the cost of providing that care (Dennis and Blanchard 2013). Consequently, the financial survival of abortion-providing clinics necessitated sustaining a high volume of patients served per facility allowing better economies of scale.

But by 2000 the number of annual abortions was dramatically declining. After peaking in 1990 at 1.6 million, the number of abortions had dropped to 1.3 million in 2000, representing a 20 percent decline in patient volume (Jones et al. 2008). The characteristics of the patient population (i.e., majority low-income) meant raising abortion prices was an untenable solution, and in the case of Medicaid payment not impactful. The inability to offset revenue declines threatened the survival of the existing facilities (Kolata 2000).

Given this background, there was little incentive for the abortion advocacy community to prioritize the diffusion of medication abortion beyond the existing abortion providers. By this time in the trajectory of the pro-choice movement, feminist activists and abortion providers had aligned their interests (Joffe, Weitz, and Stacey 2004). Protecting abortion clinics' survival had become synonymous with protecting abortion rights (McCaffrey and Keys 2000). These efforts were bolstered by anti-abortion activists' threats to physicians who were not currently abortion providers. For example, during the early efforts to stop mifepristone's diffusion, anti-abortion extremist Joseph Scheidler, author of *Closed: 99 Ways to Stop Abortion*, warned in the press, "We will probably know which physicians are dispensing it. . . . We'll send in women to ask for RU 486. . . . We'll go to [providing doctors'] homes, to their offices, to their hospitals" (Van Biema 1993). Ultimately, internal pro-choice movement pressure to prioritize abortion clinics and external pressure by the antiabortion movement through threats against prospective prescribers ensured medication abortion's place only within abortion clinics.

The first research study of access to mifepristone confirmed this reality. As of 2007, almost all providers of mifepristone were located close to existing centers of abortion provision (Finer and Wei 2009). Shockingly for the anticipated promise of mifepristone to address geographic-related access barriers, only five mifepristone-only providers who had offered ten or more abortions a year were located farther than fifty miles from any provider of 400 or more abortions that offered procedural abortion.[3] Even more disappointingly, the number of medication abortions done by private physicians' offices actually declined between 2005 and 2008 from 4,800 to 4,000 (accounting for less than 2 percent of all medication abortions) (Jones and Kooistra 2011). It was clear that even though medication abortion was routinely available as an alternative to procedural abortion in abortion clinics, it had not expanded access to abortion outside of that arena of care.

Beyond the business interests and oppositional intimidation, a few features of abortion care delivery added additional constraints on medication abortion diffusion. When mifepristone was approved, abortion services in the United States routinely used ultrasound to determine patient eligibility for medication abortion (to confirm pregnancy and determine gestational duration). One study of abortion practices conducted in 2002 found that over 90 percent of all providers assessed eligibility with ultrasound (O'Connell et al. 2009). Private physicians, especially primary care practitioners, rarely had this technology immediately available in their practice. The contemporary alternative to ultrasound was a series of blood tests that measured changing levels of pregnancy hormones before and after the abortion. Scientists interested in greater use of medication abortion had called for expanded use of this alternative as well as overall simpler protocols (Clark et al. 2007), but ultrasound both before and after medication abortion remained the standard of care. This discouraged the prospective medication abortion providers who did not have readily accessible ultrasound capabilities in their everyday practice setting.

Still, although medication abortion had failed to change the landscape of abortion care delivery, more abortion seekers were beginning to opt for medication abortions. In the first year after FDA approval, only 6 percent of abortions were performed with mifepristone and misoprostol. However, by 2011 that number had risen to 24 percent and by 2017 to 39 percent (Jones and Jerman 2017; Jones, Kirstein, and Philbin 2022). The reasons for this rapid change have not been well studied, but most countries where medication abortion has been formally introduced into the abortion delivery sector have seen similar increased utilization rates by women over time (Popinchalk and Sedgh 2019).

This change in the service-use landscape in turn engendered a shift in the organization of abortion-providing facilities: increasingly they only offered medication abortion. By 2017, 30 percent of the 808 stand-alone facilities providing abortions in the United States exclusively offered medication abortion (Jones, Kirstein, and Philbin 2022). The prioritization of a medication-abortion-only service delivery model for some abortion-providing institutions related to both the greater ease of offering nonprocedural abortion and the availability of philanthropic resources to develop this type of service.

The Limits of the Pro-Choice Imagination
for What Mifepristone Could Do

The containment of medication abortion within the existing highly stigmatized care delivery model (Augustine and Piazza 2022) hampered its potential as a radical challenge to contemporary understandings of abortion. More specifically, when medication abortion was absorbed into the existing model of abortion care, its potential to remake normative understandings of abortion as inherently undesirable (Abrams 2014) went unrealized.

From the beginning, the potential of mifepristone to increase the overall number of abortions in the United States was most evocatively imagined by the anti-abortion movement. When the drug was first discovered, pro-life advocates feared that the ease of taking a pill to end a pregnancy would make abortion easier—physically, psychologically, and emotionally—for women, thereby negating abortion opponents' efforts to socially stigmatize and discourage its use (Ehrlich and Doan 2019). In responding to the 2000 FDA decision to approve mifepristone, anti-abortion leaders focused on how the number of abortions would increase and expressed horror at that possibility. As Texas governor and Republican presidential candidate George W. Bush articulated this sentiment, "I fear that making this abortion pill widespread will make abortions more and more common" (Gottlieb 2000, 854).

Paradoxically, while supporters of mifepristone heralded the appeal of medication abortion to eliminate encounters with protesters, increase points of access, reduce moral conflict due to its earlier use, and give women greater control over the process (Brodie 2002; Kolata 2002; Simonds et al. 1998), they stopped short of suggesting that these benefits might actually lead more people to choose abortion or even slow the ongoing decline in the U.S. abortion rate. Their silence on this possibility—which was raised publicly by abortion opponents on a regular basis—hints that they perceived the claim to be politically and socially destructive. It suggests that the prospect of raising the abortion rate through the expanded availability of medication abortion was so far outside the realm of acceptability as to be unmentionable.

When the news stories and abortion rights advocates at the time did address the possibility of an increased number of abortions, they overtly rejected it. For example, the author of the 1999 *New York Times Magazine* article enumerating the wonders of the drug concluded, "The evidence that it is 'easier' or that it will raise the overall abortion rate isn't especially compelling. . . . In the United States, the incidence of abortion has been falling anyway for a variety of reasons . . . and this trend is unlikely to be reversed" (Talbot 1999, 61). The American Civil Liberties Union's (ACLU) advocacy material about the drug in 2000 staked out this position even more definitively: "MYTH: With mifepristone available, more women will have abortions. FACT: In countries where mifepristone has been available for many years, the overall abortion rate has not increased" (ACLU 2000).

Mifepristone's potential to increase the number of abortions in the United States was also ignored by the scientists publishing on the declining abortion rate in the years after the drug's approval. An article reporting on another 8 percent decline in the abortion rate between 2000 and 2008 included attention to the negative consequences of abortion stigma on the people who have abortions; the intervention offered was greater counseling about pregnancy prevention (Jones and Kavanaugh 2011). Even as it was not being framed as increasing abortions, medication abortion was positively viewed as potentially reversing the declining number of abortion *providers*, a decrease that had made abortion access more challenging (Jones et al. 2008). Within this context, greater access and thus more use was never publicly conceptualized as a response to the declining abortion *rate*. To have done so would have been to remake the meaning of the declining number of abortions in the United States—which at the time was only normatively understood as a good thing (Kaye et al. 2014; *New York Times* Editorial Board 2008).

Rather than calling for greater access to medication abortion as a means of reversing the declining rate of abortions, prominent research organizations tracking and reporting on changes in the national numbers pivoted to calling for more contraceptive access, which theoretically would accelerate the decline (Jones, Darroch, and Henshaw 2002). The U.S. federal government continued its long practice of abortion aversion by examining the outcomes of unintended pregnancies without any attention to abortion (Mosher, Jones, and Abma 2012).

TELEMEDICINE BRINGS NEW PROMISE

Although there was not sufficient pressure to move medication abortion outside the abortion clinic during mifepristone's first two decades of availability, abortion providers were interested in finding ways to offer the service that maximized care delivery efficiency. Beginning in 2008, the Planned Parenthood affiliate in Iowa began experimenting with medication abortion via telemedicine using a site-to-site model. In this model, a person seeking an abortion would go to one clinical location where they would receive counseling and an ultrasound from a non-abortion-providing member of the clinical care team. Then the patient would visit via video with the abortion-providing clinician who was physically located at a second clinical location. The clinician would remotely dispense the medication abortion pills (by entering an electronic code that opened a locked drawer) to be taken by the patient under video observation (Grossman et al. 2011). This model allowed one clinician to serve patients at multiple locations simultaneously, thereby limiting the need to pay clinicians to travel to less populated locations.

However, this model was not necessarily the most efficient for the patients. It still required them to travel to a brick-and-mortar clinical facility and undergo a preabortion ultrasound. Research found these models to be safe and acceptable to patients (Endler et al. 2019; Kohn et al. 2019), with some evidence of decreased time to schedule an appointment and slightly improved access for people who were living in previously geographically unserved areas (Grossman et al. 2013; Kohn et al.

2021). Unfortunately, although the model made more efficient use of the clinicians' time, it required significant financial investment to set up the infrastructure. As such, the price of these services remained identical to the price of in-person medication abortion care. Given its potential to maximize clinician use, the model was adopted by several other abortion providers, but it never became a large part of the provision landscape.

Starting in 2016, an FDA-approved study of telemedicine medication abortion conducted by Gynuity Health Projects iterated on this model. Rather than obtaining the ultrasound and bloodwork at a specified clinic, patients were allowed to seek these services from a willing healthcare facility in their community. Patients transmitted those results to a study physician who conducted a health assessment and counseling over the phone or via video. The pills were then mailed to the patient from the study's physician. Like the site-to-site models, research found this provision method safe and acceptable to patients (Kerestes et al. 2021; Raymond et al. 2019), although one study found that separately performed ultrasounds did lead to a delay in mifepristone initiation when compared to abortion clinic-provided services (Beardsworth et al. 2021).

Although these efforts to offer medication abortion through new pathways afforded some expanded access, they failed to meaningfully transform the overall model for the provision of medication abortion. The abortion seeker still needed multiple preabortion tests, needed to find and interact with one of a limited number of specialty abortion providers, had to pay high out-of-pocket costs, and potentially experienced anti-abortion stigma expressed either by clinic-based protesters (Carroll et al. 2021; Cohen and Joffe 2020) or by sonographers at the outside facility (Hutchens 2021; Mitchell and Georges 2013; Vinekar et al. 2023; Warren et al. 2022). It would take an endogenous shock to the system to finally challenge the idea that preabortion assessment requires a physical clinical encounter.

That shock came in 2020 in the form of the COVID-19 pandemic. Because COVID-19 was respiration-based and highly transmissible, all healthcare providers were forced to reevaluate the need for in-person contact to obtain medical care, especially when contactless options were available. Surprisingly, given their long endorsement of ultrasound as a core component of abortion care, the professional societies that oversee abortion care—including the American College of Obstetricians and Gynecologists (ACOG), the Society of Family Planning, and the National Abortion Federation—quickly endorsed new protocols for the provision of medication abortion through telemedicine without a clinical examination (ACOG 2020; National Abortion Federation 2020; Raymond et al. 2020)

With the constraints removed, for the first time since *Roe* a new type of abortion provider entered the market. These new providers were internet-based, and they only offered medication abortion via telemedicine; the patients did not need to physically present themselves anywhere. Yet despite their innovative structure, these new providers still behaved like the existing abortion providers in ways that were consequential to patients. Namely, they charged fees that were cost prohibitive to low-income abortion seekers, and they reaffirmed that a medical practitioner was required for safe provision of care. Further, the public discourse about these new providers tended to rehash an old story: rather than embrace these new options, the media reports often focused on how these disrupters threatened the financial survivability of traditional brick-and-mortar abortion facilities (Baker 2020; Littlefield 2021). Abortion provision was constructed in the public imagination (and by abortion rights advocates) as a zero-sum game: the rise of one kind of provision necessitated losses for another.

However, more challenging for abortion seekers were the many ways care from these new providers failed to address the needs of those most impacted by structural inequalities. First, none of these new providers accepted Medicaid public insurance (Weitz 2023). Although restricted by federal law, at the time of the market launch of these new abortion providers, sixteen states allowed state resident Medicaid enrollees to pay for abortion that way (Guttmacher Institute 2021). In those states, more than 62 percent of all abortions were covered by state Medicaid (Jones 2024). Prior research had demonstrated that when Medicaid is restricted, between 20 and 25 percent of Medicaid-eligible people do not obtain a desired abortion (Roberts et al. 2019). By not accepting Medicaid, use of the telemedicine medication abortion innovation was restricted to those people willing and able to pay out-of-pocket for care. Second, the states where abortion was least available due to highly restrictive abortion laws also specifically prohibited access to medication abortion via telemedicine (Anderson, Salganicoff, and Sobel 2021). It was in these states that lower abortion rates suggested a greater need for improvements in abortion access (Brown et al. 2020). As a result of both nonacceptance of Medicaid in abortion-supportive states and telemedicine prohibitions in abortion-hostile states, the people most in need of improved access to abortion care were left out of this innovation.

PUSHING TELEMEDICINE EVEN FURTHER

Fortunately for American women, not everyone followed these norms for organizing medication abortion distribution. Running parallel to the U.S.-based expansion of telemedicine was an international telemedicine provider, Aid Access, which began serving U.S. clients in 2018 (Aid Access, n.d.). This service had two significant differences over the U.S. providers, both of which made it appealing to abortion seekers. First, the cost was significantly lower at $150 for the service including the pills, compared with a median cost of $239 for the telemedicine-only providers and $580 for the brick-and-mortar clinics (Upadhyay et al. 2024). Second, Aid Access offered care to residents of states where telemedicine abortion was prohibited under state law. In these ways, Aid Access notably innovated from the model other telemedicine providers offered.

It is worth clarifying that, even with these differences, Aid Access was still fundamentally a telemedicine provider. Reflecting a conflation of legality with clinical involvement, some called using Aid Access "self-managed abortion" (SMA), but this phrase is meant to define the use of medication drugs without the involvement of a clinical provider (Pizzarossa and Skuster 2021). To obtain the medication abortion pills, Aid Access patients did interact with a medical practitioner—just not one licensed to provide this particular care in the U.S. state where the patient was being served. Ironically, U.S. licensed health care providers were often the people behind the Aid Access service, just operating outside the scope of their U.S. license (e.g., providing care to patients who resided in a different state than they were licensed in or where the care was legally prohibited). This convolution perhaps explains some of why Aid Access services were not as controversial to abortion advocates and physicians (Kerestes et al. 2019) as when patients simply ordered the pills on the internet from a pharmacy in India—a means to obtain abortion pills that was typically effective, safe, and much less expensive (Calkin 2023). The patients, however, understood what Aid Access was. In a qualitative study, users described Aid Access as a "godsend" and preferred this service over traveling to a clinic because of the clinic wait times, cost, and logistical issues, and they also highlighted how the delivery model involved a personal touch, good customer service, and a *prescription from a physician* (Madera et al. 2022). Thus, this model of care, while an important innovation, was still clearly tethered to the normative model of clinician-overseen abortion care.

Demand for Aid Access services grew quickly at the onset of the COVID-19 pandemic when abortion seekers (and, really, everyone) feared face-to-face contact. One study documented a 27 percent increase in overall demand between March 20 and April 11, 2020 (Aiken et al. 2020) when COVID-19 cases first began skyrocketing in the United States. Anti-abortion state governments also took advantage of the pandemic to hinder access to abortion, calling it "elective" care, for example, and requiring abortion providers to cease offering services (Carson and Carter 2023). Abortion seekers themselves responded by pursuing care that was not based in a clinic. Demand for Aid Access services was greater from residents of states whose government actively used the pandemic as a means to shut down abortion services. For example, in Texas an executive order prohibited most abortions for thirty days in 2020 under the justification that abortions were not essential health care. The result was the number of in-state abortions declined precipitously (White et al. 2021), accompanied by a significant increase in abortion seekers traveling hundreds of miles out of state to obtain abortions (Sierra et al. 2023). Concurrently, Aid Access saw a 94 percent increase in requests from Texas residents (Aiken et al. 2020). However, even states without governmental abortion hostility but with extensive COVID-19 protections saw significant increases; for example, requests from Massachusetts residents to Aid Access increased 65 percent (Aiken et al. 2020).

While Aid Access's service met the needs of many people, it was not a panacea. Abortion seekers experienced a time delay in receiving their medications, which could be problematic. Because the service operated outside the U.S. healthcare system—a pharmacy in India filled the prescriptions—it usually took three weeks for the medications to be received by the U.S. client (Madera et al. 2022). The mailing of medications was also disrupted briefly during the pandemic (Aiken et al. 2022), revealing the limitations of relying on extranational suppliers.

Initially, the Aid Access model effectively made it a rogue provider of care, but that changed over time. In the aftermath of the *Dobbs* decision, Aid Access was reintegrated into the formal U.S. health system through the passage of a particular type of state shield law. In general, shield laws ensure protection for providing abortion care that is legal within a state to a resident of a state where abortion is banned (Cohen et al. 2023). Eight states, including California, Colorado, Maine, Massachusetts, New York, Rhode Island, Vermont, and Washington explicitly extend this protection to telemedicine services, protecting care that is being provided by a clinician located and licensed in the state where they are operating regardless of where the patient is located (Reproductive Health Initiative for Telehealth Equity and Solutions 2024). Clinicians in states with broad shield laws began to provide telemedicine medication abortion services to people residing in states where abortion is banned. These shield laws and the U.S.-based providers who leveraged them to provide telemedicine medication abortion to any U.S. patient represented a phenomenal act of resistance against abortion bans. Beginning in July 2023, the national abortion-use documentation project known as #WeCount (see the Jenny O'Donnell's chapter in this volume for more on this project) recognized abortions obtained from shield law telemedicine abortion providers as having been provided within the formal health care system. Correspondingly the monthly number of abortions counted as provided by legally sanctioned U.S. telemedicine providers rose from approximately 7,000 to 14,000 from June to September 2023 (Society of Family Planning 2024). By mid-2024, telehealth medication abortions (provided by the newer and existing providers of the service) comprised 17 percent of all U.S. abortions performed by the formal health care system. This growth is remarkable and important, but the Aid Access and other shield law providers' telemedicine model nonetheless left intact the idea that abortion necessitates interacting with a licensed healthcare provider.

ACCEPTING SELF-MANAGED ABORTION OUTSIDE THE FORMAL HEALTH CARE SYSTEM

As abortion in the United States continued to center the role of the clinician, the global trajectory of SMA was evolving. In 2020, in recognition of the strength of clinical outcomes studies, the World Health Organization endorsed the use of SMA medication abortion without the involvement of a health care provider up through 12 weeks of pregnancy (WHO 2022b).

In the United States, activists dedicated to disseminating information about how to access medication abortion pills launched websites and on-the-ground campaigns to raise the visibility of using mifepristone and misoprostol or misoprostol alone independent of the formal healthcare system. In April 2023, 10 months after *Dobbs*, a front-page story in the *New York Times* presented the many ways people in states with abortion bans could access pills beyond the use of Aid Access, including ordering directly from an Indian pharmacy or using a community distributor (McCann 2023). Community distributors include individual activists who obtain and distribute medications within a confined geography. The term also refers to formal programs such as Self-Managed Abortion Safe and Secure (SASS) that systematically train volunteers to support people using self-sourced medications for abortion (SASS, n.d.) and feminist accompaniment models (modeled on networks in Latin America) that support people through the abortion process (McReynolds-Pérez et al. 2023). These community-focused efforts have organized networks of suppliers, distributors, and supporters of information and medicines. In a historical twist of irony, the largest of these community distributors, Las Libres, originally was founded to serve abortion seekers in Mexico when abortion was illegal and/or inaccessible there; now that abortion has been decriminalized in Mexico but rendered illegal in some U.S. states, Las Libres has been offering that same service on the other side of the border between the countries. All these entities might identify as "abortion providers," reflecting a shared identity that is no longer restricted to those with professional clinical licensure or working in a formal health care setting.

Early evidence suggests that these new alternative models of care are being utilized. A study of the provision of medication abortion via some of these alternative options found increased use after the *Dobbs* decision. From July to December 2022, over 18,000 people received care from a community network, and another 4,000 people were served by an international online vendor of medication abortion (Aiken et al. 2024). To date, there is no evidence that such widespread practices are resulting in medical harm. Rather, it is likely that these practices are safe, which is consistent with the robust evidence from around the world on the use of medication abortion outside formal health care settings (Akinyemi et al. 2022; Foster, Arnott, and Hobstetter 2017; Jacobson et al. 2024; Kapp et al. 2023; Moseson et al. 2022).

As further evidence of the perhaps begrudging acceptance of SMA as a practical means to end a pregnancy, the health care abortion provider Planned Parenthood, which had long been resistant to SMA as an option for people, added information on the practice to its website in 2023 (Marcela@Planned Parenthood 2023). Additionally, in 2023 guidance for physicians on how to positively engage with the issue of SMA with medications was released from key U.S. physician leaders (Verma and Grossman 2023). Finally, professional organizations, while falling short of encouraging this option, have stood collectively against criminalizing the practice or legally reporting patients whom they suspect of performing their own abortions (ACOG 2022; Verma and Grossman 2023).

LEVERAGING THE MOMENT TO RECONCEPTUALIZE ABORTION

This book asks the reader to examine not only what harm *Dobbs* did, but what possibilities it opened up that had been foreclosed by the *Roe* regime. Toward this challenge, I posit that the slow progression away from highly medicalized medication abortion was accelerated by two major events: the COVID-19 pandemic, which eliminated the belief that the in-person clinical encounter was required, and the *Dobbs* decision, which forced a reckoning with the necessity of new ways to access abortion. However, the transition yet to be made, but now afforded by this moment, is the reconceptualization of abortion as an autonomous act separate and distinct from both clinical approval and legal sanction (Braine 2020). The fall of *Roe* forced—or has the potential to inspire—abortion rights advocates to move beyond pro-choice activists' acceptance of abortion under specific conditions (i.e., clinician supervised and legally allowed). Abortion is better conceptualized as an autonomous *decision*—one that is not served by health care control nor legal involvement.

Legal scholars have highlighted the many ways in which the *Roe* decision privileged the rights of physicians over the rights of women (Abrams 2013). Further, when it specified that the government had a legitimate interest in developing fetal life, states were allowed to prohibit abortion after the point of "potential fetal viability" (approximately the end the second trimester). Physicians were initially given the authority to determine what constituted viability under the threat of criminal sanction for violation of state laws (*Colautti v. Franklin*),[4] but they abdicated discretion in favor of concretized gestational age limits for abortion care (Kimport and Weitz 2024). The result was that these limits worked as de facto bans on abortion care later in pregnancy.

The legitimation of the state's interest in potential life and the location of that understanding within systems of carceral control had negative consequences for all pregnancies, especially those of the populations marginalized by racism (Goodwin 2020; Kaplan 2023). An analysis of the arrest records of people prosecuted while pregnant shows that the state's interest in fetal life, as articulated in *Roe*, can be used to incarcerate or punish women for drug use while pregnant or to force women to have an unwanted cesarean delivery (Paltrow and Flavin 2013). Neither of these outcomes are abortion related, but abortion law has made them legal. The *Roe* framework, in practice, has allowed medicine in combination with criminal law to decide who can have an abortion and what the consequences will be for anyone whose behavior while pregnant is outside normative standards. Because of structural oppressions, these outcomes have been more negative for women of color. Yet despite a growing understanding of the negative externalities of *Roe*, replacing that regime seemed too risky for the U.S. pro-choice movement that had come to see "saving *Roe*" as its priority (Staggenborg 1995).

Taking a positive view, when *Dobbs* dislodged *Roe* in 2022 it opened up a space to imagine a future beyond *Roe* that could center the needs and preferences of people who seek to abort their pregnancy. But what does that mean? Let's start with what it does not mean. It does not mean recodifying physician authority over abortion. Such a dislocation of the importance of physicians may seem antithetical to the long-standing pro-choice argument that abortion is "routine health care." Proponents of this healthcare framing believe that it helps to secure the legitimacy of abortion (Lindgren 2012). Further, they believe that the authority power of physicians can destigmatize abortion by separating it from ideological debates (Manian 2024). Studies of abortion attitudes have demonstrated the success of this approach:

some people report abortion being more socially acceptable because it is provided by a physician (Becker et al. 2024).

But one can conceptualize abortion as health care without understanding control over abortion as exclusively (or even primarily) the purview of the formal medical system. This is already the case for other health issues. For example, a person with allergies might first try an over-the-counter medication or an alternative intervention like bee pollen or nasal flushing. Should those prove inadequate, the individual might then seek care from a primary care provider and eventually a specialist if still unsatisfied with the results. Or a person may start with the specialist. In any of these cases, health insurance is expected to cover the care trajectory opted for. What is most instructive from this analogy is that none of these pathways is mandated by law—nor criminalized when it is (not) pursued. The management of pregnancy trajectories should be afforded the same possibilities. Abortion drugs as over-the-counter medication or alternative interventions like herbs should be routinely available. Abortion care from primary care or specialists should also be available and should be covered by insurance. And at no stage should the options be mandated or criminalized in law.

Although *Dobbs* enabled state abortion bans that have caused acute harm, in overturning *Roe* it also created a blank slate on which abortion can be reimagined. As was its initial promise, medication abortion holds the potential to radically reconfigure the meaning of abortion in the United States: assessing and determining the outcome of a pregnancy can be solely the domain of the pregnant person. It could, therefore, actually "change everything." As a safe and easy-to-use option for pregnancy termination now released from the yoke of *Roe*, medication abortion has the potential to realize the promise set forth by feminists of the 1960s in their claim for the liberation of abortion: abortions on demand and without apology (Baehr 1990). Medication abortion can help create a future in which the desire to become unpregnant only involves others when the pregnant person chooses. It opens up the possibility of envisioning not the reinstatement of *Roe* but the abolition of all abortion laws, fully severing pregnancy decision-making from what has been termed the "medico-legal paradigm" (Assis and Erdman 2022). When abortion is freed from medical and legal control, it can be rightsized in the larger struggle for reproductive justice, which calls for the human right to maintain personal bodily autonomy, to have children, not have children, and parent children in safe and sustainable communities, and which itself cannot be separated from the struggles for economic, environmental, and other forms of social justice (Ross et al. 2017).

Positioning abortion as part of a larger liberatory agenda affords one more possibility related to the micro-realm of medication abortion: the ability to examine the number of abortions with new clarity. As noted earlier in this chapter, early advocates for medication abortion could not conceptualize it as raising the abortion rate. Yet today, in the wake of *Dobbs*, abortion numbers are on the rise, and likely it is due to more use of medication abortion both inside and outside the formal health care setting (Aiken et al. 2024; Society of Family Planning 2024). Does this increase reflect that it is now easier to become unpregnant than it was before *Dobbs*? Or does it reflect the constrained existence of people who find themselves pregnant in a country without an adequate social safety net (Matthiesen 2021)? Both are likely true. The struggle for reproductive justice, in which a liberatory framework for abortion is embedded, conceptually allows for the dual pursuit of more abortions and less social inequality—a goal pursued together when reproduction is untethered from the control of and meaning-making by medicine and law.

NOTES

1. Medication abortion differs from emergency contraception (EC). Medication abortion disrupts an established pregnancy, but the goal of EC is to act before the implantation of a fertilized egg, which is necessary to establish a pregnancy. The U.S. over-the-counter option for EC uses a progestin drug and cannot disrupt an established pregnancy. Another drug used for EC, ulipristal acetate (UP), is being tested for use in medication abortion, but the dosage is different, and UP has not been approved for that use by the U.S. Food and Drug Administration. By contrast, mifepristone is being studied as an EC option but is not approved in the United States for that purpose.

2. The organization that used the NARAL acronym underwent several name transitions. Originally founded as the National Association for the Repeal of Abortion Laws in 1969, it changed its name in 1973 after the *Roe* decision to the National Abortion Rights Action League. It again renamed itself in 1993 to the National Abortion and Reproductive Rights Action League and in 2003 to NARAL Pro-Choice America. In 2023 it formally resigned the NARAL acronym when it adopted the new name Reproductive Freedom for All.

3. Historically referred to as "surgical abortion," the clinical intervention does not involve cutting or suturing, so scholars prefer the phrases aspiration, procedural, or instrumentation abortion (Upadhyay, Coplon, and Atrio 2023; Weitz et al. 2004).

4. Colautti v. Franklin, 439 U.S. 379 (1979).

REFERENCES

Abrams, Paula. 2013. "The Scarlet Letter: The Supreme Court and the Language of Abortion Stigma." *Michigan Journal of Gender and Law* 19 (2): 293–337.

———. 2014. "Abortion Stigma: The Legacy of *Casey*." *Women's Rights Law Reporter* 35 (3/4): 299–328.

Aid Access. n.d. "Who Are We." Accessed February 23, 2025. https://aidaccess.org/en/page /561/who-are-we.

Aiken, Abigail R. A., Jennifer E. Starling, Rebecca Gomperts, Mauricio Tec, James G. Scott, and Catherine E. Aiken. 2020. "Demand for Self-managed Online Telemedicine Abortion in the United States during the Coronavirus Disease 2019 (COVID-19) Pandemic." *Obstetrics & Gynecology* 136 (4): 835–837.

Aiken, Abigail R. A., Jennifer E. Starling, James G. Scott, and Rebecca Gomperts. 2022. "Requests for Self-managed Medication Abortion Provided Using Online Telemedicine in 30 US States before and after the *Dobbs v Jackson Women's Health Organization* Decision." *JAMA* 328 (17): 1768–1770.

Aiken, Abigail R. A., Elisa S. Wells, Rebecca Gomperts, and James G. Scott. 2024. "Provision of Medications for Self-managed Abortion before and after the *Dobbs v Jackson Women's Health Organization* Decision." *JAMA* 331 (18): 1558–1564.

Akinyemi, Akanni, Onikepe Oluwadamilola Owolabi, Temitope Erinfolami, Melissa Stillman, and Akinrinola Bankole. 2022. "Quality of Information Offered to Women by Drug Sellers Providing Medical Abortion in Nigeria: Evidence from Providers and Their Clients." *Frontiers in Global Women's Health* 3: 899662.

American Civil Liberties Union (ACLU). 2000. "Mifepristone (RU-486): Myths and Facts." https://www.aclu.org/documents/mifepristone-ru-486-myths-and-facts.

American College of Obstetricians and Gynecologists (ACOG). 2020. "Medication Abortion Up to 70 Days of Gestation." ACOG Committee on Practice Bulletins—Gynecology and the Society of Family Planning, October 2020. https://www.acog.org/clinical/clinical-guidance /practice-bulletin/articles/2020/10/medication-abortion-up-to-70-days-of-gestation.
———. 2022. "Opposition to the Criminalization of Self-Managed Abortion." July 6, 2022. https://www.acog.org/clinical-information/policy-and-position-statements/position -statements/2022/opposition-to-the-criminalization-of-self-managed-abortion.
Anderson, Emma, Alina Salganicoff, and Laurie Sobel. 2021. "State Restrictions on Telehealth Abortion." KFF, modified December 2, 2021. https://www.kff.org/womens-health -policy/slide/state-restrictions-on-telehealth-abortion/.
Assis, Mariana Prandini, and Joanna N. Erdman. 2022. "Abortion Rights beyond the Medico-Legal Paradigm." *Global Public Health* 17 (10): 2235–2250.
Augustine, Grace L., and Alessandro Piazza. 2022. "Category Evolution under Conditions of Stigma: The Segregation of Abortion Provision into Specialist Clinics in the United States." *Organization Science* 33 (2): 624–649.
Baehr, Ninia. 1990. *Abortion without Apology: A Radical History for the 1990s.* South End Press.
Baker, Carrie N. 2020. "How Telemedicine Startups Are Revolutionizing Abortion Health Care in the U.S." *Ms. Magazine,* November 16, 2020. https://msmagazine.com/2020/11/16 /just-the-pill-choix-carafem-honeybee-health-how-telemedicine-startups-are-revolutioni zing-abortion-health-care-in-the-u-s/.
Beardsworth, Kathleen Marie, Uma Doshi, Elizabeth G. Raymond, and Maureen K. Baldwin. 2021. "Miles and Days until Medical Abortion via TelAbortion versus Clinic in Oregon and Washington, USA." *BMJ Sexual & Reproductive Health* 48 (e1): e38–e43.
Becker, Andréa, M. Antonia Biggs, Chris Ahlbach, Rosalyn Schroeder, and Lori Freedman. 2024. "Medicalization as a Social Good? Lay Perceptions about Self-Managed Abortion, Legality, and Criminality." *SSM-Qualitative Research in Health* 5: 100444.
Blanchard, Dallas A. 1994. *The Anti-abortion Movement and the Rise of the Religious Right: From Polite to Fiery Protest.* Twayne.
Braine, Naomi. 2020. "Autonomous Health Movements: Criminalization, De-medicalization, and Community-based Direct Action." *Health and Human Rights* 22 (2): 85–97.
Brodie, Janet Farrell. 2002. "Mifepristone in the Context of American Abortion History." *Women and Politics* 24 (3): 101–119.
Brown, Benjamin P., Luciana E. Hebert, Melissa Gilliam, and Robert Kaestner. 2020. "Association of Highly Restrictive State Abortion Policies with Abortion Rates, 2000–2014." *JAMA Network Open* 3 (11): e2024610.
Calkin, Sydney. 2023. *Abortion Pills Go Global: Reproductive Freedom across Borders.* University of California Press.
Carroll, Erin, Klaira Lerma, Alexandra McBrayer, Teairra Evans, Sacheen Nathan, and Kari White. 2021. "Abortion Patient Experiences with Protestors While Accessing Care in Mississippi." *Sexuality Research and Social Policy* 19: 886–893.
Carson, Saphronia, and Shannon K. Carter. 2023. "Abortion as a Public Health Risk in COVID-19 Antiabortion Legislation." *Journal of Health Politics, Policy and Law* 48 (4): 545–568.
Charo, R. Alta. 1991. "A Political History of RU-486." In *Bio-Medical Politics,* edited by Kathi E. Hanna, 44–93. National Academies Press. https://www.ncbi.nlm.nih.gov/books/NBK234199/.
Clark, Wesley H., Marji Gold, Daniel Grossman, and Beverly Winikoff. 2007. "Can Mifepristone Medical Abortion Be Simplified? A Review of the Evidence and Questions for Future Research." *Contraception* 75 (4): 245–250.
Cohen, David S., Greer Donley, Rachel Rebouché, and Isabelle Aubrun. 2023. "Understanding Shield Laws." *Journal of Law, Medicine & Ethics* 51 (3): 584–591.
Cohen, David S., and Carole Joffe. 2020. *Obstacle Course: The Everyday Struggle to get an Abortion in America.* University of California Press.
Cook, Philip J., Allan M. Parnell, Michael J. Moore, and Deanna Pagnini. 1999. "The Effects of Short-term Variation in Abortion Funding on Pregnancy Outcomes." *Journal of Health Economics* 18 (2): 241–257.

Dennis, Amanda, and Kelly Blanchard. 2013. "Abortion Providers' Experiences with Medicaid Abortion Coverage Policies: A Qualitative Multistate Study." *Health Services Research* 48 (1): 236–252.

Ehrlich, J. Shoshanna, and Alesha E. Doan. 2019. *Abortion Regret: The New Attack on Reproductive Freedom*. Bloomsbury USA.

Endler, Margit, Antonella Lavelanet, Amanda Cleeve, Bela Ganatra, Rebecca Gomperts, and Kristina Gemzell-Danielsson. 2019. "Telemedicine for Medical Abortion: A Systematic Review." *BJOG* 126 (9): 1094–1102.

Finer, Lawrence B., and Junhow Wei. 2009. "Effect of Mifepristone on Abortion Access in the United States." *Obstetrics & Gynecology* 114 (3): 623–630.

Foster, Angel M., Grady Arnott, and Margaret Hobstetter. 2017. "Community-based Distribution of Misoprostol for Early Abortion: Evaluation of a Program along the Thailand–Burma border." *Contraception* 96 (4): 242–247.

Fried, Marlene. 2007. "Hyde Amendment: The Opening Wedge to Abolish Abortion." *New Politics* 11 (2): 82.

Goodwin, Michele. 2020. *Policing the Womb: Invisible Women and the Criminalization of Motherhood*. Cambridge University Press.

Gottlieb, Scott. 2000. "Abortion Pill Is Approved for Sale in United States." *British Medical Journal* 321 (7265): 854.

Grossman, Daniel, Kate Grindlay, Todd Buchacker, Kathleen Lane, and Kelly Blanchard. 2011. "Effectiveness and Acceptability of Medical Abortion Provided through Telemedicine." *Obstetrics & Gynecology* 118 (2): 296–303.

Grossman, Daniel, Kate Grindlay, Todd Buchacker, Joseph E. Potter, and Carl P. Schmertmann. 2013. "Changes in Service Delivery Patterns after Introduction of Telemedicine Provision of Medical Abortion in Iowa." *American Journal of Public Health* 103 (1): 73–78.

Guttmacher Institute. 2021. "State Funding of Abortion under Medicaid." Guttmacher Institute, July 1, 2021. https://www.guttmacher.org/state-policy/explore/state-funding-abortion-under-medicaid.

Haussman, Melissa. 2013. *Reproductive Rights and the State: Getting the Birth Control, RU-486, Morning-After Pills and the Gardasil Vaccine to the U.S. Market*. Praeger.

Heisler, Gregory. 1993. "The Pill That Changes Everything" cover photo. *Time Magazine*, June 14, 1993. https://content.time.com/time/magazine/0,9263,7601930614,00.html.

Henshaw, Stanley K. 1998. "Abortion Incidence and Services in the United States, 1995–1996." *Family Planning Perspectives* 30 (6): 263–270, 287.

Hutchens, Kendra. 2021. ""Gummy Bears" and "Teddy Grahams": Ultrasounds as Religious Biopower in Crisis Pregnancy Centers." *Social Science & Medicine* 277: 113925.

Jackman, Jennifer. 2002. "Anatomy of a Feminist Victory: Winning the Transfer of RU 486 Patent Rights to the United States, 1988–1994." *Women and Politics* 24 (3): 81–99.

Jacobson, Laura E., Sarah E. Baum, Erin Pearson, Rezwana Chowdhury, Nirali M. Chakraborty, Julia M. Goodman, Caitlin Gerdts, and Blair G. Darney. 2024. "Client-reported Quality of Facility-managed Medication Abortion Compared with Pharmacy-sourced Self-managed Abortion in Bangladesh." *BMJ Sexual & Reproductive Health* 50 (1): 33–42.

Joffe, Carole E., and Tracy A. Weitz. 2003. "Normalizing the Exceptional: Incorporating the "Abortion Pill" into Mainstream Medicine." *Social Science & Medicine* 56 (12): 2353–2366.

Joffe, Carole E., Tracy A. Weitz, and Clare L. Stacey. 2004. "Uneasy Allies: Pro-choice Physicians, Feminist Health Activists and the Struggle for Abortion Rights." *Sociology of Health & Illness* 26 (6): 775–796.

Jones, Rachel K. 2024. "Medicaid's Role in Alleviating Some of the Financial Burden of Abortion: Findings from the 2021–2022 Abortion Patient Survey." *Perspectives on Sexual and Reproductive Health* 56 (3): 244–254.

Jones, Rachel K., Jacqueline E. Darroch, and Stanley K. Henshaw. 2002. "Patterns in the Socioeconomic Characteristics of Women Obtaining Abortions in 2000–2001." *Perspectives on Sexual and Reproductive Health* 34 (5): 226–235.

Jones, Rachel K., and Jenna Jerman. 2017. "Abortion Incidence and Service Availability in the United States, 2014." *Perspectives on Sexual and Reproductive Health* 49 (1): 17–27.

Jones, Rachel K., and Megan L. Kavanaugh. 2011. "Changes in Abortion Rates between 2000 and 2008 and Lifetime Incidence of Abortion." *Obstetrics & Gynecology* 117 (6): 1358–1366.

Jones, Rachel K., Marielle Kirstein, and Jesse Philbin. 2022. "Abortion Incidence and Service Availability in the United States, 2020." *Perspectives on Sexual and Reproductive Health* 54 (4): 128–141.

Jones, Rachel K., and Kathryn Kooistra. 2011. "Abortion Incidence and Access to Services in the United States, 2008." *Perspectives on Sexual and Reproductive Health* 43 (1): 41–50.

Jones, Rachel K., Mia R. S. Zolna, Stanley K. Henshaw, and Lawrence B. Finer. 2008. "Abortion in the United States: incidence and access to services, 2005." *Perspectives on Sexual and Reproductive Health* 40 (1): 6–16.

Kaplan, Sara Clarke. 2023. "After *Roe*: Race, Reproduction, and Life at the Limit of Law." *WSQ: Women's Studies Quarterly* 51 (12): 117–130.

Kapp, Nathalie, Bunsoth Mao, Jamie Menzel, Elisabeth Eckersberger, Vonthanak Saphonn, Tung Rathavy, and Erin Pearson. 2023. "A Prospective, Comparative Study of Clinical Outcomes Following Clinic-based versus Self-use of Medical Abortion." *BMJ Sexual & Reproductive Health* 49 (4): 300–307.

Kaye, Jennifer Appleton Gootman, Alison Stewart Ng, and Cara Finley. 2014. "The Benefits of Birth Control in America: Getting the Facts Straight." National Campaign to Prevent Teen and Unplanned Pregnancy. https://powertodecide.org/sites/default/files/resources/primary-download/benefits-of-birth-control-in-america.pdf.

Kerestes, Courtney A., Rebecca Delafield, Jennifer Elia, Erica Chong, Bliss Kaneshiro, and Reni Soon. 2021. "'It was close enough, but it wasn't close enough': A Qualitative Exploration of the Impact of Direct-to-Patient Telemedicine Abortion on Access to Abortion Care." *Contraception* 104 (1): 67–72.

Kerestes, Courtney A., Colleen K. Stockdale, M. Bridget Zimmerman, and Abbey J. Hardy-Fairbanks. 2019. "Abortion Providers' Experiences and Views on Self-managed Medication Abortion: An Exploratory Study." *Contraception* 100 (2): 160–164.

Kimport, Katrina, and Tracy A. Weitz. 2024. "Regulating Abortion Later in Pregnancy: Fetal-Centric Laws and the Erasure of Women's Subjectivity." *Journal of Health Politics, Policy and Law* 50 (1): 47–68.

Kohn, Julia E., Jennifer L. Snow, Daniel Grossman, Terri-Ann Thompson, Jane W. Seymour, and Hannah R. Simons. 2021. "Introduction of Telemedicine for Medication Abortion: Changes in Service Delivery Patterns in Two US states." *Contraception* 103 (3): 151–156.

Kohn, Julia E., Jennifer L. Snow, Hannah R. Simons, Jane W. Seymour, Terri-Ann Thompson, and Daniel Grossman. 2019. "Medication Abortion Provided through Telemedicine in Four US States." *Obstetrics & Gynecology* 134 (2): 343–350.

Kolata, Gina. 2000. "As Abortions Rate Decreases, Clinics Compete for Patients." *The New York Times*, December 30, 2000, A1, A13. https://www.nytimes.com/2000/12/30/us/as-abortion-rate-decreases-clinics-compete-for-patients.html.

———. 2002. "Abortion Pill Slow to Win Users among Women and Their Doctors." *New York Times*, September 25, 2002, A1. https://www.nytimes.com/2002/09/25/us/abortion-pill-slow-to-win-users-among-women-and-their-doctors.html.

Lader, Lawrence. 1991. *RU 486: The Pill That Could End the Abortion Wars and Why American Women Don't Have It*. Addison-Wesley.

———. 1995. *A Private Matter: RU 486 and the Abortion Crisis*. Prometheus Books.

Lindgren, Yvonne. 2012. "The Rhetoric of Choice: Restoring Healthcare to the Abortion Right." *Hastings Law Journal* 64: 385–422.

Littlefield, Amy. 2021. "Telemedicine Abortions Offer Cheaper Options but May Also Undermine Critical Clinics." *KFF Health News*, September 3, 2021. https://kffhealthnews.org/news/article/telemedicine-abortions-offer-cheaper-options-but-may-also-undermine-critical-clinics/.

Madera, Melissa, Dana M. Johnson, Kathleen Broussard, Luisa Alejandra Tello-Pérez, Carol-Armelle Ze-Noah, Aleta Baldwin, Rebecca Gomperts, and Abigail R. A. Aiken. 2022. "Experiences Seeking, Sourcing, and Using Abortion Pills at Home in the United States through an Online Telemedicine Service." *SSM-Qualitative Research in Health* 2: 100075.

Manian, Maya. 2024. "A Health Justice Approach to Abortion." *Health Matrix* 34: 261.

Marcela@Planned Parenthood. 2023. "Let's Talk about Self-managed Abortion." Planned Parenthood Federation of American, July 11, 2023. https://www.plannedparenthood.org /blog/lets-talk-about-self-managed-abortion.

Matthiesen, Sara. 2021. *Reproduction Reconceived: Family Making and the Limits of Choice after Roe v. Wade.* University of California Press.

McCaffrey, Dawn, and Jennifer Keys. 2000. "Competitive Framing Processes in the Abortion Debate: Polarization-Vilification, Frame Saving, and Frame Debunking." *Sociological Quarterly* 41 (1): 41–61.

McCann, Allison. 2023. "Inside the Online Market for Overseas Abortion Pills." *New York Times*, April 14, 2023. https://www.nytimes.com/interactive/2023/04/13/us/abortion-pill -order-online-mifepristone.html.

McReynolds-Pérez, Julia, Katrina Kimport, Chiara Bercu, Carolina Cisternas, Emily Wilkinson Salamea, Ruth Zurbriggen, and Heidi Moseson. 2023. "Ethics of Care Born in Intersectional Praxis: A Feminist Abortion Accompaniment Model." *Signs: Journal of Women in Culture and Society* 49 (1): 63–87.

Mitchell, Lisa M., and Eugenia Georges. 2013. "Baby's First Picture: The Cyborg Fetus of Ultrasound Imaging." In *Cyborg Babies: From Techno-Sex to Techno-Tots*, edited by Lisa M. Mitchell and Eugenia Georges, 105–124. Routledge.

Moseson, Heidi, Ruvani Jayaweera, Ijeoma Egwuatu, Belén Grosso, Ika Ayu Kristianingrum, Sybil Nmezi, Ruth Zurbriggen, Relebohile Motana, Chiara Bercu, and Sofía Carbone. 2022. "Effectiveness of Self-managed Medication Abortion with Accompaniment Support in Argentina and Nigeria (SAFE): A Prospective, Observational Cohort Study and Non-inferiority Analysis with Historical Controls." *Lancet Global Health* 10 (1): e105–e113.

Mosher, William D., Jo Jones, and Joyce C. Abma. 2012. "Intended and Unintended Births in the United States; 1982–2010." *National Health Statistics Reports* 55: 1–28.

National Abortion Federation. 2020. "Clinical Policy Guidelines for Abortion Care." National Abortion Federation (Washington, DC). https://prochoice.org/wp-content /uploads/2020_CPGs.pdf.

New York Times Editorial Board. 2008. "Behind the Abortion Decline." *New York Times*, January 26, 2008, A16. https://www.nytimes.com/2008/01/26/opinion/26sat2.html.

O'Connell, Katharine, Heidi E. Jones, Melissa Simon, Vicki Saporta, Maureen Paul, and E. Steve Lichtenberg. 2009. "First-Trimester Surgical Abortion Practices: A Survey of National Abortion Federation Members." *Contraception* 79 (5): 385–392.

Paltrow, Lynn M., and Jeanne Flavin. 2013. "Arrests of and Forced Interventions on Pregnant Women in the United States, 1973–2005: Implications for Women's Legal Status and Public Health." *Journal of Health Politics, Policy and Law* 38 (2): 299–343.

Pizzarossa, Lucía Berro, and Patty Skuster. 2021. "Toward Human Rights and Evidence-based Legal Frameworks for (Self-managed) Abortion: A Review of the Last Decade of Legal Reform." *Health and Human Rights* 23 (1): 199.

Popinchalk, Anna, and Gilda Sedgh. 2019. "Trends in the Method and Gestational Age of Abortion in High-income Countries." *BMJ Sexual & Reproductive Health* 45 (2): 95–103.

Raymond, Elizabeth G., Erica Chong, Beverly Winikoff, Ingrida Platais, Meighan Mary, Tatyana Lotarevich, Philicia W Castillo, Bliss Kaneshiro, Mary Tschann, and Tiana Fontanilla. 2019. "TelAbortion: Evaluation of a Direct to Patient Telemedicine Abortion Service in the United States." *Contraception* 100 (3): 173–177.

Raymond, Elizabeth G., Daniel Grossman, Alice Mark, Ushma D. Upadhyay, Gillian Dean, Mitchell D. Creinin, Leah Coplon, Jamila Perritt, Jessica M. Atrio, and DeShawn Taylor. 2020. "Commentary: No-Test Medication Abortion: A Sample Protocol for Increasing Access during a Pandemic and Beyond." *Contraception* 101 (6): 361–366.

Raymond, Elizabeth G., Alice Mark, Daniel Grossman, Anitra Beasley, Kristyn Brandi, Jen Castle, Mitchell D. Creinin, Caitlin Gerdts, Laura Gil, and Melissa Grant. 2023. "Medication Abortion with Misoprostol-Only: A Sample Protocol." *Contraception* 121: 109998.

Reproductive Health Initiative for Telehealth Equity and Solutions. 2024. "Map of State Policies Impacting the Provision of TMAB." Reproductive Health Initiative for Telehealth

Equity and Solutions, September 10, 2024. https://static1.squarespace.com/static
    /637e5bcdbfee712c3baf45b8/t/65fdef6cc17bd6699ddd5428/1711140716893/State+Lmpa
    cting+Telehealth+for+Medication+Abortion+Care+Map+Resource.pdf.
Roberts, Sarah C. M., Nicole E. Johns, Valerie Williams, Erin Wingo, and Ushma D. Upad-
    hyay. 2019. "Estimating the Proportion of Medicaid-eligible Pregnant Women in Louisiana
    Who Do Not Get Abortions When Medicaid Does Not Cover Abortion." *BMC Women's
    Health* 19: 78.
Ross, Loretta, Erika Derkas, Whitney Peoples, Lynn Roberts, and Pamela Bridgewater. 2017.
    Radical Reproductive Justice: Foundation, Theory, Practice, Critique. Feminist Press at
    CUNY.
Scheidler, Joseph M. 1985. *Closed: 99 Ways to Stop Abortion.* Tan Books.
Self-Managed Abortion Safe and Secure (SASS). n.d. "About SASS, a Project of Women Help
    Women." Women Help Women. Accessed April 15, 2024. https://abortionpillinfo.org/en
    /about-sass.
Sierra, Gracia, Nancy F. Berglas, Lisa G. Hofler, Daniel Grossman, Sarah C. M. Roberts, and
    Kari White. 2023. "Out-of-State Travel for Abortion among Texas Residents Following an
    Executive Order Suspending In-state Services during the Coronavirus Pandemic." *Interna-
    tional Journal of Environmental Research and Public Health* 20 (4): 3679.
Simonds, Wendy, Charlotte Ellertson, Kimberly Springer, and Beverly Winikoff. 1998.
    "Abortion, Revised: Participants in the U.S. Clinical Trials Evaluate Mifepristone." *Social
    Science & Medicine* 46 (10): 1313–1323.
Society of Family Planning. 2024. "April 2022 to September 2023." *#WeCount Public Report,*
    February 28, 2024. https://societyfp.org/wp-content/uploads/2024/02/SFPWeCountPub-
    licReport_2.28.24.pdf.
Staggenborg, Suzanne. 1995. "The Survival of the Pro-choice Movement." *Journal of Policy
    History* 7 (1): 160–176.
Talbot, Margaret. 1999. "The Little White Bombshell." *New York Times Magazine,* July 11,
    1999, 38–43, 48, 61–63, 66. https://www.nytimes.com/1999/07/11/magazine/the-little-white
    -bombshell.html.
Upadhyay, Ushma D., Leah Coplon, and Jessica M. Atrio. 2023. "Society of Family Planning
    Committee Statement: Abortion Nomenclature." *Contraception* 126: 110094.
Upadhyay, Ushma D., Rosalyn Schroeder, Shelly Kaller, Clara Stewart, and Nancy F. Berglas.
    2024. "Pricing of Medication Abortion in the United States, 2021–2023." *Perspectives on
    Sexual and Reproductive Health* 56 (3): 282–294.
Van Biema, David. 1993. "But Will It End the Abortion Debate? Protesters Will Have a Hard
    Time Finding Targets, but They Won't Give Up." *Time Magazine,* June 14, 1993. https://
    time.com/archive/6723332/but-will-it-end-the-abortion-debate/.
Verma, Nisha, and Daniel Grossman. 2023. "Self-Managed Abortion in the United States."
    Current Obstetrics and Gynecology Reports 12: 70–75.
Vinekar, Kavita, Marian Jarlenski, Leslie Meyn, Beatrice A. Chen, Sharon L. Achilles, Sara
    Tyberg, and Sonya Borrero. 2023. "Early Pregnancy Confirmation Availability at Crisis
    Pregnancy Centers and Abortion Facilities in the United States." *Contraception* 117: 30–35.
Warren, Evangeline, Alexandra Kissling, Alison H. Norris, Priya R. Gursahaney, Danielle
    Bessett, and Maria F. Gallo. 2022. "I felt like I was a bad person . . . which I'm not": Stigma-
    tization in Crisis Pregnancy Centers. *SSM-Qualitative Research in Health* 2: 100059.
Weitz, Tracy A. 2023. "Fixing Medicaid Reimbursements to Provide Access to Telehealth Medi-
    cation Abortion." *Center for American Progress,* June 23, 2023. https://www.americanprogress
    .org/article/fixing-medicaid-reimbursements-to-provide-access-to-telehealth-medication
    -abortion/.
Weitz, Tracy A., Angel Foster, Charlotte Ellertson, Daniel Grossman, and Felicia H. Stewart.
    2004. "Medical" and "Surgical" Abortion: Rethinking the Modifiers." *Contraception* 69 (1):
    77–78.
White, Kari, Bhavik Kumar, Vinita Goyal, Robin Wallace, Sarah C. M. Roberts, and Daniel
    Grossman. 2021. "Changes in Abortion in Texas Following an Executive Order Ban during
    the Coronavirus Pandemic." *JAMA* 325 (7): 691–693.

Wilson, Joshua C. 2013. *The Street Politics of Abortion: Speech, Violence, and America's Culture Wars.* Stanford University Press.

World Health Organization (WHO). 2022a. *Abortion Care Guideline.* Edited by the Human Reproduction Programme: World Health Organization.

———. 2022b. *WHO Recommendations on Self-care Interventions: Self-management of Medical Abortion.* Edited by the Human Reproduction Programme: World Health Organization.

Wu, Limei, Wanchun Xiong, Manman Zeng, Aihua Yan, Ling Song, Meng Chen, Tianqin Wei, Qian Zu, and Jiayin Zhang. 2021. "Different Dosing Intervals of Mifepristone-Misoprostol for Second-Trimester Termination of Pregnancy: A Meta-analysis and Systematic Review." *International Journal of Gynecology & Obstetrics* 154 (2): 195–203.

CHAPTER 9

"We're Living in a Really Alternative Universe Right Now"

THE LIMITS OF PHYSICIANS' CULTURAL AUTHORITY PRE-*DOBBS* AND WHAT THAT MEANS FOR A POST-*DOBBS* WORLD

Danielle Bessett, B. Jessie Hill, Meredith J. Pensak,
and Michelle L. McGowan

> *It is no longer clear whether physicians can intervene to prevent progression to critical scenarios, as is the standard in critical care medicine, or instead, if a physician must withhold evidence-based care until a patient develops an unambiguous emergency with significantly increased morbidity and mortality, such as septic shock and multisystem organ failure.*
> —MacDonald, Gershengorn, and Ashana 2022, emphasis ours

In 2022, doctors Andrea MacDonald and colleagues joined a chorus of concern at the near-total state abortion bans implemented after the *Dobbs* decision. In medical publications and the wider media, patients described being turned away from care while in various conditions of physical hazard, and physicians recounted harrowing scenes in emergency rooms and surgical units as they struggled to interpret the new laws while saving lives (e.g., see Moseley-Morris 2023; Schladen 2022). Many publications acknowledged that such bans prohibited most "ordinary abortions" provided in stand-alone clinics (Watson 2018), but commentators also highlighted how the new bans—some lacking medical exceptions and others with vague parameters for exceptions—constrained hospital-affiliated obstetrician-gynecologists, maternal-fetal medicine specialists, and emergency room physicians. Such doctors typically provide abortion care in more "exceptional," medically complex cases in which the pregnant person's life or health is endangered and/or where problems with the fetus are diagnosed.

As Whitney Arey and Klaira Lerma (in this volume) describe, cases involving medically complex pregnancies are felt to be more "legitimate" abortions, elevating "'medical' reasons for termination that are, in effect, out of a woman's control" (Kimport, Weitz, and Freedman 2016, 513). Public opinion polls commonly show significant support for abortion access required for conditions such as maternal or fetal health or rape (Jozkowski et al. 2023; Pew Research Center 2022, 9). The "stratified legitimacy of abortions," as Katrina Kimport, Tracy Weitz, and Lori Freedman have put it, helps to explain why cases involving medical exceptions garnered headlines in the wake of the *Dobbs* decision: the abortion seekers were usually sympathetic and often socially privileged, and their loss and grief were compounded by the callous treatment from the state. But these media accounts were not only supportive of patients; they also portrayed the injustice of skilled doctors helplessly watching patients suffer, waiting for conditions to worsen and thereby remove any legal doubt regarding the urgent need for their intervention.

For those of us studying, litigating, and providing abortion in the states that heavily restricted abortion before *Dobbs*, confusion about when and how abortion restrictions limit physicians' care in medically complex pregnancies is all too familiar. The fall of *Roe* pushed physicians' constraints onto the front page and, in the process, revealed how the medical profession has struggled to assert its professional authority over what constitutes a medical exception. At the same time, post-*Roe* media coverage has amplified hospital-based physicians' voices and experiences to an unprecedented degree. In this chapter, we describe the logic by which hospital-affiliated physicians who work in abortion-restrictive states tried to assert their authority over abortion in the years leading up to *Dobbs*. When their authority was not assumed, these physicians used various strategies to address the gap between their professional responsibilities and the imposed limits.

PROFESSIONAL AUTHORITY

Physicians are paradigmatic of a professional occupation, which sociologist Andrew Abbott has defined as "exclusive occupational groups applying abstract knowledge to particular cases" (1988, 8). Extensive training and apprenticeship lie at the heart of a profession's claims to exclusivity, and professional authority emanates from the skills and expertise that a member acquires through training and occupational experience (Hirst 1982). Professions must collectively self-govern because outsiders do not possess the requisite specialized technical knowledge (Hughes 1963).

Sociologist Paul Starr applied these insights to medicine, differentiating between the *social* authority and *cultural* authority of physicians. Social authority "involves the control of action through the giving of commands" (1982, 13). By this, Starr means that physicians enact social authority when they issue a prescription, advise a patient on a course of treatment, or oversee the work of other medical staff. By contrast, cultural authority captures the power to define reality, create meaning, and assign value to matters that fall within the profession's competence: "the capacity to judge the experience and needs of clients" (1982, 15). The two forms of authority are distinct, with cultural authority serving as foundation for social authority: the idea is that because physicians are the best judge of patients' medical situations, they alone can determine the best course of action or judge the work of other physicians.

Self-regulation takes a variety of forms in medicine, from professional associations' codes of ethics and practice guidelines to institutional review of a particular case. Starr argues this kind of "occupational control" often functions as a monopoly on medical services, but the control is far from total. For example, state medical boards are an especially important regulatory body, overseeing licensing, interpreting regulations, and disciplining clinicians. In their ideal type, these boards are composed of physicians, but in some states, governors appoint nonphysicians to medical boards, which can threaten medical autonomy with partisan political agendas (Wojcieszak 2021). Sociologists Steven Epstein and Stefan Timmermans (2021) point to the politicization of health expertise as an important challenge to physicians' cultural authority. They observe that while considerable research has examined how state regulation, insurers, pharmaceutical companies, and even patients have impinged on physicians' social authority, scholars have paid much less attention to changes in cultural authority in medicine. They ask "whether medicine as an institution is losing ground in the competitive struggle to frame and interpret medical and social realities—and what social and health costs and opportunities follow from a potential loss of medical cultural authority" (2021, 241).

Abortions, Moral Legitimacy, and Medical Exceptions

To increase their professional authority in the nineteenth century, physicians sought support from the state for their monopoly on the practice of medicine, including by controlling abortion (also see the chapter by Kelly Marie Ward and Barbara A. Alvarez in this volume). As historian Leslie Reagan points out, criminalization of abortion also put physicians further under the purview of the state: "State officials demanded that the profession police the practices of its members. The duty of self-policing and physicians' fears of prosecution for abortion created dilemmas for doctors who at times compromised their duties to patients in order to carry out their duties to the state" (Reagan 1997, 3–4).

Because physicians would control when, how, for whom, and why legal abortions would be performed, they maintained broad discretion over the implementation of the standard exception for preserving the life of the pregnant person. At the turn of the twentieth century, physicians "utilized widely varying definitions of what constituted proper grounds for abortion," including physical and mental health (Halfmann 2011, 8). This discretion was facilitated by professional solidarity, which became most clear as medical care shifted to hospitals (Luker 1984). By the mid-twentieth century, hospital abortion boards, staffed by medical experts, arbitrated which abortions would be performed legally in the formal medical system. Individual physicians certainly performed abortions, both approved and illicit, but without accord with their colleagues, they could not be certain their credentials would protect them from prosecution (Edelin 2007). Ultimately, physicians' liability, coupled with the number of patients seeking formal care after unsafe abortions, contributed to the growing support for legalized abortion in medical circles. During the reforms of the 1960s, organized medicine supported the expansion of grounds for exceptions, which they hoped would balance their autonomy to practice without "removing the necessity of diagnoses" lest doctors become, as the American Medical Association put it, "mere technicians" carrying out women's demands for abortion (Halfmann 2012, 196).

The U.S. Supreme Court decision in *Roe v. Wade* legalized abortion across the United States in 1973. Allowing "abortion on demand" gave pregnant people more say over their care, tempering physician authority. Yet medical exceptions were built into the *Roe v. Wade* decision: states were never allowed to prohibit abortion care necessary to preserve maternal health or life, even as they were allowed to significantly restrict abortion later in pregnancy.[1] Such exceptions centered a physician's cultural authority to determine what was—and was not—necessary care, and *Roe*'s legal privacy framework did not establish an affirmative right for patients to access abortion care. Many physicians largely continued to use their discretion over abortion provision in the decades that followed *Roe*. This discretion contributed to segregation in abortion care such that stand-alone abortion clinics provided most abortions in the United States and clinicians in other settings typically provided care only when there was a "medical indication" (Freedman 2010).

From the beginning, the exception framework proved unreliable. Under the federal Hyde Amendment, first passed in 1976, programs such as Medicaid and the Indian Health Service cannot use federal funds to cover abortion care; these laws include exceptions for cases where there is a threat to the pregnant person's life or in cases of rape or incest (Ranji et al. 2024, 16). Yet research evaluating these laws found that stand-alone abortion clinics were unable to obtain reimbursement from Medicaid in more than half of eligible cases involving rape, incest, and life endangerment in the study period (Kacanek et al. 2010). For decades, the government exerted its authority as payer to arbitrate which claims to funding were legitimate, reserving the right to ignore not only patients' accounts of the circumstances of conception that would justify a rape exception but also abortion providers' expertise when it came to medical conditions endangering patient well-being.

Some states leveraged exceptions in their efforts to reduce access to abortion by restricting the locations where services could be provided. For example, in 2011 the state of Ohio enacted House Bill 153, which prohibited public facilities, such as public and university hospitals, from providing "nontherapeutic abortions," which—echoing many existing exception clauses—they defined as "an abortion that is performed or induced when the life of the mother would not be endangered if the fetus were carried to term or when the pregnancy of the mother was not the result of rape or incest reported to a law enforcement agency."[2]

Physicians have sometimes been complicit with the moral hierarchy that underlies abortion exceptions. Countless reports from before *Roe* document how medical boards favored more privileged women over those against whom they were socially biased. Reflecting on how obstetrician-gynecologists differentiated among reasons for abortion after *Roe*, Kimport, Weitz, and Freedman point out how "the narrative of stratified legitimacy" not only perpetuates the moral hierarchy but also "weakens the claim that abortion care decision making requires medical expertise. This opened the door for legislators and voters who lack medical knowledge to nonetheless claim authority to regulate and restrict abortion through recourse to social knowledge" (2016, 513). Following from this logic, exceptions served as a wedge, framed as sympathetic to those whom public opinion favors while moving decision-making from clinicians and pregnant people to lawmakers.

Ohio's incursion on physician authority preceded the *Dobbs* decision by more than a decade and, as we will show below, prefigured the post-*Dobbs* concerns about operationalizing exceptions. Yet evidence of physician's cultural authority over abortion persisted alongside these prohibitions. For example, Lisa Harris and colleagues (2024) found that doctors speaking publicly about the complexities of providing abortion care could decrease support for abortion restrictions in small but meaningful ways.

How Abortion-Adjacent Physicians Perceived Ohio's Abortion Restrictions

In 2019–2020, prior to *Dobbs*, we conducted focus groups and interviews with thirty-five Ohio obstetrician-gynecologists about their experiences with state abortion regulations. These physicians provided reproductive health care in hospital and clinical settings where abortion was not regularly offered, yet their work inevitably intersected with abortion regulations, albeit with some unpredictability (Czarnecki et al. 2023; Field et al 2022; Gyuras et al 2023).[3] The physicians identified the abortion regulations that generated uncertainty for them in their practice, including a twenty-one-week and six-day gestation ban, a viability ban, and a partially enacted ban on the dilation and evacuation abortion method. The further enacted and proposed state laws that frustrated and bewildered physicians in how they counseled patients and practiced medicine included the ban on provision of nontherapeutic abortion by facilities that receive public funds (as described previously), a ban on state Medicaid funding covering abortion, and proposed requirements about reversing medication abortions and transferring ectopic pregnancies into the uterus. Here we briefly describe how our participants, with near unanimity, perceived these restrictions to be impinging on their cultural authority in the following ways (see also McGowan et al. 2024):

- *Abortion restrictions assert that abortion is different from other kinds of health care.* Abortion restrictions have distinguished abortion from other forms of health care, thus removing it from physicians' sphere of authority.
- *Abortion restrictions do not reflect medical evidence.* Several legal mandates or proposed practice requirements demand actions that are not medically possible, among them "viability" testing, "reversal" of medication abortion, and uterine reimplantation of ectopic pregnancies. Multiple laws have not

been grounded in evidence and thus, for physicians, have constituted unnecessary—and unworkable—interference with their work.

- *Abortion restrictions misunderstand the potential for certainty about morbidity and mortality outcomes.* Abortion regulations have presumed more certainty—in particular, a more definitive assessment of "life-threatening" conditions—than physicians have deemed appropriate in dynamic clinical cases.
- *Abortion restrictions require translation by legal experts.* The mere existence of abortion restrictions often puts distance between physicians and their ability to exercise their professional judgment. The study participants varied considerably in how well-versed they were in the abortion restrictions that influenced their practice; some were very knowledgeable while others had, to quote one participant, "no idea what the laws are." But even those who were quite well-informed about the existing abortion laws recognized that there are limits to their legal knowledge—several participants were emphatic that they were trained in medicine, not law. The institutional legal counsel has been charged with interpreting abortion restrictions for their practice, which has often resulted in more conservative institutional interpretations of state and federal laws and policies than required by law.

In short, the physicians who participated in our research overwhelmingly found these regulations were not grounded in the specialized technical knowledge of their profession. *Contra* the claim by MacDonald and coauthors that opened this chapter, our research shows that abortion exceptions have long been difficult for clinicians to operationalize. In the rest of this chapter, we take up Epstein and Timmerman's charge to interrogate physicians' cultural authority, particularly "the hybrid spaces where health institutions intersect with other arenas, such as the law . . . [where] the viewpoints of health authorities on the nature of social reality may compete with or be advisory to the authoritative claims of other parties that invoke different epistemologies, values, and goals" (2021, 250). We first explore how physicians who worked outside the facilities dedicated to providing abortion have tried to assert cultural authority over abortion; we argue that their logic anticipates the discourse of the post-*Dobbs* period. We then describe how physicians' authority has informed the strategies they employ to provide care in a restrictive setting.

How Physicians Assert Cultural Authority Over Abortion
Abortion Is Health Care

One primary way physicians have asserted cultural authority over abortion has been by defining abortion as health care. In doing so, our research participants tied abortion care to their traditional control over what counts as medicine, in line with what sociologists would consider the scope of physicians' cultural authority. Importantly, our participants treated this framing of abortion as a self-evident truth. For example, reflecting on how clinicians who do not or cannot perform abortions rely on their colleagues who do provide abortion care, our participant Sandy argued, "this is not such a bright line, and also even if you're not personally doing these things, you're referring patients to this. This is still part of medical care."

Because many of our research participants practiced in Ohio's public facilities where "nontherapeutic" abortion was banned or in religiously affiliated healthcare systems that restricted abortion care even further (see the chapter by Lori Freedman in this volume), their examples frequently centered on the medically complex cases that were allowed in their institutions. Nevertheless, they often emphasized the continuity between the care they provided and that of their colleagues in stand-alone clinics, which was evident in Sandy's emphasis on the health care ecosystem of which abortion was a regular, if often segregated, part.

Another way in which physicians asserted their cultural authority over abortion care was by painting abortion as necessary in life-threatening or life-altering conditions in ways that paralleled news stories about medical exceptions to abortion laws. As our participant Dylan asserted, "we've seen cases where this is a life-saving procedure. . . . it's a very important, necessary thing." Reflecting on her hospital's past policy not to terminate pregnancies with serious pregnancy complications in the second trimester, interview participant Judy explained, "the chance of the fetus surviving, you know, not only to delivery but long-term survival, is quite low, whereas the chance of maternal morbidity and even mortality is reasonably high. They can get infected. They can lose their uterus. They can die. I've seen a woman die from that [condition]. Um, and we weren't able to offer termination for it." She later concluded that abortion "is a medical procedure that does not need to be legislated." Physicians repeatedly emphasized that abortion could save lives and consequently was a necessary tool of medical practice.

One physician, Heather, emphasized this point to her colleagues on the state medical board during discussions of efforts to regulate abortion care more than comparable practices: whenever the word "abortion" would have been used, she would swap in "hernia surgery." She reported that her colleagues came to recognize the equivalency: "Now that you've put it that way, this is not an abortion issue, this is an access issue, and we can get on board with access." By asserting that abortion is just "another medical procedure," physicians sought to reclaim their ability to practice without abortion-specific restrictions constraining them.

Invoking Medical Expertise, Education, and Evidence

In a second rhetorical practice, our participants contrasted physician characteristics with lawmakers', asserting that physicians held "the capacity to judge the experience and needs of clients" (Starr 1982, 15) by invoking their training and expertise, their professional experience and judgment, and their relational experiences serving patients, a background the lawmakers did not have. In addition to trying to control the meaning of abortion, our study participants also grounded their claim to oversight of abortion in their own professional knowledge and skill. Charlotte declared, "I have been trained to serve society, and I should do that; to save this woman's life because I have the skills to." Having "skills" meant that she should use them to protect her patients.

Participants such as Pamela frequently emphasized their own medical training and contrasted lawmakers' lack of such: "I think in general policymakers should stay out of my exam room. [Participant Carla laughs.] Like, unless you go to medical school, you don't get to have a say of what happens between me and my patient." Other participants posed rhetorical questions to their focus group such as "Why are people who don't know anything about medicine making these laws?" and "Why are people who don't understand medicine making these laws?" These questions were paired with comments like "ridiculous" and general disparagement of lawmakers' inadequate understanding of medical realities.

Because she had specialized expertise in obstetrics and gynecology, Lynne felt compelled to testify against proposed restrictions at the statehouse as often as she could. In her view, anti-abortion legislators seeking political gains through abortion lawmaking lacked both the motivation to engage with relevant evidence and the necessary expertise to understand the implications of their proposals. She believed that expert advocates, as defined by their medical training and experience, should influence health policy, especially when existing policy conflicted with her ability to provide optimal care to her patients. Lynne concluded with a rueful laugh, "If you as a legislator can pass a bill that has no scientific basis to it . . . then we're living in a really alternative universe right now." For her and many participants, facts and evidence should carry the day, and physicians are the best positioned to arbitrate those facts.

Invoking Professional Medical Judgment

In addition to medical expertise acknowledging abortion as a component of comprehensive reproductive health care, physicians also pointed to the importance of medical judgment when clinical situations were dynamic or uncertain and the outcomes not fully known. There was strong resistance to what the participants perceived as a uniform, universal proscription in abortion law that did not acknowledge nuance, variation among cases, and the resulting need for clinician improvisation. Deb spoke to this collective perception: "There's so many nuances that occur for many different patients and individual clinical scenarios that some of these laws make things a lot more dangerous for patients."

Implicit in these examples was the physician's invocation of professional experience: *they* had managed fluid situations in pregnant patients' care, and thus they had earned the ability to judge the appropriate action for the situation at hand. It was not only that the restrictive laws were wrong, but that they, as physicians, understood the complexities of pregnancy management better than lawmakers.

Authority Grounded in Clinical, Relational Experience

Finally, several physicians centered their relational experiences serving patients—and the legislators' lack thereof—in their claim to authority over abortion:

LEIGH: Unless you're sitting there, face to face with a woman with that decision or a family talking about a lethal fetal anomaly, I just don't think you're equipped to make rules about it.

ANDREA: When I pulled them [nurses and other staff posting online in support of abortion restrictions] aside and explained to them what it meant and how it felt to talk to these women, they finally were like, "Oh, we had no idea." . . . The education for everyone, for the public, and the legislature who isn't used to talking about reproductive issues—they just don't know half the time.

With her emphasis on both "what it meant" (presumably both their interpretation of the laws and its consequences) and "how it felt to talk to these women," Andrea captured both the importance of expertise and engagement with pregnant people as important credentials in claiming authority over abortion care, especially against lawmakers whom physicians saw as being more distant from these interpersonal relationships.

Notably, our participants did not compare or rank the factors they believed entitled them to claim authority over abortion. All the various characteristics they possessed—and interfering legislators lacked—were essential to why the medical profession (and specifically their subspecialty of obstetrics and gynecology) was uniquely prepared for this role. Participants also acknowledged and were sympathetic to people who chose abortion for reasons other than health indications, and they volunteered examples of how state restrictions also put abortion out of reach for those seeking care for "non-medical" reasons, such as economic need. However, it is worth noting that by emphasizing abortion as lifesaving and using medical exceptions as examples to showcase the need for their superior knowledge and experience, these physicians centered the medical exceptions that came up regularly in their own work—and thereby tacitly limited their authority to these types of cases.

CLINICAL STRATEGIES PHYSICIANS EMPLOYED
IN RESPONSE TO ABORTION RESTRICTIONS
Practicing Defensive Medicine

The physicians who participated in our research felt strongly that they should be able to exert their authority over "medically indicated" abortion care but that they often could not do so in practice because of abortion restrictions or conservative institutional interpretations thereof. As a result, three years before the Dobbs decision, the participants in our study described engaging in practices of defensive medicine that have since been reported in so much of the post-Roe abortion news coverage.

The term "defensive medicine" has generally been applied to clinical behavior resulting from concerns of malpractice liability and is especially salient to obstetrics and gynecology as a medical specialty (Morris 2013). Tammy distilled the motivation behind defensive medicine in the following way: "It comes down to knowing the nuances of Ohio law and who is going to stand next to you if you get charged. So you want to know that your lawyers . . . would be able to say, 'Yes, this is defensible in the court that this would go to.' And I hate to say that, but that's where we are right now."

Like Tammy, we extend the term defensive medicine to cover compliance with restrictions because our study participants described altering their clinical practice due to regulations and institutional policies in ways that parallel liability-focused descriptions of defensive medicine. We note that physicians often experienced negligent malpractice and compliance with restrictions as contemporaneous, if opposing, forces. Defensive medicine is often linked to "intervention bias," with the suggestion that liability is more likely to be perceived in inaction than in unsuccessful efforts to resolve a condition (Foy and Filippone 2013). Echoing the observations by Reagan (1997) of doctors' dilemmas before *Roe*, the physicians we interviewed often described abortion restrictions as creating potential for patient harm through inaction, which they experienced as a conflict between regulatory compliance and the ethical standards of their profession (see also Field et al. 2022).

Institutional legal counsel, risk management, ethics committees, and other institutional leaders translated and enforced abortion restrictions. In some cases, uncertainty about the interpretations led to institutional rules that were more restrictive than the laws necessarily required (Czarnecki et al. 2023). Further, institutions rationally favored the risk of civil malpractice liability (for failure to provide care) over that of providing care when criminal liability (for violating abortion restrictions) was at play. Mary said, "You call [counsel] and you feel like you're pleading for someone's life, and then they're just like sitting there, they don't come down and like say, 'Hey, let's talk about this.' They're like, 'No.' . . . It just feels strange to make a phone call for a woman's life and then, and then just get an answer that you just have to obey, and you're like, this is life?" Mary's bewilderment illustrates her inability to exercise authority over her medical practice, even in what she believed were life-and-death circumstances, when her in-house counsel declined to grant permission to provide abortion care.

Examples of defensive medicine volunteered by our study participants evoked fear and worry about the legal consequences of withholding care a doctor knew was required to resolve the problem. As Karen explained, "we had this one patient that was like having like hemorrhaging, but like not quite enough that it was like emergent. . . . So we just like waited till her hemoglobin was like below seven, which is what was considered like more dangerous until you like move forward with the procedure. . . . Everyone knew what they wanted to do, but you couldn't like legally do that." Although these physicians felt they had the requisite skills and expertise about the likely outcome when it came to medical emergencies—the very qualities they asserted made them the appropriate party to have authority over abortion care—they felt unable to enact them in these settings.

By contrast, some participants were able to incorporate legal support into their defensive practices. For example, Lynne worked at a hospital that allowed "medically indicated" abortions. She explained that her institution's legal team respected her and her colleagues' authority to arbitrate which pregnancies fit these criteria: "I would say they've been very much, 'We're going to treat you as professionals; we're going to support you as professionals. Just put the documentation in.' I did not get any sense of 'No, you can't do this.'" Maintaining patient records is a routine part of medical practice; in this sense, the institution was placing little demand on Lynne to practice defensively, and the clinicians could rely on their professional judgment to determine which cases fit within the allowed scope of practice. At the same time, the lawyers' reminder to discharge this routine practice of documentation in relation to abortion also served as a signal to Lynne and her colleagues: they could be called upon to account for their rationale at a future time. The documentation would presumably weigh heavily in retrospectively adjudicating the abortion's acceptability.

Referring to the extensive documentation that institutions use to ensure physician compliance with laws, which includes attending physicians having to review and sign off on each completed form, Jamie exclaimed, "The paperwork is terrifying." In this way, being treated as a professional is not absolute, and the documentation practices are not neutral. Physicians anticipate that their institutions and state actors could interrogate their decisions; the formidable abortion-specific paperwork itself could also function as punishment for abortion providers (Heymann et al. 2023).

An important part of physician authority is positionality as leader of a team with distinct roles and responsibilities. Physicians are responsible for the conduct and outcome of each case and thus are charged with providing direction to nurses and other staff (Starr 1982); physicians typically exert authority not only over what to do but—in their managerial role—over who will do what. As Erin observed, deference to the law can also be a management challenge in an emergency:

> A lot of nurses do not want to be involved in what they perceive as an abortion . . . and you have to work with nurses. I mean, you need instruments; you need medication. I mean, I don't know how to get these things out of the medicine system. I guess I could figure it out, but, and if it's always this delay, . . . instead of that we're doing the thing that's the right thing for the person, [it becomes] how to convince somebody that we're not doing the wrong thing. There's never—it's never easy. It's never safe. It's never efficient. It's never kind of a straightforward thing. It's always a battle of who's interpreting what to be what.

State restrictions have disrupted physicians' social authority over their team members, especially with those who may be reluctant to be associated with abortion.

To be sure, in some cases the physicians were able to leverage their clinical authority to redefine interpretations of cases. Erin explained that, although her institution's legal counsel was conservative when it came to the interpretation of abortion restrictions, "a strong clinical push" from her or her colleagues could sometimes result in being allowed to perform the abortion. Practicing medicine in line with clinical guidelines is not defensive medicine on the part of the physicians, but a strong clinical recommendation push may activate in legal counsel the well-known intervention bias to protect the institution from wrongful death or malpractice claims.

Seeking Support Through Consultations with Other Clinicians, Ethics Committees, Collective Societies, or Clinical Guidelines

Our study participants leveraged medicine's cultural authority by turning to other medical professionals for confirmation of their assessment and planned course of action. In cases such as Ohio's twenty-two-week ban and postviability ban, consultations were required by their institutions or by law. Mary described the typical consultations that were needed to provide an abortion in her institution:

> At our institution, if you decide that a patient needs a termination for some reason like a medical, medically indicated termination, whatever that may be, typically you have two providers confirm that that's what needs to happen. . . . Then we usually talk to the person who's kind of in charge of the labor and delivery unit or the chair of the department, some, some sort of 'higher-ups' situation. And then, you know, if all three agree and it seems fine, then we'll just proceed. But then if there's any questions, we've talked to legal as well. . . . But if you have someone who needs a therapeutic abortion for a medical indication, there's an ethics committee if it's not an emergency.

Physicians at this hospital always had to confirm their decision with at least two departmental colleagues, and nonemergent cases would require additional review. Our participants did not tend to describe the same kind of consternation about their departmental consultations as they did about the lawyers or the ethics boards. This may be because their fellow clinicians shared a common understanding of the situation, even if they disagreed with the approach, or because cases over which there was disagreement were ultimately arbitrated by legal counsel. It also seemed that, due to the uncertain legal landscape, our participants took some comfort in sharing responsibility for abortion decisions with fellow physicians.

Our study participants also described increasingly invoking existing professional society guidance as the legal landscape became more restrictive. As Judy put it in her interview, "We've just had some people who are more vocal about saying this [restriction] isn't in line with what ACOG [American College of Obstetricians and Gynecologists] says. ACOG is kind of our governing board. I don't know how we can say that we're practicing evidence-based medicine, but then be completely against an ACOG recommendation. So people have fought the fight."

Professional society recommendations epitomize collective, cultural authority; by citing these guidelines, the physicians were better able to exert their own authority on institutional and, they hoped, state interpretations. Professional self-regulation, whether voluntary or required, worked best when the physicians received professional support through consultations with other clinicians, professional societies, and clinical guidelines. Engagement with those who did not share the physicians' expertise—such as lawyers—was much more mixed, was frequently unhelpful, and was described as a barrier to evidence-based care.

Indirectly Asserting Their Authority Through Creative Compliance with Institutional and Legal Requirements

Although the study participants were not consistently able to provide abortion care when they believed it was medically necessary (or otherwise), they described instances in which they exerted authority over other dimensions of their practice in ways that facilitated better access to abortion care for their patients. For example, Carla explained that when she felt caught between her institution's legal interpretations and her professional obligations, she chose to compromise on the lesser obligation: "I'm vague in my documentation and just say 'options reviewed' and don't really go into the options or the fact that a referral [for abortion care] was made. I feel like I fulfill my clinical and ethical obligations, but don't necessarily [fulfill] my medical and legal documentation." Carla would have preferred to meet all her obligations, but when she found she was unable to do so, she exercised her professional discretion.

Clinicians with supervisory or leadership positions could also set policies for other clinicians to help facilitate abortion access within the confines of the restrictions. One such interview centered around the anatomy scan ultrasound, which Judy recommended moving from twenty-weeks' gestation to eighteen-weeks' gestation; this would give patients who might discover fetal anomalies more opportunity to receive their results, seek specialized medical expertise, and explore their options before Ohio's ban on abortion after twenty-two weeks applied:

> INTERVIEWER: Your response . . . is responsive to this particular regulation—
> JUDY: That's correct.
> INTERVIEWER:—to try to work within the limits but still use the available technology.
> JUDY: That's exactly it.
> INTERVIEWER: Okay. That's really interesting. So has there been—what kind of reaction was there to you recommending this kind of change?
> JUDY: Not much, honestly. I mean, eighteen weeks is well within the established range of when we can do an anatomy ultrasound. No, some people would be concerned that we are going to have to bring other people back for additional imaging because [we] can't always see what we want to at eighteen weeks.
> INTERVIEWER: Right.
> JUDY: But insurance usually doesn't give us a hassle about that.

Judy was able to exert her authority over the recommended schedule for ultrasound within the evidence-based guidelines, even against one of the commonly described limits on physician authority generally: the ability of doctors to secure payment for services from insurance companies (Skinner 2019). However, she did realize that this discretion could be used by other physicians with opposite intent: "I know that there are providers who will not send patients for detailed anatomy ultrasounds until twenty-one weeks or after, and while I've never asked them, I can almost guarantee that they're doing it to restrict their patients, the availability of abortion for patients."

These examples of physicians working creatively within the law differed from the practice of defensive medicine because here physicians used their authority to try to expand access to abortion care. They recognized that they would frequently be unsuccessful in directly challenging the prohibitions on abortion, but they could exert control over the system of care in other ways to create more flexibility and opportunity. By contrast, when physicians engaged in defensive medicine in relation to abortion restrictions, they typically seemed almost paralyzed by the limits placed on them and the moral distress they experienced (Rivlin et al 2024).

WHAT ABORTION TEACHES US ABOUT PHYSICIAN AUTHORITY

Our research reveals the ambiguous status of physicians' cultural authority when it comes to contested topics like abortion. Abortion care is never structured only by clinical guidelines but must also be responsive to the regulatory environment. While doctors may be effective spokespersons for the legalization of abortion (Harris et al. 2024), medical professionals struggled to operationalize medical exceptions to abortion bans in Ohio well before *Dobbs* and despite federal protections for abortion provision under *Roe*. Physicians responded by asserting their cultural authority over abortion as a form of health care, deploying various clinical strategies to balance legal compliance with their duty to patients, and leveraging their authority to respond creatively. Yet the participants in our research firmly believed that their reduced cultural authority in their own practices under Ohio's regulations increased the risks for pregnant people in the state.

Cultural authority in medicine is a collective endeavor, one vested in groups, symbols, and institutions. Individuals must rely on others to share their expertise and to understand the logic governing their practice. Given that the Ohio state medical board includes a non-physician leader of the group that has sought to curb abortion by limiting its provision, it is no surprise that physicians fear they would not have the support of the institutions that are supposed to uphold evidence-based medical practice. As Epstein and Timmermans have observed, "the increasingly sharp battle lines forming around the cultural authority of health thus threaten to impair the capacity of health institutions to rescue us from the most pressing threats to health and well-being" (2021, 250). Our data point to a divergence in the salience in physicians' cultural authority—one in which physicians influence public debates while being less authoritative in day-to-day clinical practice—and raise questions about the long-term prospects for physicians' cultural authority if doctors are unable to deliver a standard of care that patients—and the public—expect of them.

Although we might expect that hospital counsel would defend physicians' rights to practice to the full scope of their professional judgment and skill, instead we see that institutional lawyers are a primary enforcer of the limits on physicians' cultural authority (Field et al. 2022). Though their actions are conservative, institutions act rationally when they deny care, even to the point of risking patient death: the civil malpractice liability of failing to provide care is preferable to criminal liability for violating restrictions. Our data show how abortion restrictions transfer risk from hospitals to clinicians and from clinicians to patients.

By contrast, abortion providers who work in stand-alone clinics may be better able to exert authority over their practice. These abortion providers are more likely to be knowledgeable about state restrictions, thus needing less translation from legal counsel, compared with hospital-based physicians (Heymann et al. 2023). Their institutional missions may be more abortion-focused, altering the balance of risk to the clinic. Additionally, abortion clinics in Ohio were not subject to the same public facilities ban on abortion provision that affected many of the physicians in our sample. Restrictive state laws and policies certainly limit the care that abortion clinics can provide, and sometimes even put them out of business (McGowan, Norris, Bessett 2020), but the clinics may better acknowledge that abortion is health care in ways that facilitate physician authority, albeit in service of patient demand.

The physicians who participated in our study recognized that abortion restrictions are threats to their professional authority, and they enumerated reasons why they—not lawmakers or lawyers—were the best positioned group to "judge the experience and needs of clients" in medically complex cases (Starr 1982, 15). While our participants acknowledged that most abortion care in the United States is not provided in hospitals or under emergency conditions, they nevertheless provided examples consonant with the medical exception frames that appeal to sympathy for some patients. However, when clinicians elevate cases that emphasize distinctions among abortions, they may inadvertently stigmatize "ordinary" abortions and implicitly limit their cultural authority over abortions to the pregnancies where there is a medical issue.

Similarly, when the physicians emphasized their unique medical competence as integral to their authority, they were frequently responding to anti-abortion lawmakers whom they saw as impinging on their ability to provide health care. Yet their assertions of cultural authority—and justifications for it—at times implicitly denied that authority to abortion seekers. Equally important was that these assertions were ineffective against anti-abortion doctors. If physicians are to advance their authority over medically complex cases, they must also consistently and explicitly pair those claims with abortion seekers' need for reproductive autonomy.

In the years immediately following the *Dobbs* decision, heartbreaking stories centering medical exceptions claimed headlines, and we expect abortion care for medically complex pregnancies will remain a flashpoint. These prominent cases illustrate how much control physicians have lost over the framing of medical realities in pregnancy care and over the scope of their abortion practice more broadly. Yet their very prominence also reveals that physicians' invocations of their cultural authority remain salient in both medicine and in the public sphere. As physician expertise is increasingly politicized, the case of abortion care reveals the great irony that physicians' cultural authority may be more salient in political realms and media representations than it is in their everyday clinical practice.

ACKNOWLEDGMENTS

We gratefully acknowledge the contributions of our team members Hillary Gyuras, Jessica Sinclair, Danielle Czarnecki, and Meredith Field and of our research participants. We also benefitted greatly from editor Katrina Kimport's feedback. This research was funded by the Charles Phelps Research Center at the University of Cincinnati and an anonymous philanthropic organization.

NOTES

1. Roe v. Wade, 410 U.S. 113 [1973].
2. Ohio Revised Code, Section 5101.57, "Use of Public Facilities for Nontheurapeutic Abortions Prohibited," effective September 29, 2011 (legislation: House Bill 153, 129th General Assembly), https://codes.ohio.gov/assets/laws/revised-code/authenticated/51/5101/5101.57/9-29-2011/5101.57-9-29-2011.pdf.
3. Twenty participants were attending physicians, and fifteen were fellows or residents. All had practiced in Ohio for at least six months between 2010 and 2020. The interviews and focus groups covered the impact of Ohio's several abortion restrictions, both current and proposed by the state legislature. All quotes herein are from focus groups unless noted, and all names are pseudonyms.

REFERENCES

Abbott, Andrew D. 1988. *The System of Professions: An Essay on the Division of Expert Labor.* University of Chicago Press.

Czarnecki, Danielle, Danielle Bessett, Hillary Gyuras, Alison H. Norris, and Michelle L. McGowan. 2023. "State of Confusion: Ohio's Restrictive Abortion Landscape and the Production of Uncertainty in Reproductive Health Care." *Journal of Health and Social Behavior* 64 (4): 470–485. https://doi.org/10.1177/00221465231172177.

Edelin, Kenneth C. 2007. *Broken Justice: A True Story of Race, Sex and Revenge in a Boston Courtroom.* Pondview Press.

Epstein, Steven, and Stefan Timmermans. 2021. "From Medicine to Health: The Proliferation and Diversification of Cultural Authority." *Journal of Health and Social Behavior* 62 (3): 240–254. https://doi.org/10.1177/00221465211010468.

Field, Meredith P., Hillary Gyuras, Danielle Bessett, Meredith J. Pensak, Alison H. Norris, and Michelle L. McGowan. 2022. "Ohio Abortion Regulations and Ethical Dilemmas for Obstetrician–Gynecologists." *Obstetrics & Gynecology* 140 (2): 253–261. https://doi.org/10.1097/AOG.0000000000004870.

Foy, Andrew J., and Edward J. Filippone. 2013. "The Case for Intervention Bias in the Practice of Medicine." *Yale Journal of Biological Medicine* 86 (2): 271–280. https://pmc.ncbi.nlm.nih.gov/articles/PMC3670446/.

Freedman, Lori. 2010. *Willing and Unable: Doctors' Constraints in Abortion Care.* Vanderbilt University Press.

Gyuras, Hillary J., Meredith P. Field, Olivia Thornton, Danielle Bessett, and Michelle L. McGowan. 2023. "The Double-edged Sword of Abortion Regulations: Decreasing Training Opportunities While Increasing Knowledge Requirements." *Medical Education Online* 28 (1): 2145104. https://doi.org/10.1080/10872981.2022.2145104.

Halfmann, Drew. 2011. *Doctors and Demonstrators: How Political Institutions Shape Abortion Law in the United States, Britain, and Canada.* University of Chicago Press.

———. 2012. "Recognizing Medicalization and Demedicalization: Discourses, Practices, and Identities." *Health* 16 (2): 186–207. https://doi.org/10.1177/1363459311403947.

Harris, Lisa H., Amy Simon, Meghan Seewalda, Sara Knight, and Lisa Martin. 2024. "Doctors' Voices Generate Support for Abortion Care: Results from a Nationally Representative Survey." *Contraception* 140: 110535. https://doi.org/10.1016/j.contraception.2024.110535.

Heymann, Orlaith, Danielle Bessett, Alison H. Norris, Jessie Hill, Danielle Czarnecki, Hillary J. Gyuras, Meredith Pensak, and Michelle L. McGowan. 2023. "Unlimited Discretion: How Unchecked Bureaucratic Discretion Can Threaten Abortion Availability." *Journal of Health Politics, Policy, and Law* 48 (4): 629–647. https://doi.org/10.1215/03616878-10449914.

Hirst, Paul H. 1982. "Professional Authority: Its Foundation and Limits." *Society for Educational Studies* 30 (2):172–182. https://doi.org/10.2307/3121550.

Hughes, Everett C. 1963. "Professions." *Daedalus* 92 (4): 655–668. https://www.jstor.org/stable/20026805.

Jozkowski, Kristen N., Xiana Bueno, Ronna C. Turner, Brandon L. Crawford, and Wen-Juo Lo. 2023. "People's Knowledge of and Attitudes toward Abortion Laws before and after the *Dobbs v. Jackson* Decision." *Sexual and Reproductive Health Matters* 31 (1): 2233794. https://doi.org/10.1080/26410397.2023.2233794.

Kacanek, Deborah, Amanda Dennis, Kate Miller, and Kelly Blanchard. 2010. "Medicaid Funding for Abortion: Providers' Experiences with Cases Involving Rape, Incest and Life Endangerment." *Perspectives on Sexual and Reproductive Health* 42 (2): 79–86. https://doi.org/10.1363/4207910.

Kimport, Katrina, Tracy A. Weitz, and Lori Freedman. 2016. "The Stratified Legitimacy of Abortions." *Journal of Health and Social Behavior* 57 (4): 503–516. https://doi.org/10.1177/0022146516669970.

Luker, Kristin. 1984. *Abortion and the Politics of Motherhood.* University of California Press.

MacDonald, Andrea, Hayley B. Gershengorn, and Deepshikha Charan Ashana. 2022. "The Challenge of Emergency Abortion Care Following the *Dobbs* Ruling." *JAMA* 328 (17): 1691–1692. https://doi.org/10.1001/jama.2022.17197.

McGowan, Michelle L., Megan A. Allyse, Niamh A. Condon, Jason P. Wheatley, and Meredith J. Pensak. 2024 "From the Front Lines: The Need for Stakeholder Coalitions in Preserving Reproductive Autonomy." *American Journal of Bioethics* 24 (2): 46–48. https://doi.org/10.1080/15265161.2023.2296405.

McGowan, Michelle L., Alison H. Norris, and Danielle Bessett. 2020. "Care Churn—Why Keeping Clinic Doors Open Isn't Enough to Ensure Access to Abortion." *New England Journal of Medicine* 383 (6): 508–510. https://doi.org/10.1056/NEJMp2013466.

Morris, Theresa. 2013. *Cut It Out: The C-Section Epidemic in America.* New York University Press.

Moseley-Morris, Kelcie. 2023. "Most Americans Want Health Exceptions in Abortion Bans. Political Infighting Keeps Blocking Them." *Ohio Capital Journal*, November 8, 2023. https://ohiocapitaljournal.com/2023/11/08/most-americans-want-health-exceptions-in-abortion-bans-political-infighting-keeps-blocking-them/.

Pew Research Center. 2022. "America's Abortion Quandary." *Pew Research Center* (blog), May 6, 2022. https://www.pewresearch.org/religion/2022/05/06/americans-views-on-whether-and-in-what-circumstances-abortion-should-be-legal/.

Ranji, Usha, Karen Diep, Ivette Gomez, Laurie Sobel, and Alina Salganicoff, 2024. "Health Policy Issues in Women's Health." In *Health Policy 101*, edited by Drew Altman. Kaiser Family Foundation. https://www.kff.org/health-policy-101-health-policy-issues-in-womens-health/.

Reagan, Leslie J. 1997. *When Abortion Was a Crime: Women, Medicine, and Law in the United States, 1867–1973.* University of California Press.

Rivlin, Katherine, Marta Bornstein, Jocelyn Wascher, Abigail Norris Turner, Alison H. Norris, and Dana Howard. 2024. "State Abortion Policy and Moral Distress among Clinicians Providing Abortion after the *Dobbs* Decision." *JAMA Network Open* 7 (8): e2426248. https://doi.org/10.1001/jamanetworkopen.2024.26248.

Schladen, Marty. 2022. "While in Effect, Ohio's Abortion Ban Led to Chaos, Suffering, and Worse Health Care, Doctor Says." *Ohio Capital Journal*, November 4. https://

ohiocapitaljournal.com/2022/11/04/obstetrician-ohio-abortion-law-stymies-doctors
-endangers-patients/.

Skinner, Daniel. 2019. *Medical Necessity: Health Care Access and the Politics of Decision
Making*. University of Minnesota Press.

Starr, Paul. 1982. *The Social Transformation of American Medicine*. Basic Books.

Watson, Katie. 2018. *Scarlet A: The Ethics, Law, and Politics of Ordinary Abortion*. Oxford
University Press.

Wojcieszak, Doug. 2021. "Consumer Background and Composition on State Medical
Boards: Who Are These Citizen Members and Do They Adequately Protect the Public?"
Journal of Patient Safety and Risk Management 26 (6): 267–271. https://doi.org/10.1177
/25160435211054343.

CHAPTER 10

Physician Workforce Sensitivity and Reactions to Abortion Bans

Alexandra Woodcock and Jessica Sanders

Following the overturn of *Roe v. Wade*, a wave of local and national media shared anecdotes of obstetrician-gynecologists (ob-gyns) leaving their jobs in states that banned abortion. This chapter discusses research exploring the impact of legal and policy environments on the physician workforce and their plans for future practice. Like the stories of providers leaving restricted states, our research finds that many graduating obstetrics and gynecology (OB-GYN) residents have changed their plans or actively avoided practicing in restricted and ban states altogether following the *Dobbs* decision. Considering these emergent findings, the impact of the *Dobbs* decision on practice patterns reveals how and to what extent abortion access as part of the full spectrum of reproductive health plays—and likely has played—a role in career decision-making. Yet, although policy has a strong impact on ob-gyns' decision-making, we do not find evidence that state abortion policy influences placement preferences in other medical specialties. In this, the research also sheds light on the longer history of how abortion care has been marginalized within the medical field, illuminating what *Dobbs* has not, in effect, changed.

BACKGROUND

The OB-GYN specialty has several distinct subspecialty fields. Here, we provide a brief overview of the residency application and subspecialty certification process. In the last year of medical school, medical students electing to pursue OB-GYN as their specialty apply to OB-GYN residency programs. In 2022, at the time of our study, there were 302 Accreditation Council for Graduate Medical Education–accredited programs in the United States (ACGME 2023). Although abortion training is a required component of all OB-GYN training, about one-third of OB-GYN residency programs are designated Ryan programs. Ryan programs include a specialized abortion training curriculum and have been found to lead to improved competency in both routine and complicated abortion care (Landy et al. 2021). OB-GYN residencies with Ryan programs are attractive to medical student applicants who are interested in abortion provision, as abortion is recognized as an essential part of pregnancy care and is a skill that is necessary in treating a variety of maternal conditions. After medical students apply, the residency programs select and interview applicants. When the interview season closes each year, the applicants rank the residency programs, and the residency programs rank the applicants. Finally, the National Resident Matching Program (NRMP) accepts these ranks, and through a complex mathematical algorithm that optimizes the ranking of the program and applicant, applicants are "matched" to a residency program.[1]

Residency is a form of continued training during which physicians take on increasing responsibility. OB-GYN residency lasts four years, after which graduates either apply for jobs as an "attending" level OB-GYN generalist or apply to a subspecialty/fellowship-trained "match." This latter route includes additional specialized training and research opportunities. As of 2021, 75 percent of residents applied for a job after residency, and 25 percent entered the subspecialty fellowship match process (Rayburn and Xierali 2021). The following are the most common OB-GYN subspecialties (and their acronyms), each of which has its own match process (similar in structure to that of residency): maternal-fetal medicine (MFM), complex family planning (CFP), gynecologic oncology (GYN ONC), urogynecology (URO-GYN), and reproductive endocrinology and infertility (REI). CFP is the subspecialty dedicated to advanced abortion and contraception care, though many MFM programs also offer advanced abortion training. After completion of their subspecialty training, these providers go on to become subspecialty attendings at academic medical institutions and in clinical settings. Subspecialty programs and attending jobs, like residency options, are distributed around the country.

The location of residency training has previously been a strong predictor of where geographically physicians will work in the longer term; over half of residents (51.7 percent) of all medical specialties from 2013 to 2022 stayed in their state of residency training for their next position (AAMC 2023b). There is no literature that we could find that describes the retention—or lack thereof—of fellowship-trained individuals in their state of fellowship training. Equally, there are gaps in knowledge surrounding the patterns of movement of attending-level individuals—whether postfellowship or not—and how frequently they move states during their posttraining careers. It follows, however, that the further individuals get in their careers, the less likely they are to move, resulting from both their personal and professional lives rooting deeper in the community the longer they stay. This means that residency (and likely fellowship, too) is a primary determinant of the physician workforce in any geographic area.

Post-Dobbs OB-GYN Migration

Of course, people do move, and they do so for many reasons. Shortly after the *Dobbs* decision, news coverage began pointing to a pattern of physician relocation. The media focused on the stories of ob-gyns and the new realities (and complexities) of caring for pregnant people in states that had banned abortion. Restricting abortion not only affected individuals who sought to end their pregnancies, but also increased medical provider burdens and legal and personal risks. It altered how documentation needed to occur as well as dictated the tasks, responsibilities, and procedures that they could legally perform. For example, Texas targeted physicians through vigilante tactics and limited how they could counsel or refer patients for abortion care. In Idaho, the laws left vague language around ectopic pregnancy and banned abortion with limited exceptions and narrowly defined threats to maternal health (Center for Reproductive Rights, n.d.). Physicians who performed abortion care outside of these margins risked significant criminal penalties. For ob-gyns in Idaho, for example, this represented significant restrictions on standard medical practice.

Mainstream media outlets interviewed individuals who initially had cared for patients in these post-*Dobbs* abortion-restrictive environments but eventually decided to leave. For example, a piece in the online magazine *Slate* entitled "You Know What? I'm Not Doing This Anymore" featured providers who had hit a breaking point in Texas (Novack 2023). The piece was accompanied by an introduction graphic of mug-shot-like pictures of providers with their eventual decisions over their faces: "Moved to New Mexico," "Transferred to Boston," "Moved to Utah." A survey in 2023 by the Idaho Coalition for Safe Healthcare revealed that 40 percent of Idaho ob-gyns were considering leaving the state (Varney and Buhre 2023). *The New York Times* featured a story on the physicians left behind as other ob-gyns "fled" states with abortion bans, accompanied by a stoic photo of one of the only maternal-fetal medicine doctors still practicing in Idaho (Stolberg 2023). Together, these articles and others like them pointed to an increased area of the country without skilled OB-GYN providers.

Maternity Care Deserts

From a pregnancy safety and care standpoint, regional ob-gyn departures are concerning. The March of Dimes, an organization devoted to improving the health of "moms and babies" has defined maternity care deserts as "any county without a hospital or birth center offering obstetrics care and without any obstetric providers." Also concerning are counties with "low access," defined as having fewer than sixty obstetric providers per 10,000 births (Brigance, Lucas, and Jones 2022). The lack of general obstetricians has a direct patient impact: women who live in geographic areas with limited obstetric care are nearly two times more likely to die during childbirth and up to one year after delivery than those living in areas with adequate obstetric staffing (Petersen et al. 2019; Wallace et al. 2021).

There is another way that an exodus of ob-gyns can harm obstetric patients *during* pregnancy. Sometimes pregnancy goes wrong, and the only treatment is to perform an abortion procedure. However, not all obstetricians have the skillset or willingness to perform abortions. For example, both dilation and curettage (D&C) and dilation and evacuation (D&E) are essential abortion-related skills. D&E is a procedure to remove a pregnancy from the uterus after the first trimester of pregnancy. It is often a critical skill in managing life-threatening conditions later in pregnancy where continuing the pregnancy could lead to serious maternal morbidity or even mortality. The same skills involved in D&E are also used in the management of miscarriage and intrauterine fetal demise. Even geographic locations with seemingly sufficient obstetric workforce may not have obstetrics providers who can handle these cases if politics and policy curtail training. With this in mind, the consequences of providers with these skills, including Ryan-trained generalists and CFP and MFM providers, leaving states with abortion bans could be severe.

Although they exemplify the struggles that ob-gyns in abortion-restrictive states have experienced in the immediate aftermath of the *Dobbs* decision, the individual accounts provided in the mainstream media are not generalizable. The *Dobbs* decision's impact on the OB-GYN provider workforce nationally was unknown. Our University of Utah ASCENT Center for Reproductive Health team sought to measure this impact empirically.[2]

Measuring the Impact on OB-GYN-Trained Physicians

The ASCENT Center is a team of individuals who approach reproductive health research, advocacy, and public policy from various positions of expertise, including health care providers (including physicians, midwives, and nurse practitioners), PhDs, statisticians, and other experts in public health. Living and practicing in a state on the verge of an abortion ban after *Dobbs*, our team was interested in measuring the impact of *Dobbs* on the OB-GYN provider workforce and beyond. We elected to document the effect on the next generation of OB-GYN providers.

Starting from the assumption that it is more challenging for established providers—those settled and deeply rooted in abortion-restrictive states—to move their professional and personal lives to a different state, we focused on whether and how *Dobbs* might influence where physicians earlier in their career choose to practice. We anticipated that the desire to avoid a restrictive state at an earlier stage in training might be more actionable and more impacted by *Dobbs*. Our study would measure how the *Dobbs* decision and resulting state-based abortion bans influenced the decisions of graduating OB-GYN residents on where they would practice as an OB-GYN generalist attending or rank and pursue an OB-GYN subspecialty fellowship.

We conducted a national survey of OB-GYN residents graduating in June 2023 from residencies with Ryan abortion training programs. Although residencies with Ryan programs make up one-third of OB-GYN residencies nationwide, their larger cohorts mean that Ryan program residents comprise almost 50 percent of residents at ACGME-accredited programs (ACGME 2022). We anticipated that physicians interested in providing abortion care in the future would be motivated to train at residencies with Ryan programs. Given this, our survey was designed to understand how *Dobbs* impacted the work practice decisions of those most likely to contribute to the future abortion provider workforce.

We sent our survey to residency program directors to distribute to their residents via email and regular mail in March and April 2023. The survey included both closed- and open-ended questions. To adequately assess how *Dobbs* impacted the location where providers would practice (our primary outcome), we asked what state residents were planning on practicing in or highly ranking for fellowship. We then asked if this was different than where they had been planning before *Dobbs*; if they selected yes, they were asked to indicate the previous state (Woodcock et al. 2023). The survey also included an open-ended, optional prompt that read "Please describe how the *Dobbs v. Jackson Women's Health Organization* decision impacted your professional plans."

Study Findings

Of the 349 OB-GYN residents who responded to our survey (a response rate of 48.2 percent of a total invited population of 724), almost one in five said they had changed their state of intended future practice after the *Dobbs* decision. Those who had initially planned on practicing in a state that restricted abortion after *Dobbs* (hereafter "abortion-restrictive state") were 8.52 times more likely to have changed their future practice state. Additionally, those who were planning on providing abortion care as part of comprehensive OB-GYN care in their future practice were 4.24 times more likely to have changed their state of future practice. In the open-ended responses of those pursuing further training via a fellowship position, thirty-six of 143 indicated that they placed a lower rank or chose not to rank programs in abortion-restrictive states (Woodcock et al. 2023).

In participants' responses to open-ended questions, they tied the ability to provide abortion care to their ability to care for patients more broadly and also to the theoretical ability to use the skills they had been trained to do in a supportive environment. One wrote, "First, despite my convictions that states that restrict abortion still need fierce advocates to fight for pregnant people, I don't have enough fight left in me to stay in a state that does not support my work as a physician. I cannot see myself ever moving back to a state that restricts abortions as extensively as [the state where I completed my residency] does."

Apart from the job itself, participants highlighted that their personal (or partner's) ability to receive abortion services also impacted their decision (Woodcock et al. 2023). Notably, OB-GYN is a feminized specialty where a majority of new practitioners are pregnancy-capable individuals in their reproductive years (AAMC 2023a). This fact likely contributes to our study finding that 24 percent indicated that their access to personal (or a partner's) abortion access "very strongly" impacted their choice of state of work. Providers who endorsed this statement were four times more likely to have changed their state of future practice.

The open-ended question responses further demonstrated concerns regarding personal family planning goals, such as the risk of pregnancy complications and not being able to receive care and even the storage of embryos created through in vitro fertilization. For example, one wrote, "I was always planning to apply to urogynecology fellowship, but the *Dobbs v. Jackson* decision impacted what states I would want to live in (i.e., [I] do not want to be a pregnant patient in a state where I cannot access reasonable medical care)." In this respondent's ranking of URO-GYN fellowships, *Dobbs* mattered significantly. Even in the URO-GYN subspecialty, which less frequently manages pregnant patients, the respondent's ability to personally receive abortion care influenced the fellowship ranking.

As we have described thus far, our research lifted the narrative dilemma initially captured at the individual provider level to a more empiric workforce level. In addition to individual provider stories covered in the media, our study found that the *Dobbs* decision and resultant state-based abortion restrictions impacted where one in five OB-GYN residents chose to practice or ranked highly for a fellowship position. This means that *Dobbs* has affected both the geographic distribution of the OB-GYN workforce and the skills that are available in those geographical settings.

ADDITIONAL RESEARCH FINDINGS

Career choices at the end of residency are not the only stage in the OB-GYN trajectory where a state's abortion regulatory status might influence physician plans. Other studies illuminate the impact of the *Dobbs* decision on OB-GYN providers at different levels of the training and professional ladder. For example, in a 2023 study conducted by the Association of American Medical Colleges (AAMC) using the Electronic Residency Application Service (ERAS) database of medical students applying to residencies in the United States, there was a 5.2 percent drop of applicants to OB-GYN, with the drop most significant in states with abortion bans (Orgera, Mahmood, and Grover 2023). Another investigation examined the experiences of fifty-four OB-GYNs practicing in abortion-restrictive states in the post-*Dobbs* landscape. Of these, six providers (11 percent) had left their original practice state, and twenty-nine of the remainder had "entertained the ideas of leaving their state" (Sabbath et al. 2024). These studies support our conclusion that ob-gyns along the spectrum of career stages are sensitive to abortion restrictions in choosing their geography of practice.

The *Dobbs* decision seems to have widely exposed ob-gyns to risk in providing comprehensive reproductive health care and illuminated the role that practice location plays in professional and personal risk mitigation. That said, we also know that a state's legal environment around abortion has long been a consideration for physicians for whom abortion provision makes up a majority of their practice. Even when *Roe v. Wade* was in place, some states still substantially restricted abortion through restrictions on providers, patients, and procedures. Targeted regulation of abortion providers laws (TRAP laws) were in place in twenty-three states before *Dobbs* (Guttmacher Institute 2023). These laws could make it very difficult to offer abortion care. For example, when Texas implemented a TRAP law in 2013 that required abortion providers have admitting privileges to a nearby hospital, between 2014 and 2017 there was a 5 percent drop in abortion providers in the state (Sagar et al. 2023). It is possible and even likely that (before *Dobbs*) TRAP laws like this deterred providers—like the graduating OB-GYN residents we studied—from electing to train further or practice in abortion-restrictive states. Utah, for example, had only two licensed abortion clinics in the state prior to the *Dobbs* decision, so there were few opportunities for people who wanted to provide abortion care. This likely impacted OB-GYN recruitment to the state even when abortion was federally protected.

When considering the wider population of ob-gyns, including those who do not consider abortion provision to be central to their practice, these studies suggest that the *Dobbs* decision revealed an underlying sensitivity to the importance of abortion—and a reliance on the ability to offer and receive it. This sensitivity was not immediately obvious until *Dobbs*. It is also possible that this sensitivity was previously narrower and, following *Dobbs*, has extended to more subspecialties in OB-GYN. Abortion restrictions may not have professionally impacted the graduating resident bound for a URO-GYN fellowship, but their knowledge of the medical importance of abortion access may have increased their sensitivity to abortion restrictions in their fellowship ranking. Similarly, it is possible that *Dobbs* heightened an existing sensitivity to abortion provision for MFM providers, who are the providers who specialize in the diagnosis and care of high-risk pregnant people. The inability to counsel on and provide abortions for pregnancies with fetal anomalies and/or maternal health risk could prompt a recognition of the importance of abortion access in their work and influence their geographic preferences.

Impact Beyond OB-GYN

But how far do these sensitivities to the legal landscape extend? Do we see the same geographic preferences for other medical specialties? There are reasons to think so, especially building off the observations by graduating OB-GYN residents who do not practice abortion care yet state abortion policy could be important to them personally. Of all active medical providers, most recent studies demonstrate that 37.1 percent identify as female and over 50 percent are younger than fifty-five years old (AAMC 2023a), suggesting that this population also has a personal interest in the legality of abortion where they practice. Simply put, among medical providers at large, many are capable of pregnancy.

To answer these questions, we completed a survey of all graduating residents of all specialties graduating from the University of Utah in June 2023. Like OB-GYN residents, residents of other specialties have specialty-specific fellowship options after residency that they might elect to pursue, or they may choose a location to start their practice. Like our previously described study, this survey also included both closed- and open-ended questions, and our primary outcome of interest was a provider changing their intended state of practice before and after *Dobbs*.

Representing nineteen distinct medical specialties, eighty-six graduating residents responded to our survey (a response rate of 55 percent, of a total invited population of 155 residents). Of these, only six respondents (7 percent), three of whom were OB-GYN residents, indicated that the *Dobbs* decision changed their future state of practice or rank for a fellowship position. Noting the difference in surveyed populations between the two studies (a nationwide, large, single specialty cohort with respondents from states with and without abortion restrictions versus providers of different specialties, from a smaller, single institution cohort in an abortion-restrictive state), there does seem to be a difference in reaction to the *Dobbs* decision. Where graduating OB-GYN residents were both sensitive and reactive to abortion restrictions, we do not find the same for other specialties.

To make sense of this finding, we must look at how abortion care has been situated in medicine. From a physical perspective, most abortions do not occur within hospitals but instead in standalone clinics. In 2020, clinics "specializing in abortion care" provided 54 percent of abortions nationwide, and only 3 percent of abortions were performed in hospital settings (Jones, Kirstein, and Philbin 2022). Given this disparity, providers of other specialties (who receive their training in hospital settings) have likely not been exposed to routine abortion care or the volume of patients that these clinics care for. From a figurative perspective, abortion care has long been situated outside of mainstream medicine.

Before 1973 and the establishment of a federal right to abortion in *Roe*, abortion was illegal, and people still had abortions. Many of the providers performing these services outside of institutional medicine had been trained, but a subset, often known as "back-alley butchers," were untrained and provided dangerous, substandard care. Unfortunately, although they were not representative of most abortion providers in the pre-*Roe* era, these unsafe providers left a stain on abortion medicine that persisted through the post-*Roe* era, despite the increase in training and qualified providers (Joffe 2022). As we have seen after the *Dobbs* decision, even though there is great public attention paid to abortion, abortion care has been and continues to be marginalized within the healthcare system.

Indeed, the *Dobbs* decision may be the first time since *Roe* that physicians of other specialties have had to consider abortion policy and its practice implications. Although these various specialties do care for patients who are capable of being pregnant, it is likely that they previously did not have to be concerned about a referral for a patient. Now, with state-based bans and departing obgyns, abortion policy may start creeping into their purview and impacting their patients in unanticipated ways. Furthermore, providers in these other specialties had not previously engaged in or experienced abortion restrictions; however, now their own reproductive decision-making may be governed by them, so they may increasingly consider the implications for their own health care of living in a state with an abortion ban. It remains to be seen whether abortion remains exceptionalized in medicine or if the effects of abortion bans on patients seen by physicians in many specialties will catalyze a shift in this relationship.

Summary

In this chapter, we have shown that the *Dobbs* decision revealed an underlying sensitivity to abortion restrictions by ob-gyns as they consider their workplace. Importantly, we document that some graduating OB-GYN residents who are highly sensitive to abortion policy will change their location of practice based on state abortion bans. There is no reason to think this is a one-time anomaly. Continued OB-GYN movement out of (or never into) states that have restricted abortion and into states that have retained abortion rights is likely to have significant consequences for maternal health, including maternity care deserts, longer waits for pregnancy care, lack of trained providers to handle obstetric emergencies, and a reduced number of experienced physicians to train the next generation of OB-GYN providers in core competencies. Whether people with the capacity for pregnancy have access to robust OB-GYN health care may depend on their state's abortion policy.

Our second study shows, however, that this movement trend may not extend to the location of practice of other physicians. Additional research from both abortion-restrictive and abortion-protective states is required. Even more, it will be important to evaluate how and whether more physicians of other specialties will react to these constraints the longer that the abortion restrictions persist, as they affect their patients and/or themselves or their family members.

For now, our findings highlight the continued marginalization of abortion in health care. This research on the provider workforce should also serve as a warning more broadly. As we see an increase in politically motivated restrictions on specific areas of essential health care (e.g., gender-affirming care, vaccinations, infertility care), it is likely that there will be trickle-down effects of limiting practices that will impact broader access to expertly trained, highly skilled healthcare providers.

ACKNOWLEDGMENT

This chapter was supported by the ASCENT Center for Reproductive Health.

NOTES

1. See "Intro to The Match," https://www.nrmp.org/intro-to-the-match/.
2. See Ascent Center for Reproductive Health, School of Medicine, University of Utah, https://medicine.utah.edu/obgyn/ascent.

REFERENCES

Accreditation Council for Graduate Medical Education (ACGME). 2022. "Obstetrics and Gynecology Case Logs: National Data Report." Department of Applications and Data Analysis. https://apps.acgme-i.org/ads/Public/Reports/CaselogNationalReportDownload ?specialtyId=40&academicYearId=28.

———. 2023. "Number of Accredited Programs: Academic Year 2022–2023." ACGME Accreditation Data System. https://apps.acgme.org/ads/Public/Reports/Report/3.

Association of American Medical Colleges (AAMC). 2023a. "2022 Physician Specialty Data Report: Executive Summary." AAMC. https://web.archive.org/web/20230321004550 /https://www.aamc.org/media/63371/download?attachment.

———. 2023b. "Report on Residents: Table C6, Physician Retention in State of Residency Training, by State." 2013–2022, data through 2023. https://www.aamc.org/data-reports /students-residents/data/report-residents/2023/table-c6-physician-retention-state -residency-training-state.

Brigance, Christina, Ripley Lucas, and Erin Jones. 2022. "Nowhere to Go: Maternity Care Deserts across the U.S." March of Dimes, 2022 Report. https://www.marchofdimes.org /sites/default/files/2022-10/2022_Maternity_Care_Report.pdf.

Center for Reproductive Rights. n.d. "Idaho." https://reproductiverights.org/maps/state /idaho/.

Guttmacher Institute. 2023. "Targeted Regulation of Abortion Providers." https://www .guttmacher.org/state-policy/explore/targeted-regulation-abortion-providers.

Joffe, Carole. 2022. "Failing to Embed Abortion Care in Mainstream Medicine Made It Politically Vulnerable." *Washington Post*, January 11, 2022. https://www.washingtonpost .com/outlook/2022/01/11/failing-embed-abortion-care-mainstream-medicine-made-it -politically-vulnerable/.

Jones, Rachel K., Marielle Kirstein, and Jesse Philbin. 2022. "Abortion Incidence and Service Availability in the United States, 2020." *Perspectives on Sexual and Reproductive Health* 54 (4): 128–141. https://doi.org/10.1363/psrh.12215.

Landy, Uta, Jema K. Turk, Kristin Simonson, Katheryn Koenemann, and Jody Steinauer. 2021. "Twenty Years of the Ryan Residency Training Program in Abortion and Family Planning." *Contraception* 103 (5): 305–309. https://doi.org/10.1016/j.contraception.2020.12 .009.

Novack, Sophie. 2023. "'You Know What? I'm Not Doing This Anymore.'" *Slate*, March 21, 2023. https://slate.com/news-and-politics/2023/03/texas-abortion-law-doctors-nurses-care -supreme-court.html.

Orgera, Kendal, Hasan Mahmood, and Atul Grover. 2023. "Training Location Preferences of U.S. Medical School Graduates Post *Dobbs v. Jackson Women's Health*." AAMC Research Institute. https://www.aamcresearchinstitute.org/our-work/data-snapshot /training-location-preferences-us-medical-school-graduates-post-dobbs-v-jackson -women-s-health.

Petersen, Emily E., Nicole L. Davis, David Goodman, Shanna Cox, Carla Syverson, Kristi Seed, Carrie Shapiro-Mendoza, William M. Callaghan, and Wanda Barfield. 2019. "Racial/ Ethnic Disparities in Pregnancy-Related Deaths—United States, 2007–2016." *MMWR. Morbidity and Mortality Weekly Report* 68 (35): 762–765. https://doi.org/10.15585/mmwr. mm6835a3.

Rayburn, William F., and Imam M. Xierali. 2021. "Subspecialization in Obstetrics and Gynecology." *Obstetrics and Gynecology Clinics of North America* 48 (4): 737–744. https:// doi.org/10.1016/j.ogc.2021.06.003.

Sabbath, Erika L., Samantha M. McKetchnie, Kavita S. Arora, and Mara Buchbinder. 2024. "US Obstetrician-Gynecologists' Perceived Impacts of Post–*Dobbs v Jackson* State Abortion Bans." *JAMA Network Open* 7 (1): e2352109. https://doi.org/10.1001/jamanetworkopen .2023.52109.

Sagar, Kareena, Erica Rego, Radhika Malhotra, Amanda Lacue, and Kristyn M. Brandi. 2023. "Abortion Providers in the United States: Expanding beyond Obstetrics and Gynecology." *AJOG Global Reports* 3 (2): 100186. https://doi.org/10.1016/j.xagr.2023.100186.

Stolberg, Sheryl. 2023. "As Abortion Laws Drive Obstetricians from Red States, Maternity Care Suffers." *New York Times*, September 7, 2023. https://www.nytimes.com/2023/09/06 /us/politics/abortion-obstetricians-maternity-care.html.

Varney, Sarah, and Maea Lenei Buhre. 2023. "Idaho's Strict Abortion Laws Create Uncertainty for OB-GYNs in the State." *PBS News Hour*, May 1, 2023. https://www.pbs.org/newshour /show/idahos-strict-abortion-laws-create-uncertainty-for-ob-gyns-in-the-state.

Wallace, Maeve, Lauren Dyer, Erica Felker-Kantor, Jia Benno, Dovile Vilda, Emily Harville, and Katherine Theall. 2021. "Maternity Care Deserts and Pregnancy-Associated Mortality in Louisiana." *Women's Health Issues* 31 (2): 122–129. https://doi.org/10.1016/j.whi.2020 .09.004.

Woodcock, Alexandra L., Gentry Carter, Jami Baayd, David K. Turok, Jema Turk, Jessica N. Sanders, Misha Pangasa, Lori M. Gawron, and Jennifer E. Kaiser. 2023. "Effects of the *Dobbs v Jackson Women's Health Organization* Decision on Obstetrics and Gynecology Graduating Residents' Practice Plans." *Obstetrics & Gynecology* 142 (5): 1105–1111. https:// doi.org/10.1097/AOG.0000000000005383.

What the Fall of *Roe* Revealed About Advocacy For and Against Abortion

CHAPTER 11

Know Your Enemy

THE ETHICAL FAILINGS OF THE "EXPOSE FAKE CLINICS" CAMPAIGN AGAINST ANTI-ABORTION, CRISIS PREGNANCY CENTERS

Sara Matthiesen

When a leaked draft of the Supreme Court's *Dobbs v. Jackson Women's Health Organization* (2022) decision made clear that *Roe v. Wade*'s (1973) days were numbered in May 2022, some pro-abortion activists sought vengeance. Members of a group called "Jane's Revenge" claimed credit for numerous acts of vandalism against anti-abortion organizations across the country.[1] Most of the targeted buildings were crisis pregnancy centers (CPCs). In at least sixteen cities, messages like "fake clinic" and "Jane was here" appeared in graffiti across local CPCs' doors and walls overnight. In some cases, property damage accompanied the messages. The final communication from the group promised not to target any "anti-choice group who closes their doors" while declaring "open season" on all who refused. Republicans, pro-life activists, and conservative media swiftly condemned the group and demanded they be punished for their alleged crimes (Bukuras 2024; Jane's Revenge 2022; Noor 2023; Tiffany 2022).

But Republicans were not the only ones to come down harshly on pro-abortion activists who heeded the call for rageful revenge. While the Biden Administration was mobilizing its milquetoast defense of abortion rights in the days and weeks after the leak, its justice department conceded to conservatives' calls and brought criminal charges against four women in Florida for allegedly spray-painting crisis pregnancy centers there. The Department of Justice used the Freedom of Access to Clinic Entrances (FACE) Act—legislation passed by the Clinton Administration to protect abortion clinics from the anti-abortion violence that peaked in the 1980s and early 1990s—to prosecute the activists. They each faced up to twelve years in prison if convicted (Lennard 2023).[2] Unprecedented mainstream news coverage of every aspect of the abortion debate following the *Dobbs* leak and subsequent decision—of which the right-wing media's amplification of Jane's Revenge was a small but loud part—meant wide swaths of the American public learned for the first time about the existence of faith-based, anti-abortion crisis pregnancy centers and abortion rights activists' belief that they are better described as "fake clinics."[3]

Although the militancy of Jane's Revenge and the brutal, bipartisan crackdown may have been specific to the post-*Dobbs* moment, the strategy of combatting CPCs by labeling them "fake clinics" is nearly forty years old. Recent histories of the CPC movement show that the anti-abortion centers have been around even longer than that (Haugeberg 2017; Matthiesen 2021). However, most supporters of abortion rights who know the acronym "CPC" are far more familiar with the tactics that prompted Jane's Revenge to target CPCs across the country than they are with the complex history of the CPC movement and pro-choice efforts to oppose it. In the reproductive rights and justice world, CPCs are infamous for two things: their use of deception to obstruct abortion access and their false promise of "free pregnancy resources" offered in advertisements that appear on billboards and bus stops near college campuses.

There are an estimated 2,500 CPCs in the United States, many of which are affiliated with one of the two major CPC networks, Heartbeat International and Care Net (Swartzendruber and Lambert 2020). The stated goal of these organizations and their affiliates is to convince pregnant women who are considering an abortion to carry their pregnancies to term.[4] What Ziad Munson (2008) has described as the "individual outreach stream" of the pro-life movement is also its largest part as measured by number of volunteers, volunteer hours, and organizations—all working to render abortion obsolete through service.

CPCs use a variety of deceptive tactics to deter women from abortion, including spreading lies about the supposed medical risks of pregnancy termination, deliberately misdating ultrasounds, and calling centers things like "Choices for Women" so that individuals seeking abortion care will think they are at an abortion clinic. CPC advertisements and other outreach strategies especially target students, young women, Black and Latina women, and poor women. The pregnancy services they provide are often limited and come with strings attached, such as requiring individuals to attend Evangelical Christian-based parenting classes in exchange for things like maternity clothes (Montoya, Judge-Golden, and Swartz 2022). Despite these realities, CPCs serve the broader anti-abortion movement by deflecting public attention from the common—and accurate—charge that it does little to support pregnant women and/or families.

Abortion rights activists have for decades worked to expose the CPC movement's deceptive tactics. At both the feminist grassroots and professionalized, non-profit levels, oppositional campaigns have worked to expose the various ways the CPC movement attempts to trick women into keeping their pregnancies. This is illustrated by the rhetoric of investigative advocacy reports published by major pro-choice organizations, which for years have used titles like "The Truth Revealed" or "Crisis Pregnancy Centers Lie" to demonstrate that, as in the subtitle of one report, CPCs are "an insidious threat to reproductive freedom" (Kleder and Richmond Crum 2008; McIntire 2015). Jane's Revenge encouraged a form of politics the major pro-choice non-profits would never abide, and their missives argued such actions were necessary precisely because the largest movement players had been too acquiescent for too long.[5] Still, these otherwise oppositional corners of the abortion rights movement relied on the same rhetorical strategy of "fake clinics"—even if one advocated spray paint over glossy pages filled with Times New Roman.

This chapter argues that there is more to know about the CPC movement than merely its deceptive tactics, limited services, and too many strings. The continuous, widespread effort to document and expose their deception has obscured a finding that should make abortion rights activists think twice about the "fake clinics" strategy: by the CPC movement's own admission, its deceptive tactics by and large do not successfully trick pregnant people into visiting centers or deter them from ending their pregnancies. Both historical and sociological research on CPCs has confirmed this fact. Very few pregnant people turn to CPCs for either pregnancy or abortion support. The few who do have already decided to carry their pregnancies to term and are seeking pregnancy-related services such as diapers, maternity clothes, assistance with welfare programs, and emotional support. These clients are overwhelmingly low-income, already have children, and have nowhere else to turn. The research also has shown that the services they receive are insufficient to meet their needs. Despite this, many speak positively about feeling emotionally supported (Hussey 2020; Kelly 2014; Kimport 2020; Kimport, Kriz, and Roberts 2018; Matthiesen 2021; McKenna and Murtha 2021).[6]

The dominant pro-choice narrative that CPCs pose a major threat to pregnant people seeking abortion services has proven incredibly durable despite these findings. This framing ensures that struggling families forced to rely on CPCs for paltry care rife with anti-abortion propaganda and Evangelical Christian proselytizing disappear from view. In contrast, this chapter aims to center the individuals most likely to interact with a CPC by posing the following question to supporters of abortion rights: If the deception used by centers is by and large ineffective at getting what the CPC movement calls "abortion-minded" clients through center doors, then do pro-choice efforts to "expose fake clinics" end up strengthening a movement they claim to oppose?[7] If, as this chapter will argue, the answer to this question is yes, then even more urgent questions follow: In what ways does the "fake clinics" campaign *benefit* the pro-choice movement, and how does it *fail* those forced to engage with CPCs in hopes of obtaining the most basic of necessities?

Through an analysis of advocacy reports, media coverage, and archival records of both feminist and anti-abortion activism related to CPCs, this chapter documents how abortion rights activists and pro-choice organizations have responded to the CPC movement since the mid-1980s by repeatedly exposing its deceptive practices.[8] It also explores how leaders in the CPC movement countered these oppositional campaigns. In tracing the stories pro-choice and anti-abortion organizations tell about CPCs and one another, I illustrate how what is widely understood as an oppositional dynamic is also a mutually beneficial one. Each "side" relies on an oversimplified, adversarial characterization of the other to mobilize their respective bases. For abortion rights activists, this mobilization frequently centers around (1) encouraging donations to major pro-choice organizations so that they can continue fighting CPCs, and (2) spreading the "truth" that CPCs are "fake clinics." This activation strategy tethers a revenue stream to the *continued* existence of the very enemy pro-choice organizations claim they are trying to defeat. It also enlists individuals in perpetuating a simplistic narrative of the opposition that can garner more donations over and above involvement in a campaign that accurately identifies the threat and targets its weaknesses.

While this may periodically fill non-profit coffers, such activation does little to benefit the individuals and families most impacted by the CPC movement's involvement in reproductive services, however limited and compromised those services may be.[9] The singular focus on exposing CPCs as "fake clinics" refuses to reckon with the far more complex, structural reality: The CPC movement's claims to service provision only have purchase because of inequality that makes poor women of all racial backgrounds vulnerable to such offers. This refusal makes it harder to build more redistributive campaigns that could target the major drivers of need the CPC movement capitalizes on. For example, advocates and politicians can lead investigations into CPCs in their state, thereby establishing their pro-choice credentials, without ever having to champion universal healthcare or resources for new parents that would undercut the CPC movement's strategy of offering "free" services. The unwillingness to consider campaigns that center the individuals most likely to end up at a CPC is an ethical failing of the pro-choice movement that should concern anyone committed to reproductive justice, which includes abortion freedom (SisterSong Women of Color Reproductive Collective n.d.; Ross and Solinger 2017). Ultimately, my humble hope is that this research encourages activists working against anti-abortion CPCs to rethink their political analysis and strategic approach—a shift we urgently need if access to both abortion and the other basic necessities of life are to be won.

Know Your Enemy

The first step to developing an effective organizing strategy is learning everything you can about your opposition. The pro-choice movement first learned about CPCs in the early 1980s when pregnant women lured by centers posing as abortion clinics advertised free pregnancy tests. While women waited for their test results, center volunteers bombarded them with anti-abortion propaganda. Tactics ranged from showing clients slideshows of aborted fetuses to claiming that abortion could result in death to calling abortion murder. These women sued individual centers for deceptive advertising in several states, and the multiple lawsuits catapulted CPCs into the national spotlight for the first time since the movement's founding (Haugeberg 2017; Kelly 2012). With some exceptions, these suits overwhelmingly targeted centers affiliated with the Pearson Foundation, a CPC umbrella organization founded by Rob Pearson in 1969 (Gross 1987).[10] As a result, media coverage of CPCs regularly highlighted Pearson and his "How to Start and Operate Your Own Pro-Life Outreach Crisis Pregnancy Center" manual, which advocated many of the coercive tactics used by volunteers.[11] Despite the fact that there were other CPC umbrella organizations in operation during this period, Pearson's network also featured prominently in congressional hearings on anti-abortion violence that examined the tactics used by "bogus clinics"—the term of derision favored by CPC opponents in the 1980s (U.S. House of Representatives 1991).[12] These initial responses to the existence of CPCs helped cement Pearson's identity as the father of a movement defined by deception.

The response also established a connection between CPCs and the anti-abortion extremism that erupted during this period (Grimes et al. 1991). For example, speaking at a press conference in 1987, then-president of Planned Parenthood Faye Wattleton linked anti-abortion activists who popularized clinic blockades and sometimes used violence to obstruct access to abortion to those running CPCs. "These extremists resorted to intimidation and even violence to inflict their own views on an unwilling America. The latest effort in their campaign of deception is the creation of anti-abortion counseling centers, many of which appear to offer abortion services, but actually lure unsuspecting pregnant women into their clutches under false pretenses" (quoted in Scott 2000). Four years later, the National Abortion Federation and the Planned Parenthood Federation of America co-published a report titled "Anti-Abortion Counseling Centers: A Consumer's Alert to Deception, Harassment, and Medical Malpractice" to raise awareness about the true intentions of "antiabortion counseling centers." The report alerted readers that "these centers are designed to misinform and intimidate women—some will go to any lengths necessary to dissuade women from ending their pregnancies" (Planned Parenthood Federation of America, 1991). Importantly, sometimes the link between CPCs and anti-abortion violence was accurate. For example, James Kopp, who was convicted in 2003 for the murder of physician and abortion provider Barnett Slepian, headed a Pearson affiliate called "A Free Pregnancy Center" in San Francisco in the 1980s (Staba 2007). But as I discuss further below, pro-choice organizations and politicians misjudged the scope of their opposition when they zeroed in on Pearson and framed CPCs solely as an extension of anti-abortion violence rather than a growing movement in its own right.

Lastly, abortion rights activists' discovery of CPCs gave rise to an organizing tactic that readers well-versed in the contemporary abortion debate will likely recognize: Pro-choice groups ranging from large nonprofits to smaller grassroots coalitions began sending activists into centers as "undercover" pregnant women seeking abortion services in order to expose the centers' deception. For example, suits brought against three Pearson-affiliated centers in New York City and one in San Francisco were based on affidavits from real clients as well as "women who made undercover visits to the centers, some gathering information for advocacy groups such as Planned Parenthood and the National Organization for Women" (Gross 1987).[13] The D.C.-based Washington Area Clinic Defense Task Force also "infiltrated" clinics in order to share common tactics with its members through self-published materials.[14] The People for the American Way brought suits against multiple centers in Maryland based on reports from women sent undercover by the progressive advocacy group (Sullivan 1991; Tapscott 1991). Journalists also picked up the tactic of posing as pregnant women when covering the debate over CPCs.[15] And feminist abortion rights groups featured their reconnaissance work alongside testimonies from real clients to mobilize against CPCs in major cities ranging from San Francisco to Chicago to New York City to Ann Arbor. They organized "fake clinic" demonstrations in front of individual CPCs and circulated fliers and pamphlets that warned women away from centers.[16]

While pro-choice organizations and feminist activists were exposing CPCs through profiles of Pearson, lawsuits, investigations, and "fake clinic" demonstrations, other major players in the CPC movement were watching. Importantly, these activists enjoyed less infamy than Pearson. For example, Heartbeat International, formerly Alternatives to Abortion International, had coordinated its own affiliates since 1971. Up to this point, most Heartbeat affiliates were run by a volunteer base consisting largely of Catholic, white, lower-to-middle class women (Matthiesen 2021, chapter 5). In 1980, the Evangelical pro-life lobbying group Christian Action Council (CAC) opened its first CPC in Baltimore after establishing its "crisis pregnancy center ministry," a division dedicated to growing a network of CPC affiliates; today, that affiliate network is known as Care Net.[17] CAC's turn to CPCs brought Evangelicals into a movement that had until then been primarily composed of Catholics. This influence especially encouraged volunteers to treat client interactions as opportunities for religious conversion and to promote conservative family values regardless of the beliefs held by those seeking support (Kelly 2012; Kelly 2014).

Pearson affiliates were not the only centers to use some form of deception during the period when CPCs first came under fire, but the hyperfocus on Pearson enabled the leaders of Heartbeat and Care Net to salvage their organizations' reputation and mount a counterattack.[18] Central to their strategy was depicting CPCs as victims of the pro-choice activists who had infiltrated their centers by pretending to be pregnant women seeking abortion services. Peggy Hartshorn, president of Heartbeat International, described the tactic this way: "In the early 1980s, Planned Parenthood of New York City hired Amy Sutnick for the specific purpose of finding a way to discredit pregnancy centers. . . . Sending fake clients into our centers with hidden tape recorders and cameras in the 1980s was common" (Hartshorn 2011, 84). Tellingly, Hartshorn omitted that actual pregnant women looking for abortion services reported the same deceptive practices.

CPC leaders worked to flip the script on the pro-choice strategy of exposure by mounting a defense of their affiliates. This was the start of a major professionalization effort headed by Hartshorn and Tom Glessner, founder of the National Institute of Family and Life Advocates (NIFLA). Importantly, Glessner used his legal expertise to provide affiliates with guidance and insurance so they would be better insulated from charges of consumer deception. He also established a path by which CPCs could administer nondiagnostic ultrasounds without being sued for practicing medicine without a license, providing centers with the veneer of professional medical services (Hartshorn 2011, 85). Heartbeat, Care Net, and NIFLA were also instrumental in drafting a Commitment of Care document in the late

1990s that sought to standardize volunteers' interactions with clients (Matthiesen 2021, 174n62).

In other words, the movement undertook a major image management and liability effort in response to the pro-choice campaign to "expose fake clinics" of the mid-1980s and 1990s. As Hartshorn tells it, "So, ironically, the opposition charged us with being 'fake clinics' (fake abortion clinics). But we responded with becoming actual clinics, medical clinics that provide a medical diagnosis of pregnancy through the use of a limited ultrasound exam, and more! This has made pregnancy help centers and clinics less vulnerable to attack and stronger than ever" (Hartshorn 2011, 87). Hartshorn and other leaders narrate these various initiatives as a period of significant change for the movement, one that Kimberly Kelly (2012, 212) has described as a shift to "woman-centered strategies" formulated "consciously . . . to counter these [pro-choice] accusations" and restore "the movement's credibility." However, such changes did not signal a departure from the movement's central goal of dissuading women from abortion. Recent advocacy reports show that most CPCs do not offer robust medical services despite Hartshorn's claim, and many continue to rely on deceptive practices such as perpetuating debunked myths about the health risks of abortion (McKenna and Murtha 2021).[19]

My interest in analyzing CPC leaders' response to the "expose fake clinics" campaign is not to lend it credence or even assess whether such changes can be considered a strategic win for the movement.[20] I simply want to highlight that when confronted with an attack by their opponent, the movement *responded and adapted*. The same cannot be said for the pro-choice movement. Instead, pro-choice organizations and abortion rights supporters have consistently repeated the strategies they first developed in the 1980s: sending women to clinics undercover to expose clinics' deception; picketing CPCs with "fake clinics" signs; and disseminating materials that warn supporters about this vast but invisible threat to abortion.

For example, beginning in 2008, NARAL Pro-Choice America initiated state-level investigations into CPCs across ten different states. These investigations relied on undercover volunteers who visited centers posing as pregnant women in search of options counseling. Both the state-level reports and the 2015 national report that collated the state chapters' findings confirmed that centers are still using the same deceptive strategies. NARAL's stated aim for undertaking the investigation was to urge policymaking that would protect women by requiring CPCs to be transparent about their "anti-choice bias" (McIntire 2015, 1).[21]

Local activist groups have also continued the strategy of combatting CPCs by exposing them as "fake clinics" and attempting to pass legislation banning deceptive advertising (Thomsen and Tacherra Morrison 2020). Contemporary campaigns such as Expose Fake Clinics and ReproAction's Fake Clinic Database aim to provide activists the tools necessary for such exposure.[22] Exposés based on undercover clients' reports are routinely published (Abcarian 2015; Aslam 2014; Bancroft 2013; Cooperman 2002; Gaebe 2019; Greenberg 2018; Marty 2013). And recent scholarship on CPCs has used the "mystery shopper" method to expose center practices and emphasize the dangers of CPCs to abortion access (Frasik et al. 2023).

At this point, you may be thinking, If both advocacy and academic investigations continue to find evidence of deception at CPCs, and if CPCs continue to state that they are most interested in reaching women "at risk" of abortion, then why does it matter that abortion supporters have not changed their strategy? The trouble begins when one surveys the evidence produced by pro-choice advocacy investigations alongside research demonstrating that CPCs largely fail to get anyone through the door; as for those who do come, they are most often looking for support during a pregnancy rather than abortion services. It is more troubling still when one actually *listens* to what the CPC movement has to say about the people who do—and do not—walk through their centers' doors.

Abortion rights activists know that CPC movement spokespersons are unabashed about their belief that the "best client" is one who thinks they are walking into an abortion clinic, but far fewer also know that the leaders in the movement regularly lament how *infrequent* such clients are.[23] Additionally, they worry that centers are serving *too many* people looking for services unrelated to abortion. I have written elsewhere about the economic and political changes that have funneled this latter group toward CPCs, and how the movement's leadership identified the "services-only client" as a problem that should be rectified as early as the mid-1990s (Matthiesen 2021, chapter 5). Even without this and other evidence detailing the movement's failure to achieve its main goal (Kelly 2014), a critical observer might posit that the deceptive lengths the majority of centers go to—distributing medically inaccurate information, failing to make clear on center websites that they do not provide abortion services, using targeted ads for "abortion" google searches, locating near abortion clinics, promising free services, and providing sex education in schools—suggest in and of themselves that the movement struggles to get pregnant people seeking abortion services through center doors.

Given these facts, supporters of abortion rights must ask some difficult questions about the strategy of combatting CPCs by exposing them as "fake clinics." By repeatedly sending undercover activists to centers to obtain proof of the movement's deceptive tactics, do pro-choice advocates artificially increase centers' track record of drawing the "best" client it so desperately tries to conjure? And by publishing and circulating these findings every few years, as pro-choice organizations, investigative journalists, and activists have done since the mid-1980s, do they end up amplifying the very image the CPC movement wishes to project of its success in deterring pregnant women from abortion when the reality is otherwise? Rather than following the organizing directive to first "know your enemy," is it possible the pro-choice movement looks selectively at the opposition to sustain its own relevance—even if doing so also helps the monster grow?

Grow Your Enemy

For readers willing to answer yes to these questions, only one remains: Why keep at a campaign that is not only failing, but might even be doing public relations work for the opposition? One obvious answer is that the CPC movement has not stopped using lies, deception, and religious conversion in its battle against abortion. This coercion should not go unchallenged. Any follower of the debate over CPCs knows that in addition to the continued publication of investigative advocacy reports and journalistic exposés, first-person accounts by people who sought abortion services only to learn—sometimes too late—that they had been deceived by an advertisement or center volunteer also persist (Gerson 2019; McGuire 2018; Stack 2011; UltraViolet 2018; Winter 2015). As long as CPCs continue to evade regulation despite their role in service provision, publicizing these experiences so that others might avoid similar harms is a useful and necessary form of advocacy.

However, this does not explain why the "fake clinics" campaign remains the *only* strategy when pregnant individuals who want an abortion are the least likely to seek CPC services. To understand the dogged focus on anti-abortion deception, one must understand what keeps the pro-choice movement activated and funded.

I first learned of the lawsuits against Pearson-affiliated CPCs while conducting archival research in the National Organization for Women (NOW) records for my book *Reproduction Reconceived: Family Making and the Limits of Choice after Roe v. Wade* (2021). I came across a letter from two NOW staff attorneys asking for litigation funds to aid the California Committee to Defend Reproductive Rights in its suit against A Free Pregnancy Center in San Francisco in the 1980s. Like other feminist and pro-choice analyses of the time that understood CPCs as an outgrowth of antiabortion violence, the attorneys linked the "dishonest and disgraceful activities of the elements of the pro-life movement" on display at A Free Pregnancy Center to the growing number of "abortion clinic assailants." The attorneys requested that NOW serve as "Of-Counsel" and allocate $1,000 toward legal support. They further advised that the organization make its involvement public because it had the potential to direct donations into NOW coffers. To demonstrate their hunch that "our participation in the case could prove a useful fundraising handle," the attorneys included a draft of a mailer that could be sent out to supporters.[24]

For me, the letter illuminates the unsettling reality that pro-choice and pro-life activism is caught in a reciprocal relationship, with each side relying on an oversimplified, villainous characterization of the other in order to mobilize their respective bases. Of course, in the case of the anti-abortion movement's characterization of the abortion rights movement, this narrative is also typically an outright fabrication. This willingness to blatantly lie is the lynchpin of an overall strategy that has so successfully transformed a safe, simple procedure into a heinous transgression that abortion is "unchooseable" for many (Kimport 2021).[25] For this reason, it is all the more important that campaigns working to make abortion both "chooseable" and accessible do not rely on rhetorical distractions or partial narratives. It is necessary for abortion rights supporters to examine what function the oversimplified villains play in the pro-choice "fake clinics" campaign—especially if raising these bogeymen is not helping to limit the reach of CPCs into people's lives. The link the feminist attorneys made between CPCs and antiabortion extremist violence in their memorandum to NOW illustrates an important throughline of pro-choice opposition to CPCs that is still relevant today: white conservative men—unvarnished misogyny incarnate—have been the preferred villain of pro-choice opposition to CPCs.

For example, as I discussed above, both grassroots feminist groups and pro-choice organizations that first took on CPCs in the 1980s and 1990s consistently highlighted Rob Pearson's role in the movement. This early anointment of Pearson as founder and leader has profoundly shaped contemporary understandings of the movement. Those well versed in the contemporary debate over CPCs no doubt recognized Pearson and his infamous manual—"How to Start and Operate Your Own Pro-Life Outreach Crisis Pregnancy Center"—when I first introduced them in the prior section. Both are still routinely invoked in overviews of the CPC movement, despite scholarship demonstrating that the movement extended far beyond Pearson and has, since its inception, overwhelmingly been powered by women volunteers (Campbell 2017; McElroy 2015; Naftulin 2022; Stacey 2009; Thomsen and Baker 2022).[26]

The strategy of highlighting extremist villains as representative of the CPC movement is not limited to Pearson even if he still regularly appears as the original enemy in contemporary discussions of CPCs. For example, in New York City in the early 1990s, Women's Health Action Mobilization (WHAM!) activists pursued a multiyear campaign against CPC owner Chris Slattery, in part due to his connection to the radical, anti-abortion organization Operation Rescue.[27] The New York chapter of NARAL was still highlighting Slattery's connection in its investigative advocacy reports in 2010 (NARAL Pro-Choice New York Foundation 2010, 3).

In 2017, Planned Parenthood took aim at the ultimate contemporary manifestation of misogyny—President Donald Trump—by collaborating with the cast of Hulu's adaptation of *The Handmaid's Tale* to analogize Republican attacks on abortion rights to the Republic of Gilead, the Evangelical, authoritarian nation at the center of novelist Margaret Atwood's seminal dystopia. The collaboration resulted in an episode depicting a character who visited a CPC she thought was an abortion clinic where the clinic's staff tried to coerce her into keeping the pregnancy (Planned Parenthood 2021). This narrated to the letter the CPC movement's most desired—and least likely—scenario, in which a pregnant woman seeking abortion care is duped into walking through center doors.

Most recently, the Feminist Majority recycled 1980s era claims that CPCs were an extension of extremist anti-abortion violence. The organization's 2022 National Clinic Violence Survey found that abortion clinics in closer proximity to a CPC reported a higher prevalence of anti-abortion violence and harassment than abortion clinics not located near a CPC; the organization then used this correlation as evidence that the CPC movement is "connected to" anti-abortion violence (Feminist Majority Foundation 2022, 3).

These characterizations—played on repeat since the 1980s—reduce the CPC movement to one perpetually motored by evil, extremist misogynists who will stop at nothing to keep women from obtaining abortions. I want to be clear that my point is not to trivialize the existence of these villains or the threat they pose to abortion access. I recognize that both are real. But I also want to explore what makes them so alluring that all other aspects of the CPC movement—its participants, its infrastructure, its multiple threats, its shifting tactics, those most vulnerable to its reach—have repeatedly been ignored by the pro-choice organizations that regularly claim to be fighting the enemy.

This is not a mistake or oversight, but a logical outcome of the pro-choice campaign to expose CPCs. It should be understood as a quintessential liberal strategy—in its feminism, its mode of political analysis, and its preferred tactics. It may not be surprising that anti-CPC advocacy has inherited the broader pro-choice movement's race and class myopia, but it is still worth making plain.[28] The villainous misogynist's counterpart is a victimized woman, and for the mainstream abortion rights movement the specifically white, middle-class, liberal women voters it has long courted have repeatedly been offered as universally representative of all women under siege. Here, Sophie Lewis's observation about the handmaid protests that went viral after *The Handmaids Tale* premiered as a series in 2017 is instructive. Lewis describes the handmaid demonstrations as exposing "extremist misogyny" that is "pleasurable" and "photogenic" while crucially devoid of any analysis highlighting the racialized and systemic character of reproductive control, past and present (Lewis 2019, 14).

The history of forcing African women to reproduce slave labor in the United States was an especially loud absence. The protestors' performance as handmaids transmuted a historically specific experience of racialized gender that undergirded the transatlantic trade into a universal marker of female victimhood (Spillers 1987; Morgan 2004). Such omissions do make it easier—and more pleasurable—to rail against misogynists in Congress because liberal feminists are able to feel united against a shared enemy and feel righteous in doing so. All the while, they do not have to ask how white supremacy and class hierarchy shape the dominant gender norms they are subject to or the unequal reproductive experiences through which those norms are enforced.

The liberal feminism inherent in the villain strategy is not the only place liberalism rears its head. The handmaid protests ventured into direct-action tactics, but the major pro-choice organizations favor electoral and legislative strategies for advancing their cause. "Rallying the base" around easy to hate misogynists has by and large meant getting liberal abortion supporters to donate to pro-choice organizations and vote for pro-choice candidates.[29] If your main relationship to your members is through texts, emails, and mailers that ask for money and voter loyalty, then it is plausible that the surest way to get their attention is by emphasizing just how big and bad the enemy is. Furthermore, just as these asks comprise individual rather than collective actions, the enemy is always a singular person rather than a complex set of interlocking systems. Spectacular villains like Rob Pearson—who described women seeking abortions as "Satan . . . the girl who wants to kill her baby"—may shock members into action. Many will donate, and some may even protest CPCs with "This Is a Fake Clinic" signs (quoted in National

Abortion Federation 2006, 1). But these tactics, built from an individual-level analysis, frame people seeking abortion as individual consumers who can be supported in navigating the marketplace of reproductive health services by the right combination of pro-choice politicians, awareness campaigns, and truth-in-advertising ordinances.[30]

Instead of individual consumers pitted against singular enemies, a successful opposition campaign requires an analysis of the broader conditions that make opposing abortion through service provision possible in the first place. This approach also necessarily centers the individuals most likely to be impacted by CPCs. My prior work argued that it is only possible to understand the movement's continued relevance by accounting for the fact that if you want to raise children in the United States, you must be prepared to go it alone. The longstanding, frequently bipartisan, ethos that government should have little to no role in providing care to dependents has given CPCs a function at odds with the movement's primary goal of reaching "abortion-minded" women: the promise of free pregnancy services will draw in at least some pregnant individuals in need of the basic necessities required for pregnancy and infant care. The deception designed to lure those seeking abortion services is no match for the structural conditions that deprive people of basic resources. This reality ensures that when CPCs do dole out their limited, compromised support, it is usually to families trying to make ends meet—the very families leaders of the movement least want to support (Matthiesen 2021, chapter 5).

Replacing the fixation on individual villains with a more thoroughgoing assessment of the opposition would also make it possible to identify potential areas of weakness that could be targeted. For example, sociological research on CPCs has found that there often exists significant distance between the concerns espoused by leadership (i.e., that the so-called services-only clients are a sign the movement is failing) and the beliefs of centers' volunteers, who provide direct support to pregnant individuals and consider this in itself a win for their cause (Kelly 2012). What if, instead of amplifying the idea that a united movement is successfully obstructing access to abortion, a campaign zeroed in on the tensions between the movement's leadership and its base—to expose that the volunteers are not actually in lockstep with the most visible villains?

Research has also explored how the movement began to establish centers in predominantly Black and Latin neighborhoods in the mid-1990s.[31] It did so in part by making the thoroughly debunked claim that abortion clinics were overconcentrated in these areas (Guttmacher Institute 2014; Ross 2017).[32] Rather than being curious about what this development might reveal about the movement's weaknesses, pro-choice organizations simply highlighted how the CPC movement had begun to target poor Black and Latina communities in their advocacy reports (McIntire 2017, 7). It is important to challenge the dehumanizing, stigmatizing, and factually distorted "race-based antiabortion strategy" that reduces Black women to pawns in the abortion debate (Ross 2017, 61). But highlighting its use solely to bolster the villain narrative prevents asking and answering questions that could provide a deeper understanding of the CPC movement and uncover potential weaknesses. For example, why did CPC leaders pursue these initiatives when they did? How robust was the newly formed partnership between pro-life activists of color and the predominantly white CPC movement? And how did women of color relate to the establishment of these centers in their neighborhoods—especially those who had been providing robust reproductive health services before the arrival of CPCs?[33]

The dogged, self-serving commitment to the villain strategy has prevented these alternative approaches. And, moreover, it has even obscured or outright ignored the most glaring weakness: In the simplest terms, the research showing that those most likely to visit a CPC are looking for pregnancy support rather than abortion services is evidence that the CPC movement is *failing* at its stated aim of deterring women from abortion. This reality suggests an equally obvious campaign strategy, one dedicated to exposing the CPC movement not for its deception but for its well-documented—even self-narrated—*failure*. Instead of building a campaign around this weakness, however, major pro-choice organizations, some feminist grassroots groups, many abortion rights supporters, and some researchers examining CPCs have collectively amplified the opposite: They insist that CPC deception is an ever-looming, highly dangerous—and thus effective—threat. They consistently highlight that CPCs vastly outnumber abortion providers, thereby suggesting that CPCs and abortion clinics are competing for the same population when in fact people seeking abortion services are the *least* likely to visit a CPC. They requote the most zealous movement leaders, who are obsessed with getting more people seeking abortion care through center doors, despite evidence that movement participants hold varied beliefs on client outreach. They emphasize the harm these centers cause to pregnant people seeking abortions rather than to people seeking pregnancy support. They persist in calling CPCs "fake clinics" even when research has shown that individuals *do* make use of the pregnancy confirmation and ultrasound services offered by centers because they are often more accessible than those provided by legitimate reproductive health clinics. And they label CPCs as the greatest threat to choice despite the fact that very few pregnant people even use these centers' services. Unlike the pro-choice organizations and grassroots feminist groups who first experimented with opposing CPCs by emphasizing their villainous deception in the 1980s, those repeating their tactics now cannot say that they do not know the complex truth about CPCs.[34]

These talking points, repeated ad nauseam, have done tremendous public relations work for the pro-choice movement and its campaign against CPCs. Because this oppositional dynamic is also mutually beneficial, the same is necessarily true for the anti-abortion movement and its celebration of CPCs. After leaders of the CPC movement initiated their rebranding efforts, CPCs increasingly took on an important role within the anti-abortion movement. An arm of the movement that had been marginalized for the first fifteen years of its existence was subsequently embraced by anti-abortion activists eager for a retort to the accusation that pro-lifers care more about unborn fetuses than women and children. The story that

CPCs represent what one movement leader has described as the "compassionate approach" to the abortion debate by virtue of their promise to support pregnant women has become even more important in the post-*Dobbs* era: numerous states are successfully funneling public dollars to CPCs for the supposed purpose of meeting the increased demand for pregnancy services caused by the recriminalization of abortion (quoted in Belluck 2013; Sherman 2024).

Although this post-*Dobbs* reality is new, the strategy is not. Since the early 1990s, a handful of states have been directing public dollars toward CPCs based in part on the idea that they were funding successful anti-abortion organizations (Lin and Dailard 2002). Research has repeatedly shown that this collaboration aids a significant misuse of funds; most public dollars do not go to increasing the services offered by CPCs, but instead successfully drain the coffers of public programs meant to support poor families (Wormer 2021; Reproductive Health and Freedom Watch 2024). The idea that the "compassionate approach" of CPCs effectively obstructs access to abortion is the glue that holds this strategy together. Without it, donors, Republican legislators, and movement spokespersons would have to explain why they are investing in the infrastructure of a movement that is failing at its stated goal: deterring pregnant women from abortion.

Of course, with the *Dobbs* decision such a cover story is less necessary. In an environment where abortion is criminalized, the law does CPCs' coercive work for them, and the movement can claim that its main objective is to meet the increased demand for pregnancy services. But what if at any point since the 1990s and before *Dobbs* the major pro-choice organizations had exposed the CPC movement for its shoddy track record of successfully convincing pregnant people to not seek abortion services? Or what if pro-choice politicians had championed universal health care so that the movement's medicalization rebranding strategy and offer of free ultrasounds was rendered absurd? Or if they had championed robust, universal programs for new parents so that the centers' strategy of offering free services to lure poor families through the door was rendered impotent?[35] Would the CPC movement be enjoying such massive investment in our current moment?

As a historian, I am not supposed to entertain counterfactuals like the ones I just posed. But as someone who believes deeply in the power of social movements, I feel these questions merit reflection. They suggest that the important role CPCs are playing after *Dobbs* has been made possible in part by the past twenty-five years of pro-choice investigations, campaigns, and actions dedicated to exposing "fake clinics." This fact should be deeply troubling to anyone committed to abortion freedom and reproductive justice.

Conclusion

Other approaches are possible. In 2021, The Alliance: State Advocates for Women's Rights & Gender Equality released a report titled "Designed to Deceive: A Study of the Crisis Pregnancy Center Industry in Nine States" (McKenna and Murtha 2021). For the first time, an investigation of CPCs cited research showing that the vast majority of people who seek aid from CPCs are not considering abortion and are in need of the limited pregnancy services these centers advertise as free. Importantly, this report also relied on publicly available information about CPCs and public records requests to analyze CPC practices in different states.

This strategy avoided the problem of sending *more* of the clients the movement hopes to draw by not relying on undercover investigators posing as pregnant women seeking abortion services. These shifts resulted in a different conclusion than pro-choice advocacy investigations published over the last twenty-five years: the lack of support for pregnant people and families and widespread inequality help maintain the CPC movement's relevance by forcing individuals to rely on it for aid. This includes the surveillance, neglect, racism, and punishment poor families and families of color frequently encounter when they turn to what few welfare programs do exist (Gustafson 2011; Matthiesen 2021; Roberts 2002, 2022). The promise of free services from a charitable organization may seem like a less risky endeavor, even when those services frequently come with their own strings of stigmatizing anti-abortion propaganda and Evangelical proselytizing.

The report's authors attempted to evaluate the impact these centers have on maternal and infant health and called on policymakers to "address significant and deepening gaps in maternal and reproductive healthcare" (McKenna and Murtha 2021, 8). In other words, the report conducted a structural analysis of CPCs that exposed not only their anti-abortion tactics but also the broader conditions of exploitative deprivation that enable these centers to have a role in pregnancy support in the first place.

Notably, The Alliance's investigation was guided by a commitment to "advance gender equality at the intersection of reproductive rights, economic justice, LGBTQ+ equality, and gender-based violence." The report does not specifically invoke the term "reproductive justice," but this political framework is certainly reflected in the report's shift away from individual villains and toward the structures that constrain a broad range of reproductive rights. Most importantly, this framework ensured that the people most harmed by CPC practices *and* varied inequalities were centered in its analysis.

A year before the report's publication, reproductive justice activists also made this link. In a news article highlighting Katrina Kimport's study of women who visit CPCs, Nourbese Flint, the policy director at Black Women for Wellness, described how the centers were "unfortunately capitalizing on a gap that we have in our system in terms of responding to the actual real needs of pregnant folks and the actual real needs of families" (quoted in North 2020, Kimport, 2020). The people Flint mentions disappear underneath the stories anti-abortion and pro-choice campaigns tell about the CPC movement. CPCs either harm people seeking abortion services or save them, but neither campaign desires to link the centers to the people they most commonly encounter: struggling pregnant people and families in need of basic necessities.

The fact that CPCs exaggerate and even lie about what services they provide and make individuals jump through hoops to get them does not change the reality of people's need. That CPCs have any role to play in supporting family-making reflects just how little our society cares about poor families, especially poor families of color. This should be the source of our rage and indignation. The individuals forced to rely on CPCs deserve so much more than either movement has given them. If there was ever a time for supporters of abortion rights to imagine what a repro-ductive justice approach to combatting CPCs might look like, it is now, after *Dobbs*, when a significant portion of the abortion rights movement is obliterating the rhe-torical positions that maintain *Roe* as the political horizon.[36] We need a similar evolution of thought when it comes to CPCs. The people forced to rely on these "fake clinics" to make ends meet certainly deserve that and so much more.

ACKNOWLEDGMENTS

I am grateful to Flavia Dutra for her incredible research assistance and steadfast encourage-ment, and to Katrina Kimport, Annie Gray Fischer, Heather Berg, and two anonymous read-ers for their sharp and instructive feedback on earlier drafts. The Humanities Center at George Washington University and the 2021–2022 fellows supported and encouraged my initial exploration of these ideas.

NOTES

1. In the first of three "communiques" posted online between May 10 and June 14, 2022, the group took credit for vandalism and property destruction of a CPC in Madison, Wiscon-sin. Collectively, these statements gave anti-abortion organizations thirty days to close their doors or be targeted in a similar fashion. The communications also called on "courageous hearts to come out after dark" to defend abortion access from "evisceration" and make good on their overarching threat: "if abortion isn't safe, you aren't either." All quotes are from Jane's Revenge, "Night of Rage," May 30, 2022. The three communiques have been archived and are available here: https://theanarchistlibrary.org/category/author/jane-s-revenge.

2. In addition to the FACE charges, the Florida attorney general, Ashley Moody, and one of the CPCs brought SLAPP (strategic lawsuit against public participation) suits against the four activists. Three of the four individuals took plea deals guaranteeing that the civil suits would be dropped and that they would spend less time incarcerated. This meant plead-ing guilty to conspiracy for something—spray painting—that is typically considered a mis-demeanor. In addition to having to pay significant fines, Amber Smith-Stewart and Annarella Rivera were sentenced to thirty days in federal prison. Their co-defendant, Caleb Freestone, was sentenced to a year while the fourth activist, Gabriela Oropesa, went to trial, was found guilty, and faces up to ten years in prison. See "Jane's Revenge Defendants Share Their Experiences Inside Federal Prison," January 15, 2025, Civil Liberties Defense Center, https://cldc.org/%E2%9B%93%EF%B8%8F%F0%9F%92%A5janes-revenge-defendants-share -their-experiences-inside-federal-prison/.

3. The pro-choice movement and mainstream media use "crisis pregnancy centers" (CPCs) most often. The CPC movement itself is more likely to use "pregnancy resource" or "preg-nancy help" centers. More recently, critics of CPCs have started using "anti-abortion preg-nancy centers." In this chapter, I largely use "CPC" and "CPCs" for the sake of concision.

4. In this chapter I mostly use gender neutral language to refer to those seeking abor-tion services, but it is important to note that CPCs consider cis women their target popula-tion, and so I use that designation especially when describing their campaigns and strategies.

5. In their second communique published a month after the *Dobbs* leak, the group wrote "several weeks ago, we watched and waited as self-proclaimed 'feminist' organizations and non-profits took the lead on arranging their demure little rallies for freedom. We were told to let them handle it and defer to the political machinery that has thus far failed to secure our

liberation. . . . We cannot sit idly by anymore while our anger is yet again channeled into Democratic party fundraisers and peace parades with the police." See Janes' Revenge, "Night of Rage," May 30, 2022, https://theanarchistlibrary.org/library/night-of-rage.

6. For a rare example of in-depth reporting on CPCs that explores this angle, see Griswold (2019).

7. My intention in exploring this reality is not to trivialize or overlook the experiences of those individuals who have been deceived by CPCs. These people deserve to speak out, be defended, and have the harms they experienced be rectified to the greatest extent possible. The same is true for those individuals who turn to CPCs for pregnancy or family-related support and find limited help. Given that this is the most common way people will encounter CPCs, it is necessary to develop a political strategy that makes visible and endeavors to oppose the harms this group experiences.

8. I hope this history can engender new political approaches to CPCs, a call recently made by Thomsen (2022).

9. As evidenced by the period of "rage funds" in which supporters of abortion rights responded to *Dobbs* (2022) by briefly flooding abortion organizations with donations only to fall off months later (see also the chapter by Ophra Leyser-Whalen and Erin Johnson in this volume), it also fails to elicit sustained involvement in a fight. See Weixel, Nathaniel, "'Rage' Abortion Donations Dry Up, Leaving Funds Struggling to Meet Demand," *The Hill*, January 28, 2024, https://thehill.com/policy/healthcare/4432629-rage-abortion-donations-dry-up/.

10. See the Committee to Defend Reproductive Rights and Carla Abbotts, Plaintiffs, vs. A Free Pregnancy Center, et al., Defendants, in the Superior Court of the State of California in and for the City and County of San Francisco, December 1989, Box 448, Folder "Carla Abbotts Fake Clinics, 85–90," NOW Legal Defense Fund Records, 1968–2008, Schlesinger Library, Harvard University; and Ellen Lane, "Clinic Founder Says His Methods Are Honest, Ethical," *Gannet Westchester Newspapers*, March 23, 1986, Carton 77, Folder "Fake Clinics: pro-life pregnancy centers, 84, 86," NOW Records, Schlesinger Library, Harvard University.

11. For representative examples, see Eleanor J. Bader, "Bogus Clinics Offer Prayers, Not Abortions," *Guardian*, April 16, 1986; Susan Bolotin, "Selling Chastity: The Sly New Attack on Your Sexual Freedom," *Vogue*, n.d.; Lisa Krieger, "Just the Facts?" *City Paper*, February 21, 1986; and Ellen Lane, "Clinic Founder Says His Methods Are Honest, Ethical," *Gannet Westchester Newspapers*, March 23, 1986, all available in Carton 77, Folder "Fake Clinics: pro-life pregnancy centers, 84, 86," NOW Records, Schlesinger Library, Harvard University. Also see Gary Bergel, "A Release of Virtue: Alternatives to Abortion," *Intercessors for America*, n.d., Box 74, Folder "Fake Clinics, 1984," NOW Records, Schlesinger Library, Harvard University; and Susan Miller and Holly Hittman, "Inside a Right-to-Life 'Pregnancy' Center," *The West Side Spirit*, February 6, 1990, Box 10, Folder "WHAM! Articles, 1990," WHAM! Papers, Tamiment Library, New York University. Also see Michelle Landsberg, "Fake Abortion Clinics a Pro-Life Front for Emotional Violence," *Globe and Mail*, October 11, 1986; Mark Uehling et al., "Clinics of Deception: Pro-Lifers Set Up Shop," *Newsweek*, September 1, 1986.

12. Quoted in Susan Miller and Holly Hittman, "Inside a Right-to-Life 'Pregnancy' Center," *The West Side Spirit*, February 6, 1990, Box 10, Folder "WHAM! Articles, 1990," WHAM! Papers, Tamiment Library, New York University. Ann Menasche, a feminist attorney who successfully sued a Pearson affiliate in San Francisco, testified that Pearson "perfected the art of deception" at the hearings.

13. The undercover activists brought urine samples that would test positive for pregnancy to ensure they were subjected to volunteers' coercive tactics. Then-Attorney General Robert Abrams brought the suit against the three centers in New York City. See interview with Amy Sutnick by Sara Matthiesen, March 15, 2013, on file with author. Attorney Ann Menasche led the suit against A Free Pregnancy Center in San Francisco (Committee to Defend Reproductive Rights and Carla Abbotts).

14. For example, the New York City-based Women's Health Action Mobilization (WHAM!) reported on the Washington, D.C., group's mobilization against CPCs in its magazine, *WHAM! Frontlines*. See Neil deMause, "Fake Clinics," *WHAM! Frontlines* (Winter 1991/1992), Box 1, Folder "11th Hour Coalition," WHAM! Papers, Tamiment Library, New York University.

15. For example, see Lisa Krieger, "Just the Facts?" *City Paper*, February 21, 1986, Carton 77, Folder "Fake Clinics: pro-life pregnancy centers, 84, 86," NOW Records, Schlesinger Library, Harvard University; Susan Miller and Holly Hittman, "Inside a Right-to-Life 'Pregnancy' Center," *The West Side Spirit*, February 6, 1990, Box 10, Folder "WHAM! Articles, 1990," WHAM! Papers, Tamiment Library, New York University.

16. For Chicago, see Barker (1987). For representative feminist activism from multiple cities, see "How to Avoid Going to a Fake Clinic." undated CHOICE pamphlet, Carton 77, Folder "Fake Clinics: pro-life pregnancy centers, 84, 86," NOW Records, Schlesinger Library, Harvard University; "They Are Lying to You!" Washington Area Clinic Defense Task Force (WACDTF), undated flier, Box 4, Folder "WACDTF 90–93," WHAM! Papers, Tamiment Library, New York University; "Stop Bogus Clinics: Expose What They Really Are!" Emergency Defense Clinic Coalition of Chicago, IL, undated flier and "Defend Abortion Rights! Picket a Phony Clinic!" Ann Arbor Committee to Defend Abortion and Reproductive Rights, Box 10, Folder "Detroit Articles of Interest," WHAM! Papers, Tamiment Library, New York University; "Beware of Anti-Choice 'Pregnancy Counseling Centers,'" WomanCare Clinic, undated flier, "Fake Clinics: A Public Health Hazard," undated WHAM! pamphlet, and "Not An Abortion Clinic," undated WHAM! flier, Box 1, Folder "Fake Clinics, n.d., 1990–1992," WHAM! Papers, Tamiment Library, New York University.

17. Curtis J. Young, "Abortion, It's a Lonely Word," *Christian Action Council Newsletter*, December 1, 1984, bMS 438/3, George Hunston Williams Papers, Harvard Divinity School Repository; *Pro-Life Advocate: Magazine of the Christian Action Council* 1 (2), p. 10, n.d., Box 24, Folder "CAC," 1st Amendment Papers, Tufts University.

18. For example, a network of centers run by the Right to Life League of Southern California were also sued for deceptive advertising during this period (Oliver 1985).

19. In fact, far from providing robust medical services related to pregnancy and childbirth, professional medical organizations consider CPCs to be a risk to public health. See, for example, American College of Obstetricians and Gynecologists (2022).

20. For example, Kelly has argued that such changes not only restored the movement's legitimacy, but also ushered in its expansion: "Ironically, the attacks on the CPC movement temporarily sent it into a tailspin, but the result was a series of changes promoting successful expansion" (Kelly 2012, 212). For an alternative but complementary analysis of the movement's expansion during this period, see Matthiesen 2021, chap. 5.

21. Investigative reports from state chapters beginning in 2008 included Maryland, Texas, California, New York City, North Carolina, Ohio, Minnesota, Massachusetts, Montana, and Missouri, all on file with the author (e.g., Kleder and Richmond-Crum 2008; McIntire 2015; Moulia 2010; NARAL Pro-Choice New York Foundation 2010; NARAL Pro-Choice North Carolina Foundation 2011; NARAL Pro-Choice Texas Foundation 2009). The National Abortion Federation also relied on undercover investigators for its 2006 report, "Crisis Pregnancy Centers: An Affront to Choice."

22. For example, Expose Fake Clinics is at https://www.exposefakeclinics.com/, Repro-Action's Anti-Abortion Pregnancy Center Database is at https://reproaction.org/database/. While these are activist projects, researchers Andrea Swartzendruber and Danielle Lambert also maintain a mapping project of CPCs that is publicly available. The Crisis Pregnancy Center (CPC) Map is at https://crisispregnancycentermap.com/.

23. The quote from pro-life activist Abby Johnson is as follows: "The best client you ever get is one that thinks they're walking into an abortion clinic." Johnson was speaking at a Heartbeat International conference in 2012, and the quote became infamous when John Oliver's "Last Week Tonight" show aired a segment on crisis pregnancy centers on April 8, 2018, Episode 7, Season 5. (For another example of CPC-related activism involving Abby Johnson, see the chapter by Micki Burdick in this volume.)

24. "Memorandum to NOW LDEF Defense Committee from Marsha Levick and Alison Wetherfield," April 1, 1986, Box 448, Folder "Carla Abbotts Fake Clinics, 85–90," NOW Legal Defense Fund 1968–2008, Records, Schlesinger Library, Harvard University.

25. Katrina Kimport (2021) offers the equation "abortion=killing" to explain that the predominance of this cultural frame renders abortion "unchooseable" for some people.

26. For histories that trace women's participation in the movement, particularly during the period Pearson was most active, see Haugeberg (2017) and Matthiesen (2021, chap. 5). For work on women's contemporary role, see Kelly (2012) and Hussey (2020).

27. See "Wanted: Chris Slattery director of Manhattan Pregnancy Services," undated WHAM! flier, Box 1, Folder "Fake Clinics, 1990–1992," WHAM! Papers, Tamiment Library, New York University.

28. For a classic analysis on the early abortion rights movement's failure to confront white supremacy and capitalism, see Davis (1981, chap.12). For a history that explores how mainstream, majority-white feminist organizations refused to expand their agenda beyond abortion through the experience of Black feminist activist-scholar Loretta Ross, see Nelson (2015, chap. 4). See also Ross (2016).

29. On the professionalization of the pro-choice movement and how it came to rely on these and other electoral strategies such as lobbying, see Staggenborg (1994).

30. For a recent overview of municipal and state level efforts to educate the public about CPCs and rein in their deceptive advertising, see Baker and McKenna (2023). For the argument that abortion increasingly became a matter of consumer choice rather than rights following *Roe v. Wade* (1973), see Solinger (2001).

31. For two in-depth analyses of this development from different disciplinary approaches, see Matthiesen (2021, chap. 5) and Kelly and Gochanour (2018).

32. In addition to Guttmacher's widely cited report debunking this claim, the reproductive justice organization SisterSong countered a similar argument made about abortion clinics in Georgia by a Black spokeswoman for the "toomanyaborted.com" anti-abortion billboard campaign that targeted Black, pregnant women: "SisterSong's research revealed the actual facts: only three of the fifteen clinics in Georgia were in Black neighborhoods." See Ross (2017, 68).

33. For one example of investigative reporting that addresses these questions while illustrating how the knowledge of those most impacted—in this case, poor, Black mothers in Kansas City—can powerfully counter many of the CPC movement's claims, see Solomon (2013). For a model of opposition research into the anti-abortion movement's turn to eugenics ideology that also thinks along these lines, see Ross (2017).

34. It is only very recently that scholars writing about CPCs have begun citing research on the movement's failed effort to deter pregnant women from abortion. After acknowledging this fact, however, many immediately return to the standard pro-choice narrative that the movement's deception threatens pregnant women's access to abortion. For representative examples, see University of Wisconsin Collaborative for Reproductive Equity (2023) and Thomsen and Baker (2022).

35. For example, research has shown that, at least in the cases of pregnancy confirmation and ultrasound scans, CPCs are able to capitalize on the realities of inaccessible and insufficient reproductive health care. See Vinekar et al. (2023) and Kissling et al. (2022).

36. The most popular slogans illustrating this shift include "*Roe* is the floor, not the ceiling" and "*Roe* was never enough." See also Sherman and Mahone (2024) and Brown (2019). On the Democratic party's stubborn refusal to acknowledge this sea change, see Grant (2024).

REFERENCES

Abcarian, Robin. 2015. "California Journal: Going Undercover at Crisis Pregnancy Centers." *LA Times*, May 1, 2015. https://www.latimes.com/local/abcarian/la-me-0501-abcarian-crisis-pregnancy-20150501-column.html.

American College of Obstetricians and Gynecologists (ACOG). 2022. "Issue Brief: Crisis Pregnancy Centers." October 2022. https://www.acog.org/-/media/project/acog/acogorg/files/advocacy/issue-briefs/crisis-pregnancy-centers.pdf.

Aslam, Fazeelat. 2014. "The Fake Abortion Clinics of America: Misconception." *Vice News*, September 17, 2014. https://archive.org/details/TheFakeAbortionClinicsOfAmericaMisconception.

Baker, Carrie N., and Jennifer McKenna. 2023. "Grassroots Progress to Hold Anti-Abortion Crisis Pregnancy Centers Accountable." *Ms. Magazine*, February 7, 2023. https://msmagazine.com/2023/02/07/crisis-pregnancy-center-fake-abortion-clinic/.

Bancroft, Caitlin. 2013. "What I Learned Undercover at a Crisis Pregnancy Center." *Huffington Post*, August 15, 2013. https://www.huffpost.com/entry/crisis-pregnancy-center_b_3763196.

Barker, Teresa. 1987. "Testing Anti-Abortion Clinics." *Chicago Tribune*, March 15, 1987.

Belluck, Pam. 2013. "Pregnancy Centers Gain Influence in Anti-Abortion Arena." *New York Times*, January 4, 2013. https://www.nytimes.com/2013/01/05/health/pregnancy-centers-gain-influence-in-anti-abortion-fight.html.

Brown, Jenny. 2019. *Abortion Without Apology: The Abortion Struggle Now*. Verso.

Bukuras, Joe. 2023. "Ohio Pregnancy Center Vandalized in 'Jane's Revenge' Attack." *Catholic News Agency*, April 17, 2023. https://www.catholicnewsagency.com/news/254117/ohio-pregnancy-center-vandalized-in-jane-s-revenge-attack.

Campbell, Brittany A. 2017. "The Crisis Inside Crisis Pregnancy Centers: How to Stop These Facilities from Depriving Women of Their Reproductive Freedom." *Boston College Journal of Law and Social Justice* 37 (1): 73–105. https://lira.bc.edu/files/pdf?fileid=37b8ddfc-eeb3-4d88-8b8d-cd8ff5021317

Cooperman, Alan. 2002. "Abortion Battle: Prenatal Care or Pressure Tactics? 'Crisis Pregnancy Centers' Expand and Draw Criticism." *Washington Post*, February 21, 2002. https://www.washingtonpost.com/archive/politics/2002/02/21/abortion-battle-prenatal-care-or-pressure-tactics/cb2e711d-cf1b-4667-80eb-bc253e61e09d/.

Davis, Angela Y. 1981. *Women, Race and Class*. Vintage.

Feminist Majority Foundation. 2022. "National Clinic Violence Survey." https://feminist.org/wp-content/uploads/2023/07/2022-national-clinic-violence-survey.pdf.

Frasik, Christina, Claire Jordan, Corrine McLeod, and Rachel Flink-Bochacki. 2023. "A Mystery Client Study of Crisis Pregnancy Center Practices in New York State." *Contraception* 117: 36–38. https://doi.org/10.1016/j.contraception.2022.08.004.

Gaebe, Molly. 2019. "The Lies They Tell." *Expose Fake Clinics* (blog), February 4, 2019. https://www.exposefakeclinics.com/blog/2019/2/4/the-lies-they-tell.

Gerson, Jennifer. 2019. "Fake Health Clinics Are Tricking College Students." *Cosmopolitan*, February 1, 2019. https://www.cosmopolitan.com/health-fitness/a26062253/crisis-pregnancy-centers-college-campus/.

Grant, Melissa Gira. 2024. "'Restore *Roe*' Is a Bad Rallying Cry." *New Republic*, March 20, 2024. https://newrepublic.com/article/179961/abortion-ballot-restore-roe-biden.

Greenberg, Rachel. 2018. "Going 'Undercover' (as Myself) in a CPC." *Medium*, August 20, 2018. https://prochoicemd.medium.com/going-undercover-as-myself-in-a-cpc-77e3e365f592.

Grimes, David A., Jacqueline D. Forrest, Alice L. Kirkman, and Barbara Radford. 1991. "An Epidemic of Abortion Violence in the United States." *American Journal of Obstetrics & Gynecology* 165 (5): 1263–1268. https://doi.org/10.1016/0002-9378(91)90346-S.

Griswold, Eliza. 2019. "The New Front Line of the Anti-Abortion Movement." *New Yorker*, November 11, 2019. https://www.newyorker.com/magazine/2019/11/18/the-new-front-line-of-the-anti-abortion-movement.

Gross, Jane. 1987. "Pregnancy Centers: Anti-Abortion Role Challenged." *New York Times*, January 23, 1987. https://www.nytimes.com/1987/01/23/nyregion/pregnancy-centers-anti-abortion-role-challenged.html.

Gustafson, Kaaryn. 2011. *Cheating Welfare: Public Assistance and the Criminalization of Poverty*. New York University Press.

Guttmacher Institute. 2014. "Claim That Most Abortion Clinics Are Located in Black or Hispanic Neighborhood Is False." Guttmacher Institute, June 1, 2014. https://www.guttmacher.org/claim-most-abortion-clinics-are-located-black-or-hispanic-neighborhoods-false.

Hartshorn, Peggy. 2011. *Foot Soldiers Armed with Love: Heartbeat International's First Forty Years*. Donning Company.

Haugeberg, Karissa. 2017. *Women against Abortion: Inside the Largest Moral Reform Movement of the Twentieth Century.* University of Illinois Press.

Hussey, Laura S. 2020. *The Pro-Life Pregnancy Help Movement: Serving Women or Saving Babies?* University Press of Kansas.

Jane's Revenge. May 10, 2022. "First Communiqué." https://theanarchistlibrary.org/library/janes-revenge-first-communique.

Jane's Revenge. May 30, 2022. "Night of Rage." https://theanarchistlibrary.org/library/night-of-rage.

Jane's Revenge. June 14, 2022. "Another Communiqué." https://theanarchistlibrary.org/library/jane-s-revenge-another-communique.

Kelly, Kimberly. 2012. "In the Name of the Mother: Renegotiating Conservative Women's Authority in the Crisis Pregnancy Center Movement." *Signs* 38 (1): 203–230. https://doi.org/10.1086/665807.

———. 2014. "Evangelical Underdogs: Intrinsic Success, Organizational Solidarity, and Marginalized Identities as Religious Movement Resources." *Journal of Contemporary Ethnography* 43 (4): 419–455. https://doi.org/10.1177/0891241613516627.

Kelly, Kimberly, and Amanda Gochanour. 2018. "Racial Reconciliation or Spiritual Smokescreens? Blackwashing the Crisis Pregnancy Center Movement." *Qualitative Sociology* 41: 423–443. https://doi.org/10.1007/s11133-018-9392-0.

Kimport, Katrina. 2020. "Pregnant Women's Reasons for and Experiences of Visiting Anti-abortion Pregnancy Resource Centers." *Perspectives on Sexual and Reproductive Health* 52 (1): 51–53. https://doi.org/10.1363/psrh.12131.

———. 2021. *No Real Choice: How Culture and Politics Matter for Reproductive Autonomy.* Rutgers University Press.

Kimport, Katrina, Rebecca Kriz, and Sarah C. M. Roberts. 2018. "The Prevalence and Impacts of Crisis Pregnancy Center Visits Among a Population of Pregnant Women." *Contraception* 98 (1): 69–73. https://doi.org/10.1016/j.contraception.2018.02.016.

Kissling, Alexandra, Priya Gursahaney, Alison H. Norris, Danielle Bessett, and Maria F. Gallo. 2022. "Free, But at What Cost? How US Crisis Pregnancy Centres Provide Services." *Culture, Health, & Sexuality* 25 (8): 1024–1038. https://doi.org/10.1080/13691058.2022.2116489.

Kleder, Melissa, and S. Malia Richmond-Crum. 2008. "Maryland Crisis Pregnancy Center Investigations: The Truth Revealed." NARAL Pro-Choice Maryland Fund. https://web.archive.org/web/20141026003358/https://www.prochoicemd.org/assets/bin/pdfs/cpcreportfinal.pdf.

Landsberg, Michele. 1986. "Fake Abortion Clinics a Pro-Life Front for Emotional Violence." *Globe and Mail*, October 11, 1986.

Lennard, Natasha. 2023. "Abortion Rights Activists Face Attack from DeSantis and Conspiracy Lawsuit—for Spray Painting." *The Intercept*, May 18, 2023. https://theintercept.com/2023/05/18/abortion-conspiracy-lawsuit-florida/.

Lewis, Sophie. 2019. *Full Surrogacy Now: Feminism against Family.* Verso.

Lin, Vitoria, and Cynthia Dailard. 2002. "Crisis Pregnancy Centers Seek to Increase Political Clout, Secure Government Subsidy." *Guttmacher Report on Public Policy* 5 (2): 4–6. https://www.guttmacher.org/sites/default/files/article_files/gr050204.pdf.

Marty, Robin. 2013. "Undercover Audio Recordings Reveal False Claims Made at Virginia Crisis Pregnancy Center." *Rewire News Group*, August 12, 2013. https://rewirenewsgroup.com/2013/08/12/undercover-audio-recordings-reveal-false-claims-made-at-virginia-crisis-pregnancy-center/.

Matthiesen, Sara. 2021. *Reproduction Reconceived: Family Making and the Limits of Choice after Roe v. Wade.* University of California Press.

McElroy, Meagan. 2015. "Protecting Pregnant Pennsylvanians: Public Funding of Crisis Pregnancy Centers." *University of Pittsburgh Law Review* 76 (3): 334. https://doi.org/10.5195/lawreview.2015.334.

McGuire, Kimberly Inez. 2018. "I Love My Son, but I Was Tricked into Having Him." *Romper*, January 31, 2018. https://www.romper.com/p/i-love-my-son-but-a-crisis-pregnancy-center-tricked-me-into-having-him-7928219.

McIntire, Lisa. 2015. "Crisis Pregnancy Centers Lie: The Insidious Threat to Reproductive Freedom." NARAL Pro-Choice America. https://reproductivefreedomforall.org/wp-content/uploads/2017/04/cpc-report-2015.pdf.

McKenna, Jenifer, and Tara Murtha, for the Alliance. 2021. "Designed to Deceive: A Study of the Crisis Pregnancy Center Industry in Nine States." The Alliance: State Advocates for Women's Rights & Gender Equality, 2021. https://alliancestateadvocates.org/crisis-pregnancy-centers/.

Montoya, Melissa M., Colleen Judge-Golden, and Jonas J. Swartz. 2022. "The Problems with Crisis-Pregnancy Centers: Reviewing the Literature and Identifying New Directions for Future Research." *International Journal of Women's Health* 14: 757–763. https://doi.org/10.2147/IJWH.S288861.

Morgan, Jennifer. 2007. *Laboring Women: Reproduction and Gender in New World Slavery.* University of Pennsylvania Press.

Moulia, Danielle. 2010. "Unmasking Fake Clinics: The Truth about Crisis Pregnancy Centers in California." NARAL Pro-Choice America California Foundation. https://web.archive.org/web/20140909042546/https://prochoicecalifornia.org/assets/bin/pdfs/cpcreport2010-revisednov2010.pdf.

Munson, Ziad W. 2008. *The Making of Pro-Life Activists: How Social Movement Mobilization Works.* University of Chicago Press.

Naftulin, Julia. 2022. "Crisis Pregnancy Centers Prey on People Looking for Abortions, but Don't Offer Them. Here's How to Spot One." *Business Insider,* June 28, 2022. https://www.businessinsider.com/crisis-pregnancy-centers-prey-on-abortion-seekers-how-to-spot-2022-6.

NARAL Pro-Choice New York Foundation. 2010. "'She Said Abortion Could Cause Breast Cancer': A Report on the Lies, Manipulations, and Privacy Violations of Crisis Pregnancy Centers in New York City." 2010. NARAL Pro-Choice New York Foundation and the National Institute for Reproductive Health. https://nirhealth.org/wp-content/uploads/2015/09/cpcreport2010.pdf.

NARAL Pro-Choice North Carolina Foundation. 2011. "The Truth Revealed: North Carolina's Crisis Pregnancy Centers. October 24, 2011. https://prochoicenc.org/wp-content/uploads/2021/10/The-Truth-Revealed-North-Carolinas-Crisis-Pregnancy-Centers.pdf.

NARAL Pro-Choice Texas Foundation. 2009. "2009 Annual Report. Taxpayer Financed Crisis Pregnancy Centers in Texas: A Hidden Threat to Women's Health." https://web.archive.org/web/20250322075518/http://txpregnancy.org/wp-content/uploads/2009-CPC-Report.pdf.

National Abortion Federation. 2006. "Crisis Pregnancy Centers: An Affront to Choice." http://www.prochoice.org/pubs_research/publications/downloads/public_policy/cpc_report.pdf.

Nelson, Jennifer. 2015. *More Than Medicine: A History of the Feminist Women's Health Movement.* New York University Press.

Noor, Poppy. 2022. "Pro-Choice Militants Are Targeting 'Pregnancy Crisis Centers' across U.S." *The Guardian,* June 2, 2022. https://www.theguardian.com/world/2022/jun/11/pro-choice-militants-pregnancy-crisis-centers-attacks-us.

North, Anna. 2020. "What 'Crisis Pregnancy Centers' Really Do." *Vox,* March 2, 2020. https://www.vox.com/2020/3/2/21146011/crisis-pregnancy-center-resource-abortion-title-x.

Oliver, Myrna. 1985. "Right to Life League Sued; Woman Claims Deception." *Los Angeles Times,* January 23, 1985. https://www.latimes.com/archives/la-xpm-1985-01-23-me-14544-story.html.

Planned Parenthood Federation of America. 1991. "Anti-Abortion Counseling Centers: A Consumer's Alert to Deception, Harassment, and Medical Malpractice." Planned Parenthood Federation of America and National Abortion Federation. https://web.archive.org/web/19990202084309/https://www.plannedparenthood.org/library/opposition/antiabcenters.htm.

———. 2021. "New *The Handmaid's Tale* Episode, 'Milk,' Shows the Harm of Crisis Pregnancy Centers." Planned Parenthood Press Release, May 6, 2021. https://www.plannedparenthood

.org/about-us/newsroom/press-releases/new-the-handmaids-tale-episode-milk-shows-the
-harm-of-crisis-pregnancy-centers.

Reproductive Health and Freedom Watch (RHFW). 2024. "Why Is the Billion-Dollar Unregulated Pregnancy Clinic Industry Receiving Increasing Taxpayer Dollars?" Memo, July 2024. https://reproductivehealthfreedom.us/wp-content/uploads/2024/08/July-2024 _Memo_Taxpayer-Funding-to-UPC-Industry_updated-1-1.pdf.

Roberts, Dorothy. 2002. *Shattered Bonds: The Color of Child Welfare.* Civitas Books.

———. 2022. *Torn Apart: How the Child Welfare System Destroys Black Families—And How Abolition Can Build a Safer World.* Basic Books.

Ross, Loretta J. 2016. "The Color of Choice: White Supremacy and Reproductive Justice." In *Color of Violence: The INCITE! Anthology,* edited by INCITE! Women of Color Against Violence, 53–65. Duke University Press.

———. 2017. "Trust Black Women: Reproductive Justice and Eugenics." In *Radical Reproductive Justice: Foundations, Theory, Practice, Critique,* editors Loretta J. Ross, Lynn Roberts, Erika Derkas, Whitney Peoples, and Pamela Bridgewater Toure, 58–85. Feminist Press.

Ross, Loretta J., and Rickie Solinger. 2017. *Reproductive Justice: An Introduction.* University of California Press.

Scott, Douglas R. 2000. "The Making of Controversy: The History of the Conspiracy against Pregnancy Care Centers." *Life Decisions International* 3 (3).

SisterSong Women of Color Reproductive Justice Collective. "What Is Reproductive Justice?" Accessed April 27, 2025. https://www.sistersong.net/reproductive-justice/.

Sherman, Carter. 2024. "Anti-abortion Centers Raked In $1.4 Billion in Year *Roe* Feel, Including Federal Money." *The Guardian,* February 14, 2024. https://www.theguardian .com/world/2024/feb/14/anti-abortion-centers-funding.

Sherman, Renee Bracey, and Regina Mahone. 2024. *Liberating Abortion: Claiming Our History, Sharing Our Stories, and Building the Reproductive Future We Deserve.* Harper Collins.

Solinger, Rickie. 2001. *Beggars and Choosers: How the Politics of Choice Shapes Adoption, Abortion, and Welfare in the United States.* Hill and Wang.

Solomon, Akiba. 2013. "The Missionary Movement to 'Save' Black Babies." *Colorlines,* May 2, 2013. https://web.archive.org/web/20130611183511/https://colorlines.com/archives/2013/05 /crisis_pregnancy_centers_and_race_baiting.html.

Spillers, Hortense. 1987. "Mama's Baby, Papa's Maybe: An American Grammar Book," *Diacritics* 17 (2): 64–81.

Staba, David. 2007. "Doctor's Killer Tries to Make Abortion the Issue." *New York Times,* January 13, 2007. https://www.nytimes.com/2007/01/13/nyregion/13abort.html.

Stacey, Dawn. 2009. "The Pregnancy Center Movement: History of Crisis Pregnancy Centers," *Crisis Pregnancy Center Watch,* July 12, 2009. https://motherjones.com/wp-content /uploads/cpchistory2.pdf.

Stack, Katie. 2011. "When I Needed Help I Got Propaganda." *New York Times,* October 5, 2011. https://www.nytimes.com/2011/10/06/opinion/crisis-pregnancy-centers-and-propaganda.html.

Staggenborg, Suzanne. 1994. *The Pro-Choice Movement: Organization and Activism in the Abortion Conflict.* Oxford University Press.

Sullivan, Kevin. 1991. "Group Pickets Antiabortion 'Clinic' in MD." *Washington Post,* November 2, 1991. https://www.washingtonpost.com/archive/local/1991/11/03/group -pickets-antiabortion-clinic-in-md/2747b5fe-8838-4a26-b06e-4ae56b15150f/.

Swartzendruber, Andrea, and Danielle N. Lambert. 2020. "A Web-Based Geolocated Directory of Crisis Pregnancy Centers (CPCs) in the United States: Description of CPC Map Methods and Design Features and Analysis of Baseline Data." *JMIR Public Health and Surveillance* 6 (1): e16726. https://doi.org/10.2196/16726.

Tapscott, Richard. 1991. "5 Md. Pregnancy Clinics Accused of Deception: Abortion Rights Group Files a Complaint." *Washington Post,* July 25, 1991.

Thomsen, Carly. 2022. "Animating and Sustaining Outrage: The Place of Crisis Pregnancy Centers in Abortion Justice." *Human Geography* 15 (3): 300–306. https://doi.org/10.1177 /19427786221076154.

Thomsen, Carly, and Carrie N. Baker. 2022. "Pregnant? Need Help? They Have an Agenda."
    New York Times, May 12, 2022. https://www.nytimes.com/interactive/2022/05/12/opinion
    /crisis-pregnancy-centers-roe.html.
Thomsen, Carly, Zach Levitt, Christopher Gernon, and Penelope Spencer. 2023. "Presence
    and Absence: Crisis Pregnancy Centers and Abortion Facilities in the Contemporary
    Reproductive Justice Landscape." *Human Geography* 16 (1): 64–74. https://doi.org/10.1177
    /19427786221109959.
Thomsen, Carly, and Grace Tacherra Morrison. 2020. "Abortion as Gender Transgression:
    Reproductive Justice, Queer Theory, and Anti–Crisis Pregnancy Center Activism." *Signs*
    45 (3): 703-730. https://doi.org/10.1086/706487.
Tiffany, Kaitlyn. 2022. "The Right's New Bogeyman. *The Atlantic,* August 12, 2022. https://
    www.theatlantic.com/technology/archive/2022/08/janes-revenge-antifa-dobbs-roe
    -abortion/671098/.
Uehling, Mark et al. 1986. "Clinics of Deception: Pro-Lifers Set Up Shop," *Newsweek,* Sep-
    tember 1, 1986.
UltraViolet. 2018. "CPCs Lie." https://web.archive.org/web/20250118044231/https://weareul
    traviolet.org/cpcs-lie/.
University of Wisconsin Collaborative for Reproductive Equity (CORE). 2023. "Crisis Preg-
    nancy Centers in the U.S. and Wisconsin." *CORE Brief,* December. University of Wiscon-
    sin Collaborative for Reproductive Equity. https://core.wisc.edu/wp-content/uploads/sites
    /1349/2023/04/Crisis-pregnancy-centers_Dec-2023.pdf.
U.S. House of Representatives. 1991. *Consumer Protection and Patient Safety Issues Involving
    Bogus Abortion Clinics: Hearing Before the Subcommittee on Regulation, Business Opportu-
    nities, and Energy of the Committee on Small Business,* 102nd Cong. (1991), first session,
    Washington, DC, September 20, 1991. https://hdl.handle.net/2027/pst.000019273587.
Vinekar, Kavita, Marian Jarlenski, Leslie Meyn, Beatrice A. Chen, Sharon L. Achilles, Sara
    Tyberg, and Sonya Borrero. 2023. "Early Pregnancy Confirmation Availability at Crisis
    Pregnancy Centers and Abortion Facilities in the United States." *Contraception* 117: 30–35.
    https://doi.org/10.1016/j.contraception.2022.08.008.
Weixel, Nathaniel. 2024. "'Rage' Abortion Donations Dry Up, Leaving Funds Struggling to
    Meet Demand." *The Hill,* January 28, 2024. https://thehill.com/policy/healthcare
    /4432629-rage-abortion-donations-dry-up/.
Winter, Meaghan. 2015. "I Felt Set Up." *Type Investigations,* December 17, 2015. https://www
    .typeinvestigations.org/investigation/2015/12/17/felt-set/.
Wormer, Rachel. 2021. "Mapping Deception: A Closer Look at How States' Anti-Abortion
    Center Programs Operate." Equity Forward, June 4, 2021. https://equityfwd.org/mapping
    -deception-closer-look-how-states-anti-abortion-center-programs-operate.

CHAPTER 12

"This Right Here Is a Baby"

WHITE EVANGELICAL WOMEN
IN THE PRO-LIFE MOVEMENT

Micki Burdick

On a late spring day in the middle of Times Square in New York City, thousands of people stand around an industrial stage with a large, blank screen facing them. Suddenly, on the screen a live four-dimensional ultrasound image is shown, bringing the audience to complete silence. A full-color, moving picture of Abby Johnson's fetus in utero captivates all in the vicinity. Backstage, this ultrasound is being performed on Johnson, a former Planned Parenthood leader turned pro-life evangelist. After her ultrasound, Abby Johnson comes out and yells to the crowd, tears running down her face, fully surrounded by the moving picture of her womb still on the screen: "This is a baby! This right here is a baby. This right here is a baby! It's not a cat. It's not a parasite. This is a human being with a heartbeat, with its own DNA that is separate from my body. And this baby deserves to live" (Browder 2019). This vignette happened at a May 4, 2019, Focus on the Family event called "Alive from New York" that was part of an annual twelve-week "See Life Clearly" campaign in opposition to abortion. Each year, Alive from New York participants rally around and celebrate the life of unborn fetuses. It is popular: around 10,000 people registered for the first Alive from New York event in May 2019.

It is not just the words Abby Johnson speaks that move the crowd of mainly white women. It is the connection of emotions from the ultrasound technology to the screen to the individual audience members that creates and wields a particular *feeling* around the concept of abortion in these spaces and beyond. In common pro-life campaigns such as Alive from New York, the use of ultrasounds and sharing of sonograms creates a specific mood for the audience. And it is a mood of unease, one that is pretty common when it comes to discussions of abortion. What is not common is attention paid to the people who engender this feeling: white Evangelical women. This group tends to be ignored in lieu of focus on more male-dominated pro-life discourses and actions.

In this chapter, I show how this negative or uneasy feeling around abortion that we often name in different ways comes from the historical and contemporary performances, like those on that spring day in Times Square, of white Evangelical women. Specifically, I use Evangelical Pregnancy Resource Centers and their use of technology to explore white women's activism in the pro-life movement and its consequences for the words and feelings surrounding reproductive health care in the United States.[1]

WHY WHITE EVANGELICAL WOMEN?

White women are the backbone of the pro-life movement. Following the overturning of *Roe*, more people started paying attention to the anti-abortion movement in the United States, calling for interrogations of its (apparently) new powerful position in American political life. Many of these conversations centering on electoral politics interrogate understandings of abortion as under attack by a powerful masculinity fueled by patriarchal motivations and discursive contestations in political life (Filipovic 2019; Jong-Fast 2022). These analyses are worthwhile, but they only partially illuminate the anti-choice movement and its power. While the public face of the anti-abortion movement is (white) men focused on politicians and mainstream politics, white women focused on pregnant people seeking abortion and reproductive health care are an overlooked faction of the movement.

Overlooking these women is a problem. Evangelical women take up particular roles within conservative movements and—in keeping with gender politics writ large—do work that is often overlooked as well as taken for granted (Griffith 2000). Like Abby Johnson, whose ultrasound was projected in Times Square, the women who volunteer in the pro-life movement create and sustain its powerful anti-abortion sentiments through usages of medical reproductive technologies, such as the sonogram. In their use of medical technologies, among other activities, these women use a combination of emotion and medical discourses/performances filtered through conservative ideology to create meaning around abortion and reproductive health care. This meaning is created not only through language but also through the driving force of *affective* politics—that is, emotion used through and with structures of power to influence politics. To better understand the state of abortion politically in the United States, I argue for an understanding of anti-abortion sentiments through white pro-life women. Indeed, our paradigms for understanding the anti-choice movement and its historical significance benefit from exploration of the historical and ever-present—pre- and post-*Dobbs*—white women's activism.

A major site of white, Evangelical, pro-life women's activism is Pregnancy Resource Centers (PRCs), known popularly as Crisis Pregnancy Centers (CPCs). PRCs are almost exclusively run by women and demand the most volunteer hours out of any other branch of the pro-life movement; collectively they see around one million clients annually (Kelly 2012, 205). Their stated mission is to steer "abortion-minded women"—a pro-life term describing those seeking abortions—away from abortion care and toward parenthood or adoption.[2] Much of the persuasion work that PRCs engage in relies on medical technology such as ultrasounds, and it is premised on beliefs about the meaning and effects of these technologies. While the Matthiesen chapter in this volume offers a critique of how the abortion rights movement has conceptualized and engaged with CPCs/PRCs, I focus here on the activities of white Evangelical women *in* these centers.

I draw on four years of ethnographic fieldwork with white, Evangelical, pro-life women, including their outreach materials, interviews with PRC workers, and participant observation from technology-centered events such as See Life Clearly to understand their development and mobilization of discourses of "life"—discourses that well predate the fall of *Roe* but offer insight into the ongoing production of opposition to abortion. I contextualize these ethnographic data through archival, public, and historical research. I trace the performances of technology within PRCs that have spread into the realm of reproductive health care, illustrating the use of white femininity through examples of white women using reproductive science and technology—"medical" discourses—to promote anti-choice politics through the circulation of emotions.

Pro-Life Emotion Work

The white Evangelical women who run and volunteer in PRCs are heavily invested in politically conservative movements and respond to policies and social issues in forceful, performative ways. Among them, they utilize emotion/femininity, which is understood to be uniquely available to white women. This belief as well as these testimonies are rooted in history. Evangelical groups in American history have traditionally objectified emotion as a tool to define certain bodies as more spiritual or animated than others, tying back into who can be "saved" by God (Corrigan 2002). Building a medicalized theory to ground this Evangelical construction of emotion, these groups visualize emotion as how much blood flows through the body, and they use medical technology to "measure" it. These unscientific "measurements" of emotion and humanity purportedly evidence that white people are historically endowed with more subjectivity than Black and brown people, with white women in particular defined "scientifically" as having the greatest capacity for emotionality (Corrigan 2002).

This capacity is not without its downsides, however. Because women were seen as controlled by emotion and a woman's mind was "limited by her body," in the sense of bodily functions such as menstruation and other reproductive capacities, married white women were called to profess their public faith by choosing to use their bodies and emotions for communal praying and, more importantly, pregnancy and birth (Karant-Nunn 2022). These activities were not only in service of replicating gendered structures, but they also contributed to the reproduction of whiteness; white women were understood to occupy a unique emotional potentiality as a combination of their race and sex. Under this logic, in order to keep their unruly emotionality restrained, white Protestant women had to rely on virtuous practices of traditional femininity as well as adhere to the Protestant Christian faith and God (Welter 1966, 153). Similarly, acceptable forms of white women's activism leveraged their presumed emotionality and included praying, crying, and giving deep personal testimonies.

Starting in the 1980s, conservative women's grassroots activism, such as those opposed to the Equal Rights Amendment, joined with larger institutions to form an assemblage of relationships between the social and the political through everyday lived religion (Howard 2008, 2011). White, conservative, Protestant women became understood as protectors of the private home through, seemingly counterintuitively, a more immediate and hands-on role in the public pro-life movement. Much like earlier movements for social reform, these women activists took on roles in the "direct service" thread of the pro-life movement, which involves sidewalk counseling—that is, standing outside of abortion healthcare clinics to evangelize to those going in. Eventually this service turned into the proliferation and popularity of volunteering and working at PRCs (Hutchens 2021, 2022; Munson 2008; Taylor 2008).

PRO-LIFE WOMEN AND AFFECTIVE TECHNOLOGIES

White women in the pro-life movement's activism is animated by fervent beliefs about life—and fetal life, in particular. These metaphysical beliefs are rendered concrete through bodies and, importantly, medical technologies. Pro-life women activists define life through pregnant bodies and life signs, which are both instituted and created through medical technologies. For instance, "life signs" are defined as the material aspects of a body that, working together, render it a "human" or "living thing" (Stormer 2010). Activists use medical technologies to measure and prove the existence of these life signs. For fetuses, this includes "seeing" the body itself through ultrasound technology, defining "gender" in the womb through genitalia, and hearing fetal heartbeats (Friz 2018, 640). Although rooted in beliefs (not science, for example), these activists' understandings of fetal personhood became formalized through medical technologies like ultrasounds. They claim medical technologies as singularly able to adjudicate the truth of life and, in the case of the fetus, fetal personhood. This practice further serves to decenter the pregnant person and legitimize third-party control over the pregnant body.

So where does emotion come in? How do these women use emotion politically? They do so through *affect*. Affect is the way we experience emotion—it is a way of sense-making through assemblages of or relationships between bodies that creates and spreads a mood, energy, or movement. Emotions are those nameable (and sometimes un-nameable) feelings and ideas that exist through communication with others (Ahmed 2004, 4). For my purposes here, affect is an analytic through which to understand the activism of women in the anti-choice movement and their power in the context of the United States. It is useful in this case specifically because of white women's use of and constructed propensity for emotion historically.

The Personal as Political

Evangelical women in the anti-choice movement use personal, religious testimonies and emotional language to feed pro-life discourses, which I could very much feel as I sat in front of and talked with them. During my fieldwork, I regularly heard the words "inspiring" and "in awe," and I witnessed visible or vocal crying and praying. These were normal phenomena through which these participants used affect, through their religious convictions, to create conservative political meaning out of personal pregnancy experiences. Often, these women were recounting their own abortions. One told me, "I showed up to the abortion clinic and was moved through the process with a dozen other girls. It was an assembly line of waiting in a room crying and hearing stories about how their friends heard their babies' bones breaking during their abortions. I felt the loss of my baby like a deep hollow hole that would never be filled." In this retelling, she described a certain feeling, one that existed both physically and emotionally, and attributed its origin to her abortion. In addition to tying the physical experience of abortion to a specific, negative emotion, she asserted that this feeling was not fleeting. In fact, it is perpetual, existing within her still today.

According to many of the pro-life women with a history of abortion I observed and spoke with, these perpetual feelings led them to become volunteers or leaders of PRCs, where they believed they could find healing. One recounted, "I became an advocate at the pregnancy care center where I participated in the twelve-week Hope and Healing program. Through my own experience with abortion and now seeing what is does to the hundreds of postabortive women I've encountered, I can say I am 100 percent pro-life in all situations." This woman's healing was not just personal; it was also about connecting to and seeing her own experience reflected in others. In the process, she became ideologically rigid, opposing abortion entirely. Her personal experience metamorphosed into a political stance.

While "the personal is political" is a common refrain throughout feminist, decolonial, and race scholarship to build liberatory movements, the conversations about the personal and political within feminine-based conservative movements have different consequences. When a pro-life woman staffer at a CPC describes in emotional detail her testimony of abortion, she is cultivating a negative affect about abortion and wielding this feeling to constrain access to reproductive health care.

Similar to these personal stories, personal images of a pregnant person's fetus within the womb circulate in these spaces. Ultrasound images, rendered in PRCs as a routine part of client intake, are presented as evidence of fetal life and personhood. But it is not only the images from PRC volunteers and owners that have importance; these images are regularly sourced from PRC clients, who may be seeking CPC services for a range of reasons (Kimport 2020), and then deployed to audiences as political messaging. A PRC volunteer spoke to me about how she would ask clients if she could share the pictures of their "baby" (i.e., ultrasound image) on the website or on the walls of the CPC waiting rooms. In the language accompanying the images, fetal personhood was asserted in a tautology where the words named the image and the image was presented as evidence of the truth of the description.

Enabling the tautology was invocation of emotion, connection, and affect. The fetus is not just defined as a "baby" in these moments but is also talked about with emotional language around birthing that then creates feelings within the client and in the space of the clinic. For example, while receiving ultrasounds, patients in PRCs are accompanied by volunteers who will often become tearful at the sight of the image, pray and hold hands with patients, and feign genuine excitement at the realization that there is, in fact, a fetus in utero. These pictures are then printed out and shared with the client and passed around the space to other workers nearby. By sharing "authentic" private images in these public spaces, PRC workers create intimate bonds with imagined audiences. This sharing, like the abortion testimonies, is a religious performance. They are connecting the private and public—seemingly private acts that occur in the public realm. By locating private thoughts in a public setting and deploying their "scientific" innate emotionality, white pro-life women leverage the feeling infused within the message to render this sharing of an ultrasound image as a political act of opposition to abortion.

Just as the pro-life woman's retelling of her personal story of abortion functions politically, the use and circulation of pregnant people's bodily scans are imbued with an affective, political force. Through affective connections, the private and intimate nature of families and the bodies that receive these ultrasounds circulate as a politically charged image shared with a wider public. The circulation of these sonogram images within a mixture of the private and public, particularly in the United States, shepherded by pro-life activists who imbue the performances with associated negative emotions, creates a climate shrouded with negative affect surrounding the fetus and reproductive bodies.

Centrally, affect is the process through which these personal stories and scans become political. The everyday political resides in "affective gestures of performativity"; a context can be both personal and political at the same time (Friz 2018, 640). Affect ties the personal to ideology—making the personal political—and can do so because of the emotional histories and power that came before the present feeling (Papacharissi 2015, 15). In the case of PRC activism, these (emotional) acts wherein the personal is rendered political become intertwined with the definition of the ideal human body and being as well as what constitutes personhood and who has rights over this personhood (Doshi 2018).

Technologies like ultrasound that can be used to monitor and surveil people's bodies (particularly those who are defined as reproducers) are part of this process. PRCs/CPCs rely on medicalization for their claim-making, deploying normative practices like the "medical gaze" wherein medical issues or situations (such as pregnancy) are understood via technology and its affordances rather than from the body, voice, and agency of the individual (Friz 2018). The idea of—and trust in—a medical gaze from doctors and technologies is deeply embedded in mainstream health care today. Pro-life women invoke this trust to normalize anti-choice arguments, pairing white Evangelical women's stories and affective uses of these medical technologies to assert the "truth" of an anti-abortion position (Rose 2007).

The Production of Truth

Thinking about reproductive bodies specifically, the everyday person walking into a PRC and receiving an ultrasound from a pro-life woman or hearing their personal testimonies alone cannot be separated from the ways in which medical discourses produce "truth" about bodies, subjectivity, and experiences generally. One way of thinking about seeking medical advice is that it is a search for a truth about one's body and perhaps also the bodies of others. Medical technologies that create images and definitions around bodies are thus constructed as truth-making practices.

PRC activists deploy this association of medical technologies with "truth" in their activities. For example, they use visual and audial truth-making medical technologies to visually legitimize their centers as (pseudo) medical clinics, despite them typically being run by volunteers with no medical expertise or training. Examples of medical technologies used within PRCs include ultrasounds and fetal Doppler machines.

They also use these technologies to make claims about the "truth" of reproduction, fetal personhood, and abortion in public debate, healthcare practices, and creation of citizenship. Central to this activity is the infusion of emotion and feelings in their uses of medical technologies and interpretations of its products. Subjectivity and medical truth are formed, for both fetus and pregnant person, through the performed emotion of the PRC staff as well as through their proximity to reproductive technologies.

Kelly Rosati, vice president of Focus on the Family, has publicly stated, "Ultrasound has been described as a window to the womb. . . . It gives the woman an opportunity to see for herself and to connect with her child" (Jessen 2016). Her understanding of the sonogram and its rendering of a pregnancy takes the visual image of a fetus, constructs it as having personhood ("her child"), posits it as a truth ("see for herself"), and imbues it with an affective power ("connect"). Tied into this rendering is the undercurrent of pro-life ideology, but its inherent subjectivity is seemingly neutralized through this process to present it as singularly true.

As in this example, affect informs our sensibilities—it combines bodily movement with sense-making technology that helps us make sense of the world (Papacharissi 2015, 21). In this way, affect becomes the way in which we make "truth" out of our experiences. In the case of reproductive technology during pregnancy, PRC activists' use of these tools is immersed in their belief in a magical quality surrounding the fetus as well as an urgency to protect and fight for the unborn. In the process, the subjective status of these beliefs—which are not medical truths—is erased as they become ingrained in the ideologies and affects of anti-abortion sentiment. An initial anti-choice stance is transformed in this process into a purported objective, inevitable logic that frames termination of pregnancy as an unthinkable act after seeing a sonogram. The origin of the decision not to pursue abortion, in other words, is located in these technologies.

When this logic is echoed by PRC clients, their stories are amplified. For instance, a testimony written and publicly shared by a pregnant person who decided to keep a pregnancy after going to a CPC states, "That thing everyone wants to call 'tissue' will eventually turn into a baby that I can hold and who will look like me. I had never thought about that before. Not until seeing it" (Vincent 2015). This account, in other words, not only rebuts supposed pro-choice framings of a fetus as not yet a baby (i.e., only "tissue"), it locates the evidence for that rebuttal in the experience of seeing the ultrasound image at a PRC and suggests a conversion experience—one that is tied to emotions like connection and attachment. By publicizing this client's experience, CPCs reiterate their ideologically informed understandings of pregnancy, the fetus, and the power of affective uses of medical technologies. It is not clear, however, that such an experience is common, let alone representative of the typical PRC client experience.

One woman I spoke with who owns her own PRC described seeing pictures of three-dimensional sonograms as displaying a fetus in such great detail that it looks like a fully formed human being in the womb. She described seeing the ultrasound image as a "magical" experience. To her eyes, the fetus's smile, hands, and feet were all fully formed. In her account, fetal imaging technologies simultaneously produce and evidence the fetus as a child: they display personhood through physical features like a human outside of the womb, but also are imbued with a magical quality, or spiritual, because they are inside the womb. Life and "truth" are essentially being created right in front of people's eyes through these technologies.

Corporeal sound, often created through digital technologies, operates in similar ways to sonograms. PRCs activists use it to wield "medical truth," fundamentally rooted in their pro-life frameworks, as produced by these technologies (Edgar 2017). CPCs often accompany ultrasounds with a Doppler reading that measures a fetal heartbeat. This reading is amplified as a manufactured sound—rendered at the pace of the fetal heartbeat—and labeled as the "sound" of the heartbeat. Amanda Nell Edgar (2017) argues that this fetal sound is a force that stamps out women's voices in abortion care quite literally as well as defines pregnant people's bodies as permeable and available for inspection. Being able to "see" and "hear" the body through technology constructs personhood and medical truth in a new way: "Not only does sound traveling into the body of the pregnant woman mark a fetus as a particular kind of human agent, the sound traveling out through auscultation and amplification also marks the fetus as citizen" (Edgar 2017, 357).

As used in PRCs, the heartbeat as testimony in cases of fetal personhood overpowers the voice of the person carrying the fetus in their womb. The pregnant person's body is a part of the inhuman, inanimate technology to produce and share the rhetoric of sound while the personhood and agency is given only to the fetus inside of them. Because "there is no practical way of separating a live Doppler heartbeat reading from the body that contains that heartbeat," pregnant bodies become technologies themselves that prove a (ideologically anti-choice) point about life (Edgar 2017, 363).

Networks of Morality

Pro-life white women mobilize reproductive technologies as creating "truth" through shared experiences of emotions as well as material resources (Boyd 2010, 39). Their activities are characterized by performances and feelings of "excitement" and "awe" related to a pregnancy, with a particular focus on the fetus. With these emotions invoked, the personhood of the fetus is asserted—and between the emotion and the ostensibly neutral technology, their framing is compelling. This activity, however, is not ahistorical. Their performances around reproductive technologies align with a particular moral history of purity, whiteness, and traditional femininity. Even as they cite technology as sharing a particular truth, their invocation of this truth through white Christian ideologies imbues it with moral status. The technology thus has the ability to show the true meaning of "life" to those who need moral guidance because of its use by white Evangelical pro-life women.

Built into this logic, in turn, is the assumption that when PRC activists use this technology they change the "morality" of individuals considering abortion and, through testimonies of this occurrence, the larger culture. For example, as one pro-life activist wrote, "Pregnancy centers report that many women and their partners leaning toward abortion change their minds after ultrasound exams. The Care Pregnancy Clinic in Baton Rouge, La., reports that 98 percent of women who have ultrasounds choose to carry to term" (Malkin 2015). Missing from this summary, however, is clarity about how people were assessed to be "leaning toward abortion" and, even more importantly, how many clients this PRC saw over what period of time. This framing, however, is not aiming to meet scientific standards. Instead, it serves a (counter)messaging purpose.

Specifically, aiming to refute the assertion that PRCs offer clients less reproductive choice because of their anti-abortion stance, pro-life women use these testimonies to claim that CPC clients' choices were *expanded* by receiving an ultrasound. For example, the anti-abortion organization Focus on the Family (2011) has claimed, "Ultrasound services help a woman understand her body, her pregnancy and her baby's development. She is empowered to make choices that align with her values and priorities." By seeing the sonogram, they argue, an "abortion-minded" woman's choice becomes more than just aborting the fetus.

More than the experience of an individual "abortion-minded" woman, however, these claims must be understood through the lens of the Evangelical need to testify and share faith with others. White pro-life women's activism takes the form of testifying of the value of and sharing faith in medical technologies and discourses, motivated by their belief in moral consequences and stakes.

A common example of this distribution of morality through technology, used by many of the clinics I have studied, are sonogram technology programs. For example, Focus on the Family's "Option Ultrasound" program provided grants to

PRCs for "80% of the cost of an ultrasound machine or sonography training for your medical personnel" (Daly 2015). In order to be considered for an Option Ultrasound grant, an organization had to be located in a community with a "high abortion rate." Between January 2004 and January 2016, Option Ultrasound provided 695 grants across all fifty states and one international grant (Jessen 2016). This program is premised not only on the argument that ultrasound technology is helpful to PRCs' anti-abortion mission because it shows the "truth" of fetal personhood but also in the logic of testifying—in this case, testifying to the moral value of this technology. For example, an online pamphlet stated that "some pictures are worth a thousand words. Others leave you speechless!" implying that ultrasound images carry inherent emotional—and persuasive—power (Focus on the Family 2011). The images that leave pregnant clients speechless are supposed to create sentiments of attachment and, simultaneously, opposition to abortion, situating the personal fetus as part of a larger public discourse surrounding the sanctity of life. Pro-life women's groups see this progress in technology as "moral," as tools to distribute morality outside of their circles. By distributing ultrasound machines under the auspices that they are a form of moral technology, pro-life activists allow people to evangelize through the sharing of sonograms and sonogram images to broader audiences.

Because the larger public discourses surrounding life and morals still engage with institutional and historical power structures, even the distribution of a seemingly omnipresent morality can be applied unequally. A woman I interviewed told me about the local CPC where she volunteered: "I was so inspired to read about a local pregnancy center which was bilingual & served the community and offered resources to those in need for free. The Ultrasound room, Teaching room for Moms & Dads, organized 'New Diapers donated' on shelves, offices, and even New Baby clothes and Mom Boutique were a beautiful sight . . . just like the best of stores!" The volunteer was moved by the performance of the PRC as meeting all the possible needs of pregnant clients. Pointedly, these needs were the ones *she* (a white, Evangelical, pro-life woman) could imagine, not ones the clients identified. This CPC presumably met the needs of only some of its clients, likely ones whose pregnancies most fit this woman's normative idea of pregnancy.

Similarly, the distribution of morality comes from the PRC workers themselves and spreads through material modes of care for only particular pregnant people. A white Christian woman who runs her own CPC gave me an example of the kinds of work she does for women of color: she told me that her clinic can help women find loving homes for their babies. In so doing, she conveyed her assumption that Black mothers and parents are not able to parent their own children (with no mention that perhaps they are more in need of material resources than adoption referrals). Most of the pamphlets CPC activists offered me were resources for infant adoption to a family in the (predominantly white) church who could not have their own. PRC activists considered this effort generous. Underlying this consideration was the racist belief that morality is inherent to some (white people) and to be learned by others (Black people) (Puar 2017).

The PRC activists thought of themselves and of PRCs generally as generous and as places with resources for parenting (including by adoptive parents) instead of aborting, which points to how uses and feelings around reproductive technology are mobilized by pro-life women to have larger material consequences. The evidence that these activities change individual clients' minds is scant (Kimport, Kriz, and Roberts 2018), but CPC activists have been successful in disseminating the belief that they are effective (see the chapter by Sara Matthiesen in this book). The laws and practices engendered by that generalized belief can have significant consequences for those most marginalized in society. White women's use of emotion and medical discourses in their anti-choice activism functions not so much as a way to change individual minds about a pregnancy (i.e., to compel someone to continue it) but as a means to create and define political understandings of personhood and who inherently holds morality in a Christian worldview.

CONCLUSION

Since the Supreme Court overturned *Roe v. Wade*, there has been an understanding of the pro-life movement as having negative impacts on *all* women, regardless of their ideological beliefs. This frame paints pro-life women as victims of patriarchal anti-abortion sentiments and laws. But pro-life women are active contributors to anti-choice ideology and its adoption. They mobilize discourses of medical technology as "truth" and, through performances of white Christian femininity tied to abortion distinctly, transform pro-life beliefs into "scientific" claims. They center the supposed emotionality of their gendered and raced identities, (selectively) take personal testimonies and storytelling into public settings to claim generalizability, and hide the active work in these activities under a recourse to objective medical technologies and the "truth" of ultrasound scans and sounds. These activities long pre-dated the fall of *Roe*.

By creating certain feelings and definitions around abortion within and beyond PRCs through reproductive technologies, these sentiments of pro-life women do not stay siloed within these spaces. The histories of anti-choice politics and technologies generating emotion through contact with the object (life, sonograms, etc.) lead to larger affective moods (particularly pejorative) around abortion in the United States. Attending to how white Evangelical women use affect illustrates how personal pregnancy experiences become political, how reproductive technology is reified as the locus of truth and agency, and, lastly, how these technologies of "truth" are used by the pro-life movement to distribute morality around reproductive health care.

NOTES

1. The term "pro-life" describes a particular political movement in the United States whose aim is to ultimately ban abortion. However, the exigence to ban abortion historically comes from demographic fears and white supremacist logics. Therefore, I use the term pro-life when describing the way these women talk about their own activism and use anti-choice or anti-abortion when describing the function and intents of this movement. Using this

language of pro-life unearths the contradictions in the term with the activism of those within the movement.

2. Throughout this chapter, I often use the term "Pregnancy Resource Center" or "PRC" instead of "Crisis Pregnancy Center" or "CPC." I do this to convey the importance of words used by pro-life activists themselves so that abortion scholars can recognize these terms. Through my fieldwork with pro-life women, I have come to find that this shift in language is immediate and purposeful. However, I also understand the importance and the cultural impact of CPC as a descriptive term; therefore, I continue to interchangeably use this term.

REFERENCES

Ahmed, Sara. 2004. *The Cultural Politics of Emotion*. Routledge.

Boyd, Dannah. 2010. "Social Network Sites as Networked Publics: Affordances, Dynamics, and Implications." In *A Networked Self: Identity, Community, and Culture on Social Network Sites*, edited by Zizi Papacharissi, 39–58. Routledge.

Browder, Jenna. 2019. "'This Is a Baby!' Focus on the Family's LIVE 4D Ultrasound Largest Pro-Life Event Ever in NYC." *CBN News*, May 5, 2019. https://www1.cbn.com/cbnnews/us/2019/may/live-4d-ultrasound-highlight-of-focus-on-the-familys-alive-from-new-york-event.

Corrigan, John. 2002. *Business of the Heart: Religion and Emotion in the Nineteenth Century*. University of California Press.

Daly, Jim. 2015. "Update from Option Ultrasound." *Daily Focus* (blog). ca. 2015. https://jimdaly.focusonthefamily.com/update-from-option-ultrasound/.

Doshi, Marissa. 2018. "Barbies, Goddesses, and Entrepreneurs: Discourses of Gendered Digital Embodiment in Women's Health Apps." *Women's Studies in Communication* 41 (2): 183–203. https://doi.org/10.1080/07491409.2018.1463930.

Edgar, Amanda Nell. 2017. "The Rhetoric of Auscultation: Corporeal Sounds, Mediated Bodies, and Abortion Rights." *Quarterly Journal of Speech* 103 (4): 350–371. https://doi.org/10.1080/00335630.2017.1360510.

Filipovic, Jillian. 2019. "A New Poll Shows What Really Interests 'Pro-Lifers': Controlling Women." *The Guardian*, August 22, 2019. https://www.theguardian.com/commentisfree/2019/aug/22/a-new-poll-shows-what-really-interests-pro-lifers-controlling-women.

Focus on the Family. 2011. "Option Ultrasound Program." http://media.focusonthefamily.com/heartlink/pdf/oup-brochure-060114-web.pdf.

Friz, Amanda. 2018. "Technologies of the State: Transvaginal Ultrasounds and the Abortion Debate." *Rhetoric and Public Affairs* 21 (4): 639–672. https://doi.org/10.14321/rhetpublaffa.21.4.0639.

Griffith, Marie. 2000. *God's Daughters: Evangelical Women and the Power of Submission*. University of California Press.

Howard, Robert. 2008. "Vernacular Media, Vernacular Belief: Locating Christian Fundamentalism in the Vernacular Web." *Western Folklore* 69: 409–429. http://www.jstor.org/stable/25735255.

———. 2011. *Digital Jesus: The Making of New Christian Fundamentalist Community on the Internet*. New York University Press.

Hutchens, Kendra. 2021. "'Gummy Bears' and 'Teddy Grahams': Ultrasounds as Religious Biopower in Crisis Pregnancy Centers." *Social Science & Medicine* 277: 113529. https://doi.org/10.1016/j.socscimed.2021.113925.

———. 2022. "'People Don't Come in Asking for the Gospel, They Come in for a Pregnancy Test!' Feminizing Evangelism in Crisis Pregnancy Centers." *Gender & Society* 36 (2): 165–188. https://doi.org/10.1177/08912432211073061.

Jessen, Leah. 2016. "How This Ultrasound Program Brought Life to 358,000 Babies." *Daily Signal*, January 7, 2016. https://www.dailysignal.com/2016/01/07/how-this-ultrasound-program-brought-life-to-358000-babies/.

Jong-Fast, Molly. 2022. "The Misogyny Is the Point." *The Atlantic*, July 6, 2022. https://www
.theatlantic.com/newsletters/archive/2022/07/roe-overturned-misogyny-anti-abortion
-bills/676667/.

Karant-Nunn, Susan. 2022. *Ritual, Gender, and Emotions: Essays on the Social and Cultural History of the Reformation*. Mohr Siebeck.

Kelly, Kimberly. 2012. "In the Name of the Mother: Renegotiating Conservative Women's Authority in the Crisis Pregnancy Center Movement." *Signs: Journal of Women in Culture and Society* 38 (1): 203–230. https://doi.org/10.1086/665807.

Kimport, Katrina. 2020. "Pregnant Women's Reasons for and Experiences of Visiting Anti-abortion Pregnancy Resource Centers." *Perspectives on Sexual and Reproductive Health* 52 (1): 49–56. https://doi.org/10.1363/psrh.12131.

Kimport, Katrina, Rebecca Kriz, and Sarah C. M. Roberts. 2018. "The Prevalence and Impacts of Crisis Pregnancy Center Visits among a Population of Pregnant Women." *Contraception* 98 (1): 69–73. https://doi.org/10.1016/j.contraception.2018.02.016.

Malkin, Michelle. 2015. "Ultrasound as Abortion Block." *Project Ultrasound* (blog), ca. 2015. https://www.projectultrasound.org/ultrasound-as-abortion-block.

Munson, Ziad. 2008. *The Making of Pro-life Activists: How Social Movement Mobilization Works*. University of Chicago Press.

Papacharissi, Zizi. 2015. *Affective Publics: Sentiment, Technology, and Politics*. Oxford University Press.

Puar, Jasbir. 2017. *The Right to Maim: Debility, Capacity, Disability*. Duke University Press.

Rose, Nikolas. 2007. *The Politics of Life Itself: Biomedicine, Power, and Subjectivity in the Twenty-First Century*. Princeton University Press.

Stormer, Nathan. 2010. "Mediating Biopower and the Case of Prenatal Space." *Critical Studies in Media Communication* 27 (1): 8–23. https://doi.org/10.1080/15295030903554318.

Taylor, Janelle. 2008. *The Public Life of the Fetal Sonogram: Technology, Consumption, and the Politics of Reproduction*. Rutgers University Press.

Vincent, Lynn. 2015. "Moving Pictures." *Project Ultrasound* (blog), ca. 2015. https://www
.projectultrasound.org/moving-pictures.

Welter, Barbara. 1966. "The Cult of True Womanhood: 1820–1860." *American Quarterly* 18 (2): 151–174. https://doi.org/10.2307/2711179.

CHAPTER 13

Evolving, Innovating, Enduring

BEHIND THE SCENES ON ABORTION FUNDS CONTINUING THROUGH A POST-*DOBBS* LANDSCAPE

Ophra Leyser-Whalen and Erin R. Johnson

The 2022 *Dobbs v. Jackson Women's Health Organization* decision, overturning the right to abortion, dealt an enormous blow to abortion rights in the United States. When states banned abortion within their borders, abortion facilities closed, severely curtailing people's ability to obtain legal abortion care. But well before *Dobbs*, many patients struggled to access abortion. Only a few years after the 1973 *Roe v. Wade* decision established the federal right to abortion, federal and state laws began adding barriers to abortion care, such as bans on using public insurance funding for abortion care, forcing low-income people to pay out-of-pocket. State-level regulations limited the availability of care, for example, with burdensome guidelines for facility design that made opening and maintaining clinics difficult, putting abortion geographically out of reach for many (Adashi and Occhiogrosso 2017; Joffe 2010). Even for patients who did not have to travel, abortion could be unobtainable due to cost. As of 2016, the out-of-pocket cost for abortion care would be considered catastrophic, consuming great amounts of households' nonsubsistence income (Zuniga, Thompson, and Blanchard 2020). Along with worries about social stigma and violence from anti-abortion activists, restrictions made abortion care prohibitively costly, hard to get covered by insurance, and geographically burdensome for many patients even while the constitutional right to abortion was officially protected (Cartwright et al. 2018; Joffe 2010; Jones, Upadhyay, and Weitz 2013; Upadhyay et al. 2022).

In response to the financial and logistical challenges associated with abortion access, abortion advocates founded abortion funds across the United States starting soon after the *Roe v. Wade* decision. Abortion funds are grassroots organizations that help abortion patients overcome barriers to care. There are approximately 100 such organizations active today, though their structures and scopes vary. Most funds have a geographic catchment area, providing services to individuals living or receiving care in a particular city, state, or region. A handful of national funds serve patients with particular identities (e.g., Indigenous) or circumstances (e.g., needing to travel for care later in pregnancy).

Most of the current active funds are members of one of two umbrella organizations. The first, the National Network of Abortion Funds (NNAF), was founded by some of the earliest U.S. funds. It serves as an information hub to help abortion seekers find funds and helps member funds with fundraising, organizing, and networking. Apiary, founded in 2020, provides technical assistance, training, and community to the organizations that offer logistical support to abortion seekers.

Abortion funds have served thousands of people through offering a variety of services including providing vouchers/pledges to cover the cost of abortion care as direct payment to clinics (i.e., abortion funds) and offering logistical and economic support (i.e., practical support funds) for patient travel and lodging, which could include providing direct funds to patients or purchasing plane tickets and hotel rooms for patients. Funds may also support clinic escort teams, engage in political advocacy, and educate patients and communities about reproductive health and politics. Abortion funds' operation and success in helping abortion seekers overcome barriers, however, also masked the symptoms of a dysfunctional system, hiding the failure of the state to adequately protect citizens' bodily autonomy and right to self-determination. Appreciation of the work of funds, too, did not always highlight the people who make them successful—mostly women—and the labor—mostly uncompensated—involved in stepping in where the state failed.

Studies conducted in the 2010s found that patients receiving assistance from abortion funds were more likely to be Black or African American, seeking abortion in the second trimester, younger than the average abortion patient, and living in states with restrictions on public and/or private insurance coverage of abortion (Ely et al. 2017b). Fund clients frequently reported facing one or more hardships when seeking care such as homelessness, unemployment, or domestic violence (Ely et al. 2017a). These studies, however, focused on a limited number of funds, making it unclear how generalizable these findings were across all U.S. funds. Nonetheless, the research demonstrated that in the almost fifty years following *Roe*, abortion funds served as a vital link to care for marginalized individuals, particularly in states with hostile abortion laws. Since *Dobbs*, the need for the services that abortion funds offer has only grown.

Recent studies suggest that *Dobbs* significantly increased the travel burden for U.S. abortion seekers. Abortion volume results aggregated from provider reports in the first two years following *Dobbs* show that out-of-state travel for abortion care has doubled since the *Dobbs* decision—from one in ten patients in 2020 to one in five patients in 2023. Additionally, there is evidence that post-*Dobbs* bans on abortion will disproportionately affect Black patients, younger patients, and patients with lower socioeconomic status (Redd et al. 2023).

In the face of continuing and, indeed, mounting financial and logistical barriers after *Dobbs*, the abortion funds remained. And they have aimed to continue to serve as a key link in enabling abortion seekers to obtain the care they want. There are clear continuities in the process of abortion seeking after the fall of *Roe* and also significant changes. In this chapter, we examine how abortion funds stepped into the post-*Dobbs* landscape; what *Dobbs* has revealed about abortion funds, the work they do, and the conditions under which they operate; what is still true about the funds in the wake of the monumental legal changes *Dobbs* catalyzed; and what *Dobbs* changed for and about funds.

METHODS

Our data are a subset from a larger, institutional review board–approved study, coming from one-hour Zoom interviews conducted by the first author between March and November 2023 with nineteen abortion fund and practical support staff, volunteers, and board members, as well as two staff and one board member from national umbrella organizations. Recruitment used convenience and snowball sampling. The respondents represented funds serving the South (n = 4), Southwest (n = 2), East Coast (n = 5), Midwest (n = 4), West Coast (n = 2), and national (n = 5). The organizations provided practical support only (n = 5), abortion funding only (n = 9), practical support and abortion funding (n = 7), and legal help for minors (n = 1). Two respondents were board members at funds, and two were volunteers. The others were paid staff, including executive directors (n = 5); deputy or program directors, managers, or coordinators (n = 7); and helpline or client services coordinators, directors, or managers (n = 6). The respondents received a $30 gift card after completing their interviews. The respondents were given the option of keeping their names, choosing pseudonyms, or having the first author choose pseudonyms.

Interviews were transcribed by an undergraduate research assistant or transcription services and then deidentified and coded by the first author in NVivo software. Coding reports were generated by NVivo, and the first author subsequently manually coded these reports line by line for a thematic analysis (Braun and Clarke 2006). Here, the respondents are described by their title at the time of the interview and by the period of time they had been at their current fund, which is not necessarily the time they had been in their current position/role at the fund.

RESULTS

Although *Dobbs* worsened the conditions that the funds were already working to ameliorate, it also both intensified and expanded work that the funds were already engaged in and created new pathways for innovation. Many funds saw an increase in client volume and travel needs after *Dobbs*, which required them to strengthen existing systems for collaboration and engage in new knowledge-sharing around keeping up with existing laws, navigating risk, and values alignment. The funds represented in this sample also saw an increase in donations and national attention, which brought forth both challenges and opportunities for increasing and changing their processes and services. Finally, we found that the funds leaned into their role as information brokers for patients and providers as laws shifted in the wake of *Dobbs*, all while trying to avoid volunteer and staff burnout.

Client Volume and Increased Travel

All respondents discussed a *Dobbs*-related increase in client volume. Particularly, funds in states that protected abortion rights discussed an increase in clients coming from states that banned or severely restricted abortion who needed travel and accommodation support. Oriaku, the executive director (one year) at NNAF, estimated a "300% increase in providing practical support." This was echoed by an East Coast abortion fund that saw a threefold increase in out-of-state clients, particularly from the South or Midwest, both regions with a high proportion of states that banned abortion following *Dobbs*.

Several respondents reported that they had anticipated the fall of *Roe*, even before the draft decision was leaked two months early.[1] They had prepared by increasing staffing for helplines and hiring attorneys to challenge rulings, to advise them on interpreting the applicable law(s), and (for those in states that were expected to ban abortion) to determine the amount of risk they could handle in their fund work. Others staffed up shortly after the *Dobbs* decision. The funds with larger staff and budgets that further increased their staff capacity were better able to accommodate the increased client volume in the months after *Dobbs*; others, however, had to turn clients away. Brooke (director of strategic partnerships, two years) stated that while their fund "never had a capacity issue pre-*Dobbs*," the post-*Dobbs* client volume "just became so freaking overwhelming that finally, maybe like two months after *Dobbs*, we had to put a cap on . . . [the number of] clients" by shutting down the hotline every week.

In addition to not being able to serve all clients, the increased volume strained the staff. Brooke expressed concern for the organization's health due to the stress of increased demand, saying "it's just becoming so unsustainable. Like, we were going to collapse in on ourselves." Brooke's fund accommodated staff and volunteers by shutting down the hotline to try to avoid burnout, but for others the increased workload took its toll. Some respondents reported that their funds had lost board members and volunteers to burnout. These funds, even as they built up staff capacity, lost established workers and institutional knowledge, potentially placing more of a burden on those who remained.

Dobbs increased the postponement of abortion care for many abortion seekers due to scheduling travel, procuring money, or clinic wait times. This also meant increased coordination work for the funds. Sarah (hotline coordinator, two years) explained, "We're having to check in with people over and over again or change our pledges [amounts] . . . because people are having issues coming up with . . . money or . . . the logistics of getting to the clinic." Increased client volume also increased costs for the funds. Irene (practical support and program team manager, four years) explained that, after *Dobbs*, "now almost every single time . . . I'm booking at least one flight, lodging, transportation [for clients who live out-of-state]," although the majority of their callers are still from within the state.

These struggles reveal the immediate shock of *Dobbs* on the abortion fund system. These funds were imperative for some abortion seekers pre-*Dobbs*, but these largely grassroots organizations were not prepared to handle the increased scale of need created by *Dobbs*. The system became stressed in ways that illustrate the amazing work of these funds but also highlight that they were not set up to resolve systemic inequality. The funds are doing their best to provide clients with the resources they need to access care, but these organizations cannot fully make up for the failure of the state to protect its citizens' rights. Some clients will not receive the care they need, and both clients and fund workers will experience emotional distress.

Interfund Coordination and Collaboration

Interfund collaboration existed before *Dobbs*, both organically or through larger umbrella groups such as NNAF, but it mostly focused on more complex cases that required more money and coordination, particularly in states with severe legal restrictions on abortion (White, Leyser-Whalen, et al. 2024). These cases where clients faced significant hardship, perhaps unexpectedly, served as a microcosm of the post-*Dobbs* setting in which more clients had more complex needs. Thus, the funds and their umbrella organizations strengthened their collaborations in responding to *Dobbs* strategically and collectively.

Increased communication, regionally and nationally, brought both synergies and opportunities for conflict. As Lina (intake manager, ten months) explained, "There's always going to be tension when we're working on this scale." Sam (volunteer, eight years) reflected on their fund's increased post-*Dobbs* regional collaboration: "There's also a lot of really shared goals and commitments that bring abortion funds together. You know, and even when there's challenges . . . we get shit done." The funds still operated with their primary goal in mind: helping patients obtain abortion care.

Patient Support. Many funds sought to streamline the collaborative process in view of minimizing patients' logistical burden and emotional distress. The goal was that callers would not need to contact multiple funds to amass enough money for a procedure and travel as more patients were traveling out of state for abortion care. For the funds, that meant that clients might live in one fund's catchment area but receive care in another's. As Joy (caller services and engagement manager, two years) explained, "We'll hear from a patient first. We'll be able to provide them as much as we can, and then typically we'll start an email thread on their behalf. So we coordinate and collaborate with funds all over the country to fundraise that money."

Joy acknowledged that these collaborations "take trust building," and the fund staff reported that they appreciated these collaborations. Indeed, some respondents expressed a desire for more interfund communication, particularly around practical support, although this would also place more time commitments on the funds when time is in limited supply. Baya (director of grants and development, four years) explained, "The biggest change is . . . the level of coordination and effort it takes to get people from [a state with an abortion ban] to [a state where abortion is legal] is just a lot more complicated. And we want to ensure that our callers are always held . . . in welcoming communities when we . . . send them places."

For funds whose pre-*Dobbs* work did not require them to think about client travel and restrictions, the recent communications with other funds about patient travel have been a learning experience. For example, to help ensure clients with differing documentation statuses can travel safely, Nadirah (program manager, ten months) educated other funds, who might be sending their clients to her area on the U.S.-Mexico border, about the interior border patrol checkpoints in her area, which are located within 100 miles of country borders. Sarah (hotline coordinator, two years) particularly appreciated the funds from states that banned abortion doing "a creative job of making sure people get care and making sure people get care with privacy," even as her own fund was in a state that protected abortion and thus did not face the same challenges.

When interfund communication increased after *Dobbs*, some existing systems of collaboration were not robust enough to handle it. For example, Sam (volunteer, eight years) noted that their fund tried to coordinate with nearby funds to potentially divert some of their extra monies to the funds being inundated with callers, "but the coalition meetings sort of stopped happening because people were so overwhelmed." Sarah (hotline coordinator, two years) also reported that the demanding post-*Dobbs* environment had prevented formalization of these relationships: "From a formal perspective, I don't really think that's been anyone's focus because everyone's been in crisis with their own individual work." Before *Dobbs*, interfund collaboration was only required in the most severe cases, but after *Dobbs* it became part of the funds' everyday work to ensure safe and positive client experiences of care.

Keeping Up with Changing Laws. The funds have always played a role in digesting and sharing information for abortion seekers, in part reducing the burden on clinics to do so. For example, before *Dobbs*, Texas abortion fund staff and volunteers served as patient navigators, bridging information gaps caused by bans, policy changes, and resulting service restrictions; they helped callers gather the information and resources needed to access care and provided emotional support to help the callers overcome barriers to care (White, Leyser-Whalen, et al. 2024). Because *Dobbs* created a quickly shifting legal landscape, these funds relied on larger organizations reporting on current national laws to make sense of what was happening.

Yet the content of fund communication shifted as they worked together with the clinics to keep apprised of state-level laws after *Dobbs*. Lina (intake manager, ten months) stated, "The silver lining is . . . *Dobbs* really forced all abortion care providers, from the medical providers to the funds to community activists, . . . to really reckon with the fact that we have to find ways to work together and communicate consistently to push this work forward in a powerful way." Whereas before *Dobbs* the funds had focused primarily on their local laws and conditions, the rapidly changing national legal landscape after *Dobbs* required them to maintain a much broader awareness of the conditions in other states. An unexpected outcome of this necessity was (re)new(ed) communications with others who were committed to abortion access.

Not only did this communication help the funds keep apprised of current laws, it also facilitated sharing organizational practices to manage the chaos that followed new regulations. This was particularly apparent among the Texas funds. Alex, a helpline coordinator (nine years) at a smaller, regional Texas abortion fund, said that communication with the Texas funds with greater capacity helped them develop workable strategies as their caller volume increased. In addition, Alex's fund worked with a larger Texas fund in filing lawsuits. Shae, the executive director at the larger fund (2.5 years), also noted the necessity of maintaining these collaborations: "so that when more . . . restrictions come into place, we have ways to work."

Shae noted that the previous restrictions initially brought the Texas funds closer as they experienced "collective trauma." The groundwork that the Texas funds laid before *Dobbs* has benefited other funds nationwide, who are now in a similar post-*Dobbs* situation. Carin, a Texas fund board member, explained that, whereas Texas funds had been collaborating previously, she had not felt the same level of national collaboration that exists now. "People kind of just let us figure it out by ourselves."

After *Dobbs*, abortion funds leveraged their increased interfund communication to understand how other funds were interpreting and applying the often ambiguously written laws to their programs—these interpretations varied across funds, even in the same state. For example, several of the Texas funds implemented different internal policies in reaction to their state's abortion ban, and some of these policies hindered collaboration and communication. Joy (caller services and engagement manager, two years) explained the challenge of communicating with these funds, focusing on one particular fund that was very cautious in the post-*Dobbs* environment: "It's even to the point where they're really trying to keep it so under wraps that even in meetings with us, there's only certain things they can say. . . . One fund in particular was like, 'I can't tell you what our eligibility is . . . based on . . . what our lawyers have advised us, but what I can say is, only one-fourth of our current callers are eligible for our funding, and we're only allowed to do practical support funding. We can't fund abortion care.'"

Respondents reported that, after *Dobbs*, more of their fund's communication concerns focused on abortion surveillance and criminalization for both funds and callers. Further, they shared that call-line staff and volunteers, who are directly interfacing with clients, were fielding more and more client concerns about criminalization under these new laws. Research has shown that the media reports and shifting abortion laws before *Dobbs* could confuse the public about the legality of abortion; this led some people to choose not to attempt to obtain abortion care and caused those who did seek out care additional stress and worry (White, Arey, et al. 2024). According to respondent accounts, these fears were more widespread among the callers to the funds after *Dobbs*—and the fund workers tried to assuage those fears. As Joy (caller services and engagement manager, two years) said, "Patients being like, 'Is it—like, am I okay? Like, can I come up here and not get . . . criminalized?' And that has been a very big change for us, just in terms of even having to honestly deal with questions like that over the phone, and our volunteers not really being prepped and ready for that."

Managing these increased legal concerns created significant additional work, requiring the funds to stay current on the legal landscape, determine internal policies in response to changes, and communicate both the updated legal information and the new fund policies to staff and volunteers so that they could keep their clients informed. Carin (board member, one year) discussed the particular impact of this added work on volunteers and volunteer management: "I mean, abortion funds run on volunteers, and it's hard to keep volunteers . . . up to date when [it isn't] their full-time job." This marked a big shift in the work and responsibilities of the fund workers, even as it was within the existing fund task of being an information broker.

It was not just vague and ambiguous laws that respondents newly had to navigate. Abortion clinics also created new regulations in response to statewide legal changes, and fund staff and volunteers had to keep apprised of these as well. As Lina (intake manager, ten months) stated, "My brain is just crammed full of knowing . . . the different requirements that folks have to meet to receive funding from [different clinic organizations]." Keeping updated on these regulations was very important. Jonnette (abortion fund director, two years) recounted that when the bans came down in Utah, "Our clients in Utah had all their appointments canceled, no word on rescheduling . . . so we had to get in contact with the clinic to try to figure out what might be going on. And the clinic was like, 'We're so sorry, we are canceling left and right because of the ban . . . and we knew it was just a matter of a time, but like they [lawmakers] came up with it Friday night.' . . . We're just scrambling." In some cases, bans were temporarily blocked, which started another cycle of reshuffling appointments. Throughout all of this, the fund staff provided emotional support to their clients in addition to helping them navigate the rapidly changing landscape to access care.

Aligning Funds on Values. The two umbrella organizations were also very activated since *Dobbs*. Apiary, which started in 2020 and had to hit the ground running in dealing with COVID-19, leaned into the need for more interfund communication by creating more programming for practical support funds to gather for community building and discuss practical matters and larger philosophical questions. Oriaku (NNAF executive director, one year) explained that abortion funds are also doing this work to get more values-aligned with reproductive justice (RJ), a Black feminist framework that emphasizes "(1) the right not to have a child, (2) the right to have a child, and (3) the right to parent in safe and healthy environments" (Ross and Solinger 2017). While not all abortion funds currently consider themselves RJ organizations or engage with the RJ framework (also see Leyser-Whalen 2024), NNAF is helping lead the field in that direction.

Jonnette, the abortion fund director at Indigenous Women Rising (two years), which solely serves Indigenous abortion seekers, reported that these interfund discussions produced learning moments around the needs of Indigenous people seeking abortion care because most of the previous focus on BIPOC (Black, Indigenous, and People of Color) populations generally omitted Native Americans: "'Cause you know, there's always that question of 'Why is it necessary to have an abortion fund just for Indigenous folks?'" In Jonnette's post-*Dobbs* experience, misunderstandings that were common before *Dobbs* could be corrected and clarified through the post-*Dobbs* actions to strengthen the funding community. Perhaps counterintuitively, *Dobbs* helped the fund staff identify and address already existing gaps in how fund support (had) worked and who was less well served by the existing fund ecosystem.

Increased collaboration has also created awareness around which funds are doing particularly well and how other funds could follow their example. Anna (health-line manager, three years) believed increased fund communication directed attention to their fund as a potential RJ exemplar, noting that "some . . . [funds] are very whitewashed in the sense that they do kind of follow more of like a pro-choice approach to things where we really are centered in reproductive justice. We have a fully paid staff . . . led by people of color and Black people. And there are some other abortion funds that have had some issues with them leading by a different example, and their values being a little bit different." As the funds communicate more, they are beginning to share best practices, not only for client services but also for organizational practices and structures. This represents a huge shift from the funds previously collaborating primarily to provide abortion care to patients and being autonomous entities, to now becoming more values-aligned and interconnected.

More Attention to Abortion

Dobbs heightened public discourse around abortion, having both positive and negative effects. On the positive side, Toni (director of client services, seven years) felt that the increased attention to abortion has facilitated conversations about abortion, an arguably still stigmatized and polarizing topic, yet Toni implied that before *Dobbs* she was more cautious about discussing abortion with strangers. But now, "me and . . . my co-workers were just talking about how after *Dobbs*, we feel more willing to talk about our work just even out in the world . . . there's something emboldening. Some of it is probably the 'f-ck it' factor of like, the world's burning. Like, I'm going to tell them I fund abortion because we should be."

The increased attention to abortion also had a bright side for Brooke (director of strategic partnerships, two years), who thought that *Dobbs* helped people outside of the abortion care network understand *Roe*'s flaws, wherein *Roe* made abortion legal but not necessarily accessible, particularly for people from marginalized communities. She believes this is encouraging the public to think about progress differently, about what policies would enable access to care. Baya (director of grants and development, four years) also believed this attention could cause a paradigm shift for other organizations explicitly working in social justice to place abortion more squarely in the RJ realm:

> There's some organizations that see the interconnectedness, like, relatively easily. [For others,] for a long time for folks it's been abortion and reproductive justice as separate things. So letting folks know . . . "You may have already thought reproductive justice was relevant to the work that you do, but abortion is a piece of that, not a separate movement space." Abortion has been painted as this separate thing, and I think that's very strategic . . . because I think by painting it as a separate issue it's easier to attack. I mean, I do think it's a moment of activation for people. So when we do need to talk to other community partners . . . I think that people are listening in a way that may not have felt as urgent for them previously.

In the wake of *Dobbs*, both the general public and movement actors are increasingly understanding the role that abortion access plays in RJ and the need for policy and private programs to support a range of pregnancy and parenting decisions.

The increased attention to abortion also has had some downsides, according to respondents. For instance, it created more media interest in abortion funds, which previously had mostly flown under the radar. Carin (board member, one year) noted that the media attention and requests have been taxing on the funds, suggesting that journalists have "fetishized" fund work: "The staff doesn't have all the capacity in the world to talk to every single journalist. And the staff is not there to connect journalists to minors to be the cover story on *New York Times Magazine*." This increased attention can serve as an additional burden on overworked staff and a distraction from the core mission of helping clients.

Increased media attention to abortion also introduced many in the general public to the existence of abortion funds, including scammers. Prior to *Dobbs*, the funds were a largely unknown or overlooked part of the abortion field. Although this contributed to struggles to raise money, for instance, it also meant they were generally ignored by bad actors. They had no systematic experiences with scammers, and thus had few protections against them. This lack of experience left the funds vulnerable as they moved into the post-*Dobbs* spotlight. In the aftermath of *Dobbs*, scammers took funding allocated for clients and wasted fund staff's time. Brooke (director of strategic partnerships, two years) explained, disheartened, that funds have probably lost hundreds of thousands of dollars to scammers. These losses have been exacerbated by the increase in provision of practical support services where callers are sometimes given cash advances, hotel rooms, and flights.

Dealing with the new threat of scammers created a philosophical paradigm shift for the funds in our sample because they had to think about trust differently. Jessie (deputy director, two years) explained that funds "lead with trust. They specifically build infrastructure to not impose additional barriers on clients who call for support. And unfortunately, that means sometimes people who are not 'real' clients slip through the cracks." Anna (health-line manager, three years) lamented, "It's just so hard . . . having to have . . . that vigilance to even ask yourself, 'is this somebody that's actually needing support or not?' Because you want to trust every single caller."

More People Interested in the Cause: Volunteers. More media attention on abortion funds coupled with the realization that *Roe* had fallen brought a huge influx of people wanting to help. As Yvonne (volunteer, one year) explained, people "didn't think *Roe* was going to get overturned and just didn't see the urgency of it." She believed that, right after *Dobbs*, more people were "fired up" and "ready to risk more." Whereas the funds had relied on volunteers in the past, Vera (executive director, four years) reported that after *Dobbs* they saw ten times the amount of volunteer opportunity requests. Jessie (deputy director, two years) echoed that:

> Organizations were getting inundated with requests to volunteer from thousands of people. Everyone gets really fired up when crises happen. You know, "I work from home, I have a spare bedroom, I have a car, I can drive people to the clinic, or I can provide childcare. I live right next door to the clinic. I can escort people in and out." People felt really moved by the *Dobbs* decision and really wanted actionable ways to plug in that was more than reposting on social media or donating, which are still really worthwhile things, but they were hungry for something more. And practical support organizations had a stack of 1,000-plus volunteer applications.

This influx of volunteer requests also shows that, aside from just giving money, funds were/are one of the few nonspecialized entry points to involvement in abortion activism.

Some funds, already inundated with larger client volumes, struggled to navigate the influx of volunteer requests. Irene (practical support and program team manager, four years) relayed that they closed their volunteer sign-up form upon receiving 4,000 interest forms in one month, with only one staff person dedicated to volunteer engagement. Similarly, Nadirah's (program manager, ten months) fund did not have staff capacity to conduct background checks on the myriad volunteer applicants.

Given the overwhelming amount of volunteer offers, Apiary streamlined the process for practical support funds by hiring a full-time staff member to screen applications and train volunteers for values alignment and implementation of practical support. This was important because, according to Irene (practical support and program team manager, four years), some potential volunteers were well-intentioned but offered services that the fund did not provide or that did not match their mission or values. Upon completion of Apiary's training, volunteers could return to the practical support funds in their areas to be utilized for various volunteer opportunities. Thus, *Dobbs* spurred a more standardized, national scope for practical support volunteers.

More People Interested in the Cause: Donors. Although the funds thrived mostly on individual donations before *Dobbs*, *Dobbs* created a huge stream of donations from individuals who were either increasing their contributions or making new donations. Given that abortion funds are mission driven, more money equated to more people receiving more funding for their abortions. Carin (board member, one year) welcomed this change: "I think five years ago, the left did not consider abortion funds to be part of mainstream mutual aid. And now I hope that they do. I hope that the average person who, in general, cares about reproductive rights is going to donate to an abortion fund and not just donate to [a larger, more well-known reproductive health organization]."[2]

The increase in money meant that some funds, particularly funds that worked directly with clinics in states that banned abortion (thereby closing the clinics), were challenged with (re)allocating monies because they could no longer directly fund abortion procedures. Even in states that protected abortion, however, some funds were confronted with managing larger budgets. Sam's (volunteer, eight years) fund already had infrastructure in place to receive and allocate funds, so they did not have to "have a whole conversation about it as a board, it was just, 'We're already doing this, so let's increase it.'" Many funds, however, did not have this infrastructure, largely because before *Dobbs* their funding had been small and complex financial infrastructure had not been unnecessary.

New revenue sources also came from other organizations, including city and state legislative entities (on the West Coast and East Coast). Whereas funds found the increased funding and services helpful, this also attracted negative attention for some. Toni (director of client services, seven years) relayed that anti-abortion groups sued them for receiving city money. Although the anti-abortion groups ultimately lost, Toni's fund still had to spend time and resources on the lawsuit.

But rapid growth also requires work. As Stephanie (executive director, 6 years) stated, quoting rapper The Notorious B.I.G., "Mo' money, mo' problems." One of these problems was the challenge of sustaining those resources. Some funds wondered if the fundraising model was sustainable. As a staff member at a Midwest abortion fund noted, "Getting off of a philanthropy model that caters to a donor class would be . . . the amazing dream." Stephanie, a staff member at Indigenous Women Rising, stated, "We're crying over crumbs. I don't want crumbs. I want the full loaf of bread. And we have the opportunity to envision something better that truly serves my people, low-income folks, undocumented people, like just make abortion available. So I think there's been a lot of incredible opportunities for envisioning something better."

Sarah (hotline coordinator, two years) saw another unexpected benefit from the *Dobbs* influx of donations: faster movement toward an RJ orientation by funds that freed some monies from some of their pre-*Dobbs* framing limitations. For example, her fund did not require financial thresholds for aid qualification, but some funds did, and she associated this with a non-RJ frame. Yet she believed this might be changing based on the post-*Dobbs* values alignment. She said, "That's coming from . . . a scarcity mentality, and since *Dobbs*, at least at [her fund], we have so much money that there's no reason to put those requirements in place." Thus, *Dobbs* changed the scale of fund resources, revealing how underfunded many funds were, which had curtailed their ability to enact an RJ mission and may curtail the mission in the future as donations begin to dry up.

Change in Services

For some funds, their duties remained unchanged after *Dobbs*, yet the workload increased. For others, *Dobbs* spurred changes to organizational processes and services models. Brooke (director of strategic partnerships, two years) quipped, "Crisis is the mother of invention," and she gave examples of mobile units that distribute abortion pills and a volunteer pilot organization that provides flights; "People are doing what they need to do to take care of their community, and that's beautiful." Carin (board member, one year) also reported that her Texas fund board members had "become more dynamic in their approach to more of like a wraparound service mindset."

This mindset was also apparent in Anna's (health-line manager, three years) description of their new services to facilitate mass amounts of client travel by working with a travel agency that lets callers contact them directly 24/7: "'Cause we've seen that happen a lot where a caller misses a flight or they miss a connection, and that will make them miss their appointment in a lot of cases, because callers can sometimes only fly a certain day. There's just so many components and pieces to where travel is really hard because they have to get back on a certain day because they have to take their son somewhere. You know, things like that."

Changes were smoother for the funds who had trial runs with restrictive laws, such as the Texas funds. Still, *Dobbs* changed the landscape for abortion funds in ban states, causing some of these funds to shift from pledging funds directly to clinics to offering practical support, or as Oriaku (executive director, one year) explained, "Funds that never provided practical support . . . are now glorified travel agents because you cannot fund abortion in their state, but they're supporting people . . . going out of state." These funds, in both ban and protected abortion states, had to establish new relationships with out-of-state clinics or newly established clinics in their states.

Some funds in ban states also pivoted to increasing nonabortion programming or creating new programming such as public education campaigns. Two Texas funds discussed their comprehensive and inclusive sex education programming and contraception and pregnancy test distribution. Sasha (board member, four years), who worked with Texas funds for years, explained that after halting abortion funding because such work was now criminalized in the state, Texas funds were now engaging with other organizations to do more intersectional, multi-issue policy work. This was true for the fund where Alex (helpline coordinator, nine years) worked, which was doing more sex education programming, including some with a mutual aid organization in a neighboring state. This allowed the fund to continue doing RJ work, reach a wider audience, and get more input, people power, and funding, even though it could not support abortion seekers directly.

Providing new services may reveal that the abortion funds want to keep existing even when they are unable to enact their primary mission of abortion aid; they still can maintain their roles as activist, RJ organizations. Yet implementing new practices and scaling up existing ones was not easy, and the funds found it challenging to balance the need to meet increased demand with the need to build infrastructure to support these new practices and processes. All the while, they had to navigate staff and volunteer burnout and organizational uncertainty.

Discussion

In the United States, in the years after *Dobbs*, abortion continues to be inaccessible to many, and abortion funds continue to work to provide abortion access. The *Dobbs* decision created a both/and situation for abortion funds, wherein some aspects remained the same, some were exacerbated, and some new challenges and opportunities emerged. Our interviews with fund workers demonstrate that the funds were faced with keeping current on the changing legal landscape; increased client volume, travel, and costs; decisions about increased funding and volunteers; changing services; deterring scammers; and becoming more values aligned. The funds responded by increasing staff, changing services, and increasing interfund collaborations.

At the same time, the funds often found themselves trying to juggle too many balls at once: putting systems in place to onboard and manage new staff as well as increasing collaboration with other funds while also continuing to meet increased post-*Dobbs* demand for services and public attention. In this sense, according to our interviews, the funds were not investing in building infrastructure or capturing institutional knowledge, partially because they did not feel they had time. With the weight that the funds are shouldering, this has increased the likelihood of burnout.

Although these data were collected through convenience and snowball sampling, the sample obtained was diverse geographically and by fund type. We believe it presents a relatively coherent representation of the abortion fund landscape in the immediate aftermath of *Dobbs*. In fact, these data are not only a relevant snapshot of that moment but may also be relevant for our future as more abortion bans and criminalization are proposed by state legislators. Future research should examine how abortion funds continue to evolve and iterate, building on their decades-long histories of mutual aid work and shared values to respond to new challenges in ensuring access to abortion.

We end with a quote from Oriaku, the executive director of NNAF, who views this point in time as an opportunity to evaluate purpose, philosophy, and services:

> The work is actually the same: Building power. But it's going to look different . . . in how we show up for each other . . . truly understanding the conditions that we're in, and grounding ourselves in that, and not necessarily just always reacting or always being on the defense. This very vocal minority of people who have taken this moral high ground have made it very difficult for a majority of people to simply access basic health care, which includes abortions. How are we bold?

How do we take all of the things that we've learned in theory and put it into practice, what we've been talking about for decades at this point? How do we clearly articulate that to our membership . . . to movement partners? What are realistic expectations people can have for abortion funds? How can we harness this collective power or this cultural capital for collective change, for systemic change?

NOTES

1. On May 2, 2022, just under two months before the *Dobbs* decision was released, a news outlet published a leaked draft.

2. Mutual aid is an idea and practice based on ideas of direct action, cooperation, mutual understanding, and solidarity. Mutual aid is not charity but rather the building and continuing of new social relations where people give what they can and get what they need, outside of unjust systems of power (Spade 2020).

REFERENCES

Adashi, Eli Y., and Rachel H. Occhiogrosso. 2017. "The Hyde Amendment at 40 Years and Reproductive Rights in the United States: Perennial and Panoptic." *JAMA* 317 (15): 1523–1524. https://doi.org/10.1001/JAMA.2017.2742.

Braun, Virginia, and Victoria Clarke. 2006. "Using Thematic Analysis in Psychology." *Qualitative Research in Psychology* 3 (2): 77–101. https://doi.org/10.1191/1478088706QP063OA.

Cartwright, Alice F., Mihiri Karunaratne, Jill Barr-Walker, Nicole E. Johns, and Ushma D. Upadhyay. 2018. "Identifying National Availability of Abortion Care and Distance from Major US Cities: Systematic Online Search." *Journal of Medical Internet Research* 20 (5): e186. https://doi.org/10.2196/JMIR.9717.

Ely, Gretchen E., Travis Hales, D. Lynn Jackson, Elizabeth A. Bowen, Eugene Maguin, and Greer Hamilton. 2017a. "A Trauma-Informed Examination of the Hardships Experienced by Abortion Fund Patients in the United States." *Health Care for Women International* 38 (11): 1133–1151. https://doi.org/10.1080/07399332.2017.1367795.

Ely, Gretchen E., Travis Hales, D. Lynn Jackson, Eugene Maguin, and Greer Hamilton. 2017b. "The Undue Burden of Paying for Abortion: An Exploration of Abortion Fund Cases." *Social Work in Health Care* 56 (2): 99–114. https://doi.org/10.1080/00981389.2016.1263270.

Joffe, Carole E. 2010. *Dispatches from the Abortion Wars: The Costs of Fanaticism to Doctors, Patients, and the Rest of Us.* Beacon Press.

Jones, Rachel K., Ushma D. Upadhyay, and Tracy A. Weitz. 2013. "At What Cost? Payment for Abortion Care by U.S. Women." *Women's Health Issues* 23 (3): e173–e178. https://doi.org/10.1016/j.whi.2013.03.001.

Leyser-Whalen, Ophra. 2024. "What Is a Reproductive Justice Organization? Abortion Aid Organizations Incorporating Reproductive Justice Models." *American Studies* 63 (3): 53–71.

Redd, Sara K., Elizabeth A. Mosley, Suba Narasimhan, Anna Newton-Levinson, Roula AbiSamra, Carrie Cwiak, Kelli Stidham Hall, Sophie A. Hartwig, Johanna Pringle, and Whitney S. Rice. 2023. "Estimation of Multiyear Consequences for Abortion Access in Georgia under a Law Limiting Abortion to Early Pregnancy." *JAMA Network Open* 6 (3): e231598–e231598. https://doi.org/10.1001/jamanetworkopen.2023.1598.

Ross, Loretta J., and Rickie Solinger. 2017. *Reproductive Justice: An Introduction.* University of California Press.

Spade, Dean. 2020. *Mutual Aid: Building Solidarity during This Crisis (and the Next).* Verso.

Upadhyay, Ushma D., Chris Ahlbach, Shelly Kaller, Clara Cook, and Isabel Muñoz. 2022. "Trends in Self-Pay Charges and Insurance Acceptance for Abortion in the United States, 2017–20." *Health Affairs* 41 (4): 507–515. https://doi.org/10.1377/hlthaff.2021.01528.

White, Kari, Whitney Arey, Brooke Whitfield, Asha Dane'el, Laura Dixon, Joseph E. Potter, Tony Ogburn, and Anitra D. Beasley. 2024. "Abortion Patients' Decision Making about Where to Obtain Out-of-State Care Following Texas' 2021 Abortion Ban." *Health Services Research* 59 (1): e14226. https://doi.org/10.1111/1475-6773.14226.

White, Kari, Ophra Leyser-Whalen, Brooke Whitfield, Asha Dane'el, Alexis Andrea, Anna Rupani, Bhavik Kumar, and Ghazaleh Moayedi. 2024. "Abortion Assistance Fund Staff and Volunteers as Patient Navigators Following an Abortion Ban in Texas." *Perspectives on Sexual and Reproductive Health* 56 (3): 235–243. https://doi.org/10.1363/PSRH.12240.

Zuniga, Carmela, Terri Ann Thompson, and Kelly Blanchard. 2020. "Abortion as a Catastrophic Health Expenditure in the United States." *Women's Health Issues* 30 (6): 416–25. https://doi.org/10.1016/j.whi.2020.07.001.

Acknowledgments

In the months following the Supreme Court's 2022 *Dobbs v. Jackson Women's Health Organization* decision, many scholars found a new—or renewed—interest in abortion as a research topic. This scholarly attention was and is welcome. High-quality scholarship depends on a broad community of inquiry, on diverse perspectives and methodologies, and on collaboration. And yet, in the moment, it was not always clear what new research questions needed answering. Certainly, the landscape of abortion legality and provision was changing, but what this meant and how it mattered was not—at least to me—clear.

As I struggled to make sense of the feeling that valiant research efforts might be missing consequential opportunities, I benefited from a conversation with the ever-insightful Tracy Weitz. Tracy reframed my muddled concern about designing research questions on what had changed with the *Dobbs* decision to focusing instead on what had *not* changed. She pointed out that understanding *Dobbs* and what has come after necessitates understanding what *Dobbs* did not change. The way to capture that understanding, I realized, was through an edited volume featuring the work and hard-earned knowledge of scholars from multiple disciplines and geographies—in other words, the book you hold in your hand now.

I thank Peter Mickulas, senior editor at Rutgers University Press, for supporting this vision and enthusiastically paving the way for this book. While the chapters here aim for timelessness—capturing a moment in history—Peter's work and that of the incredible Rutgers University Press staff to get this volume in print expediently was crucial and greatly appreciated.

An edited volume is nothing without its contributors, and I offer deep thanks to the chapter authors who have shared their insights and expertise on quite tight deadlines. Many of the contributors were connected to the volume because of their role as a participant or presenter at the Abortion Researcher Incubator, an annual training event I led at Advancing New Standards in Reproductive Health (ANSIRH) at the University of California, San Francisco. This volume reaps the bounty of the work the Incubator has done to build a community of abortion scholars. I thank Nancy

Berglas, Carole Joffe, and Ushma Upadhyay for their work in creating the Incubator with me; Tiffany Green, Kelly Ward, and Tracy Weitz for co-facilitating in recent years; and Lizzy Ghedi-Ehrlich and Lisa Hernandez from the Scholars Strategy Network for their partnership on the Incubator. I also thank the larger ANSIRH community for their support of the Incubator and generous engagement with each new cohort.

My effort on this volume was supported by an anonymous foundation. The anonymous foundation had no involvement in the design, writing, revision, or publication of the volume. I am indebted to Daniel Grossman and Molly Battistelli of ANSIRH for their unflagging work to enable and support my research endeavors and those of my extraordinary colleagues.

Finally, I thank the readers of this volume for your interest and engagement. Scholars of abortion have not always enjoyed wide readership. I hope this volume is part of a broader increase in scholarly attention on the topic and how it relates to myriad facets of our social world.

Resources

ADVOCACY ORGANIZATIONS

Abortion Out Loud, Advocates for Youth, www.advocatesforyouth.org/abortion-out-loud
All Above All*, allaboveall.org
In Our Own Voice: National Black Women's Reproductive Justice Agenda, blackrj.org
Latina Institute for Reproductive Justice, www.latinainstitute.org
National Asian Pacific American Women's Forum, napawf.org
Patient Forward, www.patientforward.org
Planned Parenthood Federation of America, www.plannedparenthood.org
Reproductive Freedom for All, reproductivefreedomforall.org
SisterSong, www.sistersong.net
We Testify, www.wetestify.org

LEGAL ORGANIZATIONS

Abortion Defense Network, www.abortiondefensenetwork.org
Center for Reproductive Rights, www.reproductiverights.org
IfWhenHow Lawyering for Reproductive Justice, www.ifwhenhow.org
Reproductive Freedom Project, American Civil Liberties Union (ACLU), www.aclu.org
    /issues/reproductive-freedom
The Lawyering Project, www.lawyeringproject.org

Notes on Contributors

BARBARA A. ALVAREZ has a doctorate in information science from the University of Wisconsin–Madison and has researched the role of abortion information access. Dr. Alvarez teaches university courses and specializes in community engagement.

WHITNEY AREY is a medical anthropologist whose work focuses on abortion access and decision-making, and reproductive health policy in the U.S. South. Dr. Arey earned her doctorate in sociocultural anthropology from Brown University. She is currently a postdoctoral scholar in maternal and child health at the University of North Carolina at Chapel Hill and a sexual and reproductive health expert for Physicians for Human Rights. Her current work combines research and advocacy to examine the impacts of state abortion bans in the aftermath of *Dobbs* on experiences of, access to, and provision of reproductive health care.

DANIELLE BESSETT is a professor of sociology at the University of Cincinnati in Ohio and a faculty affiliate of both the Department of Women's, Gender, and Sexuality Studies and the Medical Scientist Training Program. Her research centers on the sociology of reproduction, including patient experiences of reproductive processes, disparities in access to care, and knowledge about reproductive health. Dr. Bessett directs the university's Kunz Center for Social Research and co-leads the Ohio Policy Evaluation Network (OPEN), which conducts and translates rigorous, forward-thinking social science research about policies and structural inequities related to abortion and contraception with a focus on Ohioans and residents of neighboring states.

MICKI BURDICK is an assistant professor of women and gender studies at the University of Delaware. They received their doctorate from the University of Iowa in Rhetoric and Communication Studies. Their work centers around conservative religious movements, reproductive justice, and medicine, with specific attunement to the affective histories of these intersections.

DIANA GREENE FOSTER is a demographer at University of California, San Francisco. She led the Turnaway Study, a nationwide longitudinal prospective study of the health and well-being of women who seek abortion, including women who both do and do not receive the abortion. Dr. Foster is leading a study of the health, legal, and economic consequences of the end of *Roe* in the United States and a Turnaway Study in Nepal. She was named a 2023 MacArthur Fellow and is the author of over 130 scientific papers as well as the 2020 book, *The Turnaway Study: Ten Years, a Thousand Women and the Consequences of Having—or Being Denied—an Abortion.*

LORI FREEDMAN is a sociologist in the Advancing New Standards in Reproductive Health program at the University of California, San Francisco. Her 2023 book, *Bishops and Bodies: Reproductive Care in American Catholic Hospitals*, won the Donald W. Light Award from the American Sociological Association. She is also a Greenwall Faculty Scholar in bioethics. Her current research centers on how new abortion laws and bans impact medical treatment for patients with a variety of obstetric complications.

JENNY HIGGINS is the Bissell Professor of Reproductive Health, Rights, and Justice at the University of Wisconsin School of Medicine and Public Health, where she directs the Collaborative for Reproductive Equity and the Division of Reproductive and Population Health. Trained in gender studies and public health, Dr. Higgins has long studied people's embodied sexual and reproductive lives, including the impact of state-based abortion restrictions on pregnancy trajectories, health and well-being, and relationships.

B. JESSIE HILL is the Judge Ben C. Green Professor of Law at Case Western Reserve University School of Law and the director of Case Western's Reproductive Rights Law Initiative. Ms. Hill's teaching focuses on constitutional law, civil rights, reproductive rights, and law and religion. She is a graduate of Brown University and Harvard Law School. Ms. Hill is a frequent lecturer and consultant on reproductive rights issues and is currently involved in litigating numerous challenges to abortion restrictions in Ohio.

ERIN JOHNSON is a postdoctoral fellow at Indiana University–Bloomington where she contributes to research on measurement of abortion attitudes. Her independent research examines how abortion funds engage communities to resist punitive anti-abortion legislation through mutual aid, community education, and political advocacy, particularly in the wake of the U.S. Supreme Court's decision in *Dobbs v. Jackson Women's Health Organization*. She also volunteers with the Online Abortion Resource Squad, which provides information, advice, and emotional support to people undergoing abortion around the world.

KATRINA KIMPORT is a professor in the Department of Obstetrics, Gynecology and Reproductive Sciences and a sociologist in the Advancing New Standards in Reproductive Health program at the University of California, San Francisco. Her research examines the (re)production of inequality in health and reproduction, with a topical focus on abortion, contraception, and pregnancy. She is the author of *No Real Choice: How Culture and Politics Matter for Reproductive Autonomy* (2021), *Queering Marriage: Challenging Family Formation in the United States* (2014), and, with Jennifer Earl, *Digitally Enabled Social Change* (2011).

KLAIRA LERMA is the associate director of the Reproductive Equity Action Lab (REAL) at the University of Wisconsin School of Medicine and Public Health, a multidisciplinary team who conduct rigorous, cutting-edge research to identify key structural inequities that stand in the way of reproductive autonomy. She holds a master of public health from the Colorado School of Public Health. Her research investigates barriers to accessing preferred contraception, the impact of legislation on abortion access, and innovative service delivery methods. Her work also explores clients' perceptions of and experiences with reproductive health services, emphasizing person-centered care.

OPHRA LEYSER-WHALEN is an associate professor of sociology at the University of Texas at El Paso. Published in both social science and clinical journals, Dr. Leyser-Whalen's research has included student and community group collaborations on reproductive health and justice topics, focusing mainly on infertility, sterilization, and abortion funds.

SARA MATTHIESEN is an associate professor of history and women's, gender, and sexuality studies at George Washington University. Her first book, *Reproduction Reconceived: Family Making and the Limits of Choice after Roe v. Wade* (2021), tells the history of family-making under state neglect to trace how mass incarceration, for-profit and racist health care, HIV/AIDS, parentage laws, and faith-based services extracted new forms of reproductive labor from families on the economic, racial, and sexual margins of society. It received the 2022 Sara A. Whaley Prize from the National Women's Studies Association. Her current project, "'Free Abortion on Demand!' After *Roe*" is a history of multiracial, feminist organizing against state and medical control of abortion during the era of choice.

MICHELLE L. McGOWAN is professor of biomedical ethics in the Mayo Clinic College of Medicine and Sciences and is codirector of the Mayo Clinic Biomedical Ethics Research Program. She is a visiting scholar in women's, gender, and sexuality studies at the University of Cincinnati and leads the Ohio Policy Evaluation Network's Abortion Clinic Closure and Care Churn Project. Her empirical bioethics research focuses on the ethical and social implications of abortion policies for clinicians and patients.

JENNY O'DONNELL is the vice president of research and evaluation at the Society of Family Planning, an academic society for over 1,800 researchers, clinicians, and partners contributing to the science and medicine of abortion and contraception. She is a social epidemiologist by training. At the Society, Jenny leads research-related strategies to respond to the shifting political landscape and in service of the vision of just and equitable abortion and contraception informed by science.

MEREDITH J. PENSAK is a volunteer associate professor of obstetrics and gynecology at the University of Cincinnati College of Medicine. She is board certified in Obstetrics and Gynecology and Complex Family Planning. Dr. Pensak provides clinical care, teaches undergraduate and graduate medical learners, and focuses her research on abortion restrictions impacting clinical practice and new contraceptive technology.

LINDSAY RUHR is an associate professor of social work at the University of Arkansas at Little Rock. She teaches evaluation research, data analysis, and social work with organizations and communities. Her research interests include abortion restrictions, period pills, contraception, access to health care, integrated behavioral health, and program evaluation. Currently, she is working on two projects. One is an evaluation of incorporating social work students into primary care clinics to better integrate behavioral health into primary health care. The other is exploring menstrual health autonomy and pregnancy intentions in red states.

JESSICA SANDERS is an assistant professor in the Department of Obstetrics and Gynecology at the University of Utah. She is the director of research for the ASCENT Center for Reproductive Health and the policy director for the Family Planning Elevated Statewide Contraceptive Initiative. Dr. Sanders approaches reproductive health research through interdisciplinary academic and clinical research, ensuring an evidence-based and person-centered approach to education, policy, and clinical care.

JANE W. SEYMOUR is a research scientist at the University of Wisconsin Collaborative for Reproductive Equity. She is an epidemiologist and abortion scholar who seeks to answer policy- and practice-relevant questions to improve reproductive health and well-being. Her current work seeks to improve the measurement of abortion accessibility, rigorously evaluate abortion preferences, and implement novel methods to understand abortion seeking trajectories in the post-*Dobbs* landscape.

KELLY MARIE WARD is an assistant professor of gender and women's studies and sociology at the University of Wisconsin–Madison. She studies the organizational features of abortion and reproductive health care with an emphasis on low-status workers. Dr. Ward is a recipient of the National Abortion Federation's Carole Joffe and Stanley Henshaw Early Achievement in Social Science Research Award and serves as the engagement hub advisor at the university's Collaborative on Reproductive Equity. Dr. Ward is a full spectrum doula who unconditionally supports the goals of pregnant people and works with community organizations focused on abortion access and birth justice.

TRACY A. WEITZ is a professor of sociology at American University with over three decades of active involvement in the abortion field as a researcher, funder, advocate, and service director. Her academic training includes specialization in medical sociology and healthcare administration, and much of her research has focused on this intersection—how health care is organized, constructed, financed, and socially understood. Dr. Weitz also directs the university's Center on Health, Risk, and Society and is an appointed member of the National Academies of Sciences, Engineering, and Medicine Standing Committee on Reproductive Health, Equity, and Society. Before joining American University, Dr. Weitz directed the U.S. programs at the Susan Thompson Buffett Foundation in Omaha, NE, and cofounded and directed Advancing New Standards in Reproductive Health at the University of California, San Franciso.

ALEXANDRA WOODCOCK is an obstetrician-gynecologist at Santa Clara Valley Medical Center. She completed her Complex Family Planning fellowship at the University of Utah, where she led the research involved in her book chapter. Dr. Woodcock is dedicated to providing family planning services clinically as well as conducting research on how these services have changed in the post-*Dobbs* landscape.

Index

Abbott, Andrew, 132

abortifacients: medications used as, 111 (*see also* medication abortion); plants used as, 87–88

abortion acceptability. *See* acceptability of abortion

abortion access. *See* access to abortion

abortion accessibility, 70, 82n2

abortion accommodation, 70, 71*t*, 75–76, 79–80

abortion affordability. *See* affordability of abortion

abortion as health care, 38, 122, 123, 136–137, 144

abortion availability. *See* availability of abortion

abortion awareness, 70, 71*t*, 78–79; new sources of information for, 96–97; relationship to other abortion access subdomains, 79–80

abortion ban. *See* gestation-based abortion bans

abortion boards: in hospitals, 89, 90, 133; in Catholic hospitals, 103–104, 106

Abortion Care Network, 62

abortion exceptionalism, 30, 31, 34, 37–38, 73

abortion funds, 11, 200–214; aligned with reproductive justice values, 207–208, 209, 211–212, 213; documentation status of clients, 205; donations to, 11, 202, 210–212; effect of restrictions on, 55; interfund coordination and collaboration, 204–208; media attention to, 209, 210; new services of, 212–213; public education campaigns of, 212; research methods on, 202, 213; research results on, 202–213; scammers targeting, 209–210; stress and burnout in,

203, 213; in Texas, 205, 206, 212; in travel assistance, 81, 201, 202, 203–205, 212; volume of clients, 202, 203–204, 206, 210

abortion incidence data. *See* incidence data on abortion

abortion legitimacy. *See* legitimacy of abortion

Abortion Provider Census of Guttmacher Institute, 59

abortion providers, 2, 9–10; abortion funds providing information on, 207; abortion incidence data from, 59–60; acceptability of services to abortion seekers, 77, 78; access to (*see* access to abortion); authority of, 131–146 (*see also* authority of physicians); availability of services, 73, 74 (*see also* availability of abortion); awareness of services, 71*t* (*see also* awareness of abortion services); in California, 9, 59, 92–95, 120; Catholic hospitals as, 9, 31, 74, 100–107; contact information on, 61–62; cost of services (*see* cost of abortion); criminalization of, 30, 56, 87–89, 106; education and training of, 156 (*see also* education and training); in exceptions to abortion restrictions, 30, 131–137, 139, 144, 145; hospital admitting privileges of, 41–42, 154; insurance reimbursement to, 91, 113, 134; in medication abortion, 6, 9–10, 93, 96, 110–124; in Missouri, 8, 41–54; number in U.S., 111–112; in Ohio, 10, 60, 134, 135–144, 145; out-of-state travel to (*see* out-of-state travel); practice location preferences, 10, 149–157; professionalization of, 9, 87–88, 89; proximity of (*see* proximity of abortion services); referral from Catholic

Available titles in the Critical Issues in Health and Medicine series:

Nursing Clio Editorial Collective, ed., *The Nursing Clio Reader*

Manon Parry, *Broadcasting Birth Control: Mass Media and Family Planning*

Alyssa Picard, *Making the American Mouth: Dentists and Public Health in the Twentieth Century*

Heather Munro Prescott, *The Morning After: A History of Emergency Contraception in the United States*

Sarah B. Rodriguez, *The Love Surgeon: A Story of Trust, Harm, and the Limits of Medical Regulation*

Jacob Rodriquez, *On the Frontlines of Crisis: Intensive Care and the Challenge of COVID-19*

David J. Rothman and David Blumenthal, eds., *Medical Professionalism in the New Information Age*

Andrew R. Ruis, *Eating to Learn, Learning to Eat: School Lunches and Nutrition Policy in the United States*

James A. Schafer Jr., *The Business of Private Medical Practice: Doctors, Specialization, and Urban Change in Philadelphia, 1900–1940*

Johanna Schoen, ed., *Abortion Care as Moral Work: Ethical Considerations of Maternal and Fetal Bodies*

David G. Schuster, *Neurasthenic Nation: America's Search for Health, Happiness, and Comfort, 1869–1920*

Karen Seccombe and Kim A. Hoffman, *Just Don't Get Sick: Access to Health Care in the Aftermath of Welfare Reform*

Leo B. Slater, *War and Disease: Biomedical Research on Malaria in the Twentieth Century*

Piper Sledge, *Bodies Unbound: Gender-Specific Cancer and Biolegitimacy*

Dena T. Smith, *Medicine over Mind: Mental Health Practice in the Biomedical Era*

Kylie M. Smith, *Talking Therapy: Knowledge and Power in American Psychiatric Nursing*

Matthew Smith, *An Alternative History of Hyperactivity: Food Additives and the Feingold Diet*

Paige Hall Smith, Bernice L. Hausman, and Miriam Labbok, *Beyond Health, Beyond Choice: Breastfeeding Constraints and Realities*

Susan L. Smith, *Toxic Exposures: Mustard Gas and the Health Consequences of World War II in the United States*

Rosemary A. Stevens, Charles E. Rosenberg, and Lawton R. Burns, eds., *History and Health Policy in the United States: Putting the Past Back In*

Marianne Sullivan, *Tainted Earth: Smelters, Public Health, and the Environment*

Courtney E. Thompson, *An Organ of Murder: Crime, Violence, and Phrenology in Nineteenth-Century America*

Barbra Mann Wall, *American Catholic Hospitals: A Century of Changing Markets and Missions*

Frances Ward, *The Door of Last Resort: Memoirs of a Nurse Practitioner*

Jean C. Whelan, *Nursing the Nation: Building the Nurse Labor Force*

Shannon Withycombe, *Lost: Miscarriage in Nineteenth-Century America*